DISEASES and DISORDERS

VOLUME 3

Occupational disorders—Yellow fever

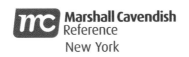

Marshall Cavendish
Reference
New York

Marshall Cavendish
99 White Plains Road
Tarrytown, New York 10591

www.marshallcavendish.us

Library of Congress Cataloging-in-Publication Data
Diseases and disorders
    p. cm.
  Includes bibliographical references and index.
  ISBN 978-0-7614-7770-9 (set: alk. paper)
-- ISBN 978-0-7614-7771-6 (v. 1) -- ISBN 978-0-7614-7772-3 (v. 2) -- ISBN 978-0-7614-7774-7 (v. 3)
  1. Diseases. 2. Medicine. I. Title.

RC41.D57 2007
616--dc22

2007060867

Printed and bound in Malaysia

12 11 10 09 08 07 1 2 3 4 5 6

Marshall Cavendish
Publisher: Paul Bernabeo
Production Manager: Michael Esposito

The Brown Reference Group
Project Editors: Anne Hildyard, Jolyon Goddard
Editor: Wendy Horobin
Development Editor: Richard Beatty
Designer: Seth Grimbly
Picture Researcher: Becky Cox
Illustrator: Darren Awuah
Indexer: Kay Ollerenshaw
Managing Editor: Bridget Giles
Senior Managing Editor: Tim Cooke
Editorial Director: Lindsey Lowe

Contents

ARTICLES IN VOLUME 1

Occupational disorders

An occupation is a trade, job, business, or career of an individual—the means by which one earns a living. An occupational disorder is any trauma injury or illness occurring at work or caused by the workplace.

There are numerous occupational disorders, but the most common are farmer's lung disease, pneumoconiosis (black lung disease), silicosis, byssinosis, asbestosis, Legionnaires' disease, latex allergy silicosis, carpal tunnel syndrome, radiation sickness, animal-to-human diseases called zoonoses, and others such as sick-building syndrome, hernias, hearing loss, and chronic back and neck pain.

Throughout the years, major attention to workplace safety has led to effective improvements in the work environment and has reduced the public health load of occupational injury and illness. However, former occupational hazards still persist, and new hazards arise as technology evolves.

The government agency responsible for monitoring workplace safety is the Occupational Safety and Health Administration (OSHA), which is a part of the U.S. Department of Labor. The mission of OSHA is to assure the safety and health of America's workers by setting and enforcing standards; providing training, outreach, and education; establishing partnerships; and encouraging continual improvement in workplace safety and health. OSHA and its state partners have approximately 2,100 inspectors, plus complaint discrimination investigators, engineers, physicians, educators, standards writers, and other technical and support personnel spread over more than 200 offices throughout the country. This agency establishes protective standards, enforces those standards, and reaches out to employers and employees through technical assistance and consultation programs. Despite these efforts, occupational hazards still persist, and new hazards arise as technology evolves.

Chronic back and neck pain are the most common complaints. The main risk of occupational back pain is lifting heavy loads from incorrect positions and working with poor posture. For example, a furniture delivery employee may lift a sofa incorrectly, which may trigger backpain. Similarly, salespeople who stand or walk for long periods of the day with poor posture can have back pain. Neck pain has emerged as a major complaint of people whose work involves long hours at the computer or many hours of driving (for example, bus or truck drivers). These risks can be reduced by health support such as exercise programs and mental stress prevention programs. Other common occupational disorders that exist affect the respiratory system, skin, and the musculoskeletal system. Information on all occupational disorders can be found at OSHA's website (www.osha.gov).

Hearing loss may occur due to occupational injury. Repeated exposure to loud noise can lead to permanent, incurable hearing loss. Prevention involves removing hazardous noise from the workplace and using hearing protectors in situations in which dangerous noise exposures have not yet been restricted or eliminated.

Hernias can also occur in the workplace. A hernia is

an opening or weakness in the wall of a muscle, tissue, or membrane that normally holds an organ in place. If the opening or weakness is large enough, a portion of the organ may be able to poke through the hole. Hernias are caused by a combination of muscle weakness and strain.

Occupational respiratory (lung) diseases

Although serious occupational respiratory disorders are now less common than they once were, some significant respiratory diseases still occur

Farmer's lung disease is an allergic disorder usually caused by breathing in the dust from moldy hay. However, dust from any moldy crop, such as straw, corn, silage, grain, or even tobacco, can also cause farmer's lung. The allergy causes shortness of breath and a feeling of general illness (malaise), either in a sudden attack or as a slow, progressive condition. If people with farmer's lung can avoid breathing in or filtering dust from moldy crops or feed, the condition can be stopped without further complicaitons. On the other hand, prolonged exposure can cause permanent lung damage, physical disability, or even death. The disease seems to occur in about 2 to 10 percent of farm workers, depending on the region. The most important factors in the diagnosis of farmer's lung are the history of exposure to dust from moldy hay or other moldy crops and the development of signs and symptoms four to eight hours later. For people suffering from acute attacks of farmer's lung, the first step in treatment is to avoid further contact with moldy dust. Certain medications provide some relief from an the allergic response, but avoidance is the only way make breathing easier.

Pneumoconiosis is a lung disease caused by inhaling coal dust for long periods of time. It is also known as black lung disease and anthracosilicosis. It predominantly affects coal workers. Pneumoconiosis occurs in two forms, simple and complicated. The simple form is usually not disabling, but the complicated form often is. The risk of developing the disease is related to the length and extent of exposure to the coal dust. The longer and more robust the exposure, the more severe the disorder. Thus, most affected workers are over the age of fifty after a lifetime of exposure. Symptoms include shortness of breath and a chronic cough. Pneumoconiosis is

diagnosed with a chest X-ray and pulmonary function tests. There is no treatment for the disorder other than treatment of complications. The best way to prevent the disease is to avoid further exposure to coal dust.

Silicosis is a lung disease caused by inhalation of silica dust, which leads to redness and scarring of the lung tissue. Silica is a common, naturally occurring crystal. It is found in most rock beds and forms dust during mining, extracting, tunneling, and work with many metal ores. Silica is a main component of sand, so glass workers and sand-blasters are heavily exposed to silica. Risk factors include mining, stone cutting, quarrying, road and building construction, work with abrasives manufacturing, sand blasting and many other occupations and hobbies that involve exposure to silica. Intense exposure to silica may result in the disease in a year or less, but it usually takes at least 10 or 15 years of exposure before symptoms develop. Symptoms are a chronic cough, fever, weight loss, and shortness of breath with exercise. Diagnostic tests such as chest X-rays and pulmonary function tests and a physical exam can confirm the diagnosis. There is no specific treatment for silicosis. Supportive treatment includes cough medications and oxygen if needed.

Byssinosis is a lung disease caused by inhalation of cotton dust or dusts from other vegetable fibers such as flax, hemp, or sisal. Sensitive individuals may have difficulty breathing after exposure to dust. Repeated exposure may lead to chronic lung disease and shortness of breath or wheezing. Symptoms include a history of exposure to dusts from textile manufacturing, worsening of symptoms at the start of the work week, improvement of symptoms while away from the workplace, chest tightness, cough, and wheezing. A physical exam, chest X-ray, and pulmonary function tests (especially repeated throughout the work day or work week during exposure) are used to diagnose byssinosis. The only treatment is to remove the source of exposure. Reduction of dust levels in the factory (by improving machinery or ventilation) can help prevent byssinosis. Some people may have to change jobs to avoid further exposure. Medications will help symptoms but will not cure the disorder.

Asbestosis is a lung disease caused by inhaling asbestos fibers, which causes scar tissue to form inside the lung. Scarred lung tissue does not expand

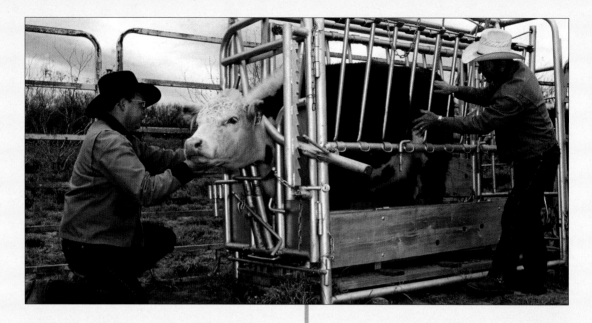

Farm workers are at risk of allergic reactions from animal feed and also from injuries caused by straining muscles when moving large animals around.

and contract normally and cannot perform gas exchange, resulting in shortness of breath. The severity of the disease depends upon the duration of exposure and the amount inhaled. Asbestos exposure occurs in asbestos mining and milling industries, construction, fireproofing, and other industries. In families of asbestos workers, exposure can also occur from particles brought home on the worker's clothing. More than 9 million workers are at risk of developing this disease. The incidence is 4 in 10,000 people. Symptoms are shortness of breath on exertion, cough, chest tightness, and chest pain. Tests that help diagnose the disease are a chest X-ray, pulmonary function tests, and a computed tomography (CT) scan of the lungs. The damage to the lungs cannot be repaired, so there is no cure available. Supportive treatment of symptoms includes removing secretions from the lungs to enable easier breathing. Preventive screening by taking chest X-rays of people exposed to asbestos may help detect asbestosis early enough to stop lung damage.

Legionnaires' disease is a severe inflammation of the lungs caused by a bacterium called *Legionella pneumophila*. There are approximately 35 *Legionella* species known to produce the disease. *Legionella* species are commonly found in any wet environment. They can survive for several months and multiply in the presence of algae and organic matter.

Legionnaires' disease usually begins with a headache, pain in the muscles, and a general feeling of sickness. These symptoms are followed by high fever, shaking chills, nausea, vomiting, and diarrhea. Dry coughing begins, and chest pain might occur, along with difficulty breathing. Most people develop pneumonia, a condition in which some of the lungs' air sacs fill with fluid or pus, so air is excluded. To distinguish Legionnaires' disease from other causes, laboratory tests are needed. The diagnosis is verified by tests that separate *Legionella* from respiratory secretions. Blood tests are usually carried out to detect whether the level of antibodies has increased in the blood. An increase indicates infection by *Legionella*. Antibodies are produced by special cells of the body's infection defense system to combat invading microorganisms. Antibiotics are usually successful in treating Legionnaires' disease. About 5 to 15 percent of known cases of Legionnaires' disease have been fatal. Workers most at risk are those with occupations that require them to work in sealed buildings, including workers who maintain water-cooling towers in air-conditioning systems. The circulated air picks up droplets of contaminated water, and bacteria can be transported throughout a building. If the droplets are small enough, they can be inhaled and infect the lungs. Some outdoor occupations are at risk as well.

Soil moved by bulldozing as well as surface or aerosolized water discharge can expose workers to the microorganism that causes Legionnaires' disease.

Occupational disorders affecting the skin

Latex is a tacky, milky sap that is produced by some types of shrubs, plants and trees. The sap is used to make latex rubber, or natural rubber. Allergies to latex rubber have been identified as a serious concern for workers who become sensitized to latex gloves and other rubber products. A common reaction to latex products is the development of dry, itchy, and irritated areas on the skin, usually the hands. Other reactions may include rashes and skin blisters, which can spread elsewhere. More severe widespread reactions may involve respiratory symptoms such as runny nose, sneezing, itchy eyes, scratchy throat, and difficulty breathing. Diagnosis involves latex-specific IgE blood testing and skin prick testing. To diagnose an allergy, a blood test and skin test are available. The blood test is performed first because of the potential severe reaction. There is no treatment for a latex allergy. The only way to prevent symptoms is to avoid latex or protect workers from latex exposure.

Occupational musculoskeletal disorders

Carpal tunnel syndrome is a condition affecting the hand and wrist. The carpal tunnel is a space in the wrist surrounded by bones and by an inflexible tendon that links the bones. The injury causes feelings of numbness, tingling, pain, and clumsiness, leading to difficulty with daily tasks, such as unscrewing bottle tops, fastening buttons, or turning keys. Carpal tunnel syndrome is mainly connected with tasks including repetitive hand motions, awkward hand positions, strong gripping, mechanical stress on the palm, and vibration. People at high risk are cashiers, hairdressers, those who work on computers for long hours, and knitters or sewers. Others at high risk are bakers who flex or extend the wrist while kneading dough and manual laborers who flex the fingers and wrist in tasks such as using a spray paint gun or hand-weeding. Excessive use of vibrating hand tools may also cause carpal tunnel syndrome. In short, anyone whose work-related tasks involve repetitive wrist movements is at risk for carpal tunnel syndrome. There may be pain not only in the hand, but also in the arm and the shoulder.

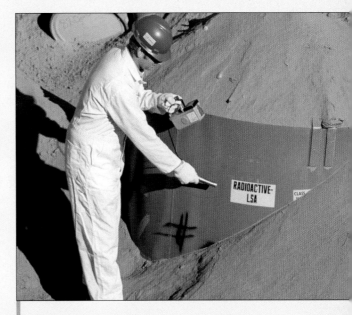

A workman points his Geiger counter at a potential occupational hazard: steel drums full of low-level radioactive waste at Hanford Nuclear Reservation, eastern Washington.

Numbness and loss of manual ability occurs in more advanced cases. Weakness of the hand also occurs, causing difficulty with pinch and grasp. The skin may dry because of reduced sweating. Diagnosis is confirmed by tests to detect damage to the median nerve. When symptoms of carpal tunnel syndrome are mild or likely to be temporary, treatment includes rest, anti-inflammatory drugs, and a metal splint. Surgery may be necessary if the symptoms are severe and if the other measures do not provide any relief. Prevention of carpal tunnel syndrome involves learning how to support the wrist during tasks that require wrist action.

Other occupational disorders

Some other occupation hazards include radiation sickness, zoonoses, and sick building syndrome.

Radiation sickness is an illness caused by excessive exposure to ionizing radiation, which produces immediate chemical effects (ionization) on human tissue. X-rays, gamma rays, and particle bombardment (neutron beam, electron beam, protons, mesons, and others) give off ionizing radiation. This type of radiation can be used for medical testing and treatment, industrial testing, manufacturing, sterilization, weapons and weapons development. Radiation exposure can occur as a single large exposure (acute), or a series of small exposures spread over time (chronic). Radiation sickness is generally associated with acute exposure and has a set of symptoms that appear in an orderly fashion. Chronic exposure is usually associated with delayed medical problems, such as cancer and premature aging, which may happen over a long period of time. Causes are accidental exposure to high doses of radiation, such as in certain occupations, or exposure to excessive radiation for medical treatments (which may include excessively high doses, excessive time of exposure, or excessive body areas exposed). Symptoms include nausea and vomiting, diarrhea, skin burns, weakness, fatigue, exhaustion, fainting, dehydration, inflammation of exposed areas (redness, tenderness, swelling, bleeding), hair loss, ulceration of the oral mucosa, ulceration of the esophagus, stomach or intestines, vomiting blood, and bloody stool. There may be bleeding from the nose, mouth, gums, and rectum, and bruising and open sores on the skin. There is no effective treatment, and the body has to heal itself. The only prevention is to avoid needless exposure to radiation sources, and to use "shields" over parts of the body not being treated or studied during X-rays or radiation treatments.

Zoonoses include any diseases or infections that can be transmitted from vertebrate animals to humans. Over 200 zoonoses have been described. They involve all types of agents: bacteria, parasites, viruses, and unusual agents. The most common route of infection related to pet contact is through bites, especially in children. Dogs bite more than 4.7 million people a year; in 2001 an estimated 368,245 persons were treated in U.S. hospital emergency rooms for nonfatal injuries related to dog bites. Some of these diseases were potentially life threatening. Others caused only short-lived, mild disease. At the time an animal appears to be ill there is no way of knowing whether or not it has a zoonosis. In addition, some diseases can be carried by animals that do not show any signs of illness. Symptoms and treatment for zoonoses depends on the disease. To prevent zoonoses, it is important to follow basic hygienic precautions such as washing hands after handling animals and not allowing animals to contaminate

plates that will be used to serve food. If an animal is ill, protective plastic gloves should be used to dispose of urine and feces as soon as possible.

Sick building syndrome (SBS) describes situations in which building occupants experience acute health and discomfort effects that appear to be linked to time spent in a building, but no specific illness or cause can be identified. The complaints may be limited to a small area in a particular room or zone, or may be widespread throughout the building. Symptoms include acute discomfort such as headache, eye, nose, or throat irritation, dry cough, dry or itchy skin, dizziness and nausea, difficulty in concentrating, fatigue, and sensitivity to odors. The cause of the symptoms is not known, and most of the symptoms decrease soon after leaving the building. Causes of or contributing factors to sick building syndrome are poor ventilation; chemical contaminants from adhesives; carpeting; upholstery; manufactured wood products; copy machines; pesticides; cleaning agents; chemical contaminants from outdoor sources (pollutants from motor vehicle exhausts, plumbing vents, and building exhausts); and biological contaminants such as bacteria, molds, pollen, and viruses. SBS may be prevented by removing the contaminants or other identified sources. Someone affected by SBS may consider avoiding the building or changing jobs.

Diagnosis, treatments, and prevention

Specialists in occupational medicine play an important role in the diagnosis of occupational disorders and the identification of new health hazards. The primary care physician, however, is usually the first health care provider to meet patients who have an occupational disease. In the workplace, occupational disorders are often dangerous and may be difficult to diagnose.

During the last century, 100,000 different chemicals with ill-defined human health risks were introduced into the work field, and health hazards persist. Primary care physicians should consider the patient's past and current workplaces as possible contributors to health problems. Employers are required to take preventive measures in the workplace to protect workers' health. People who work in high-risk occupations should wear dust masks and observe safety precautions.

Rashmi Nemade

Osteoarthritis

Osteoarthritis is a joint disorder in which the cartilage that lines the joints degenerates. It mainly affects the knee, hip, spine and shoulder joints, but may also affect any of the other movable joints. It is the most common kind of arthritis and is present to some degree in almost everyone over the age of 40. Even teenagers may be affected.

Osteoarthritis affects males and females about equally but usually appears earlier in men than in women. The name of this condition is misleading. The ending -*itis* means "inflammation," yet inflammation of the joint structures is not a basic feature of the disease. But the term has been in use for many years and is unlikely to be changed now. Inflammation, often severe and painful, is a central feature of some other forms of arthritis, such as gout and rheumatoid arthritis.

Causes and risk factors

Healthy joints that have not been unduly stressed or injured do not suffer wear. They have a good lubrication system with constant secretion of lubricating fluid and the removal of used fluid and small particles of debris. Minor damage to the bearing cartilage surfaces is effectively repaired by cartilage-secreting cells called chondrocytes. Osteoarthritis begins with abnormal production of new and excessive bone in the surfaces under the bearing cartilage. There is also an abnormal increase in cartilage production. The new bone lacks elasticity and develops many tiny fractures. Eventually small areas of protruding bone called osteophytes occur in it. These can be seen on an X-ray. The bearing cartilage and the bone under it then develop fissures through which the lubricating fluid is forced into the marrow of the bone. The result is serious loss of smoothness of the joint surfaces with roughening and pitting and then patchy loss of the cartilage surfaces.

Because the joint changes characteristic of osteoarthritis involve what appears to be a wearing-off of the smooth cartilage covering the bearing surfaces of joints, doctors have for many years assumed that this form of arthritis was no more than the result of wear and tear. However, this view did not explain the obvious fact that different people exposed to exactly the same stress factors suffered changes to very different degrees. This remained unexplained, and the real cause of osteoarthritis remained unknown until the mid-1990s, when evidence appeared of a genetic element in the disease. Careful study comparing more than 100 identical twins with more than 100 non-identical twins showed that, in a high proportion of the identical twins, when one twin had osteoarthritis the other twin also had it to a similar degree of severity. In the case of the non-identical twins, the correlation between pairs was much less. Because identical twins have identical genes, these findings suggested that a genetic element was involved. Much later research confirmed this, and it is now generally accepted that gene mutations affecting the quality of joint cartilage are a significant causal factor.

KEY FACTS

Description
The most common disease to affect joints.

Causes
Research suggests that there is a genetic basis.

Risk factors
Overweight, leading to excessive joint pressure, especially in the knees and hip joints; overuse, mechanical injury, and bone deformity.

Symptoms
Pain on joint movement, crunching or crackling sensation, limitation of joint movement.

Diagnosis
History of joint symptoms; examination of joint movement; X-ray; blood tests to exclude rheumatoid arthritis and gout.

Treatments
Keeping mobile; maintaining the strength of the muscles moving the joint; physiotherapy. Glucosamine; painkillers. In severe cases, joint replacement.

Pathogenesis
Severe, noninflammatory, degenerative changes in joints, with extensive loss of the cartilaginous bearing surfaces and damage to the bone.

Prevention
Control of weight. Avoidance of stress to joints.

Epidemiology
Affects about one person in every 13. At least 20 million people in the United States are sufficiently affected to suffer pain and disability.

Another major established risk factor is the excessive pressure that is applied to weight-bearing joint surfaces, especially the knees, hips, and ankles, when the person concerned is much overweight. Long-term obesity is likely to be associated with a significant degree of osteoarthritis.

Osteoarthritis is much more likely to occur and to be severe if any factor is present that alters the relationship of the bearing surfaces of a joint to each other. In health, joint surfaces should fit snugly together so that they move over each other smoothly and evenly, lubricated by the fluid secreted within the joint capsule. If one surface is tilted relative to the other, the pressure at one point will be increased and that at another decreased. Because of this, people with any history of injury to a joint or with any bone disease that leads to distortion (for example rickets, bowlegs, knock-knees, or congenital deformities) are much more likely to develop osteoarthritis. Traumatic injury to bones adjacent to joints is another causal factor.

HIP REPLACEMENT

A hip replacement becomes necessary when the hip joint has been damaged by arthritis and the person has stiff and painful joints, which make walking difficult. Sometimes a hip replacement is carried out if the femur is badly fractured. In both cases, the damaged joint is replaced by an artificial joint, which is usually composed of two pieces, a socket and a ball and shaft; they are pushed tightly in place or cemented.

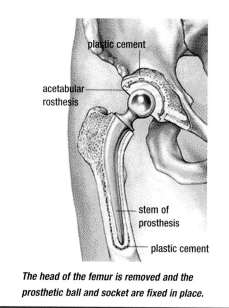

plastic cement

acetabular rosthesis

stem of prosthesis

plastic cement

The head of the femur is removed and the prosthetic ball and socket are fixed in place.

Symptoms, signs, and diagnosis

Osteoarthritis starts gradually, and the initial symptom, pain, is usually felt in one joint and is made worse by using the joint. Often other paired joints may be affected. There is relief with rest, but the affected joint or joints then become stiff. This stiffness lasts for up to half an hour but passes when the joints are again moved. Soon the affected person begins to experience a grating sensation on moving the joint, and sometimes there is tenderness on pressure over the joint. In the late stages there may be enlargement of the joint as a result of the increased bone and cartilage growth and of the soft tissues in and around the joint. It is only at this stage that inflammation may occur, and if it does, there is an increase in the level of the pain.

As the disease progresses, the joint can be moved progressively less. This reduction in possible movement may, in the absence of good treatment, have the secondary effect of tightening and shortening the muscles that move the joint. This can result in a permanently bent joint that cannot be straightened—a condition known as a flexion contracture. The prevention of flexion contractures is one of the aims of medical management of this disorder.

Treatments

Without treatment, established osteoarthritis may, in most cases, be expected to progress in severity. It will do so, however, at a rate that varies greatly from one affected person to another. The aim of treatment is to prevent or slow worsening and to relieve symptoms. It is also important to try to maintain general fitness.

The first step is to get rid of excess weight. This alone may markedly reduce the severity of symptoms. People with osteoarthritis need a daily exercise program calculated to maintain or improve general health and the state of affected joints. This program will also ensure that, by regular, deliberate stretching, the range of movement of affected joints will be increased. It will also strengthen muscles, improve posture, and maintain healthy joint cartilages. The program should be under medical or paramedical supervision. Physical therapists are trained in this work. In osteoarthritis, immobilization is dangerous. It can speed the progress and worsen the outlook of the disease. Effective pain control should be prescribed and monitored by a physician.

Robert Youngson

See also
- Arthritis • Bone and joint disorders • Gout
- Rheumatoid arthritis

Osteoporosis

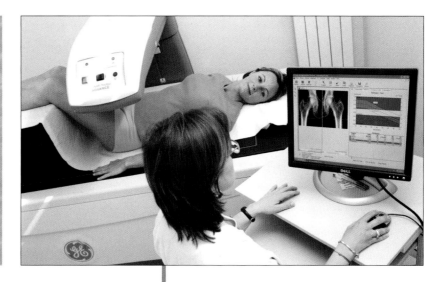

Osteoporosis is a systemic disorder characterized by loss of bone tissue and bone density, leading to skeletal fragility and an increased risk of insufficiency fractures. A fracture that results from a standing position is considered an osteoporotic fracture.

A doctor uses a bone densitometer to measure the optical density of the neck of the femur of a female patient to confirm a diagnosis of osteoporosis.

Risk factors that are associated with osteoporosis include: female gender; postmenopausal status; Asian or Caucasian race; weight less than 127 pounds (57.6 kg); history of fracture in a parent, sibling, or child; and personal history of a fracture as an adult. Modifiable risk factors associated with osteoporosis include tobacco use, alcohol abuse, low calcium or vitamin D intake, or both, and physical inactivity. Certain medical conditions predispose to osteoporosis: malabsorption states, such as celiac disease; prior gastric bypass; inflammatory disorders such as rheumatoid arthritis; primary hyperparathyroidism; and hyperthyroidism. Medications associated with bone loss include corticosteroids, intravenous heparin, lithium, depakote, and suppressive doses of thyroid replacement. Any condition that increases the risk of falls, such as decreased vision or Parkinson's disease, is associated with osteoporotic fractures.

Symptoms and diagnosis

Usually a patient does not suspect that she has osteoporosis. There is no pain unless a fracture occurs. Height loss of more than two inches may suggest vertebral compression fractures. Thoracic kyphosis (curvature) may also be a sign of multiple compression fractures and osteoporosis. Many vertebral fractures are asymptomatic when they occur and are noted incidentally on a lateral chest X-ray.

The diagnosis of osteoporosis is made after a dual X-ray absorbtiometry (DXA) scan is performed. This is the standard imaging technique that analyzes bone density (BMD, literally, "bone mass density"). It is painless and exposes a patient to less radiation than a chest X-ray. The World Health Organization (WHO) has defined osteoporosis as a T-score of 2.5 standard deviations (SD) below that expected for a gender- and race-matched control. A T-score -1.0 to -2.4 SD below that expected indicates osteopenia (decrease in bone mass). If the T-score is within one SD of that expected, the bone density is normal. The Z-score compares the patient to an age-, gender-, and race-matched control. If a patient has one or more insufficiency fractures and the bone density is not suggestive of low bone density, consideration of abnormal bone quality or of a falsely elevated BMD must be considered. Osteomalacia refers to abnormal bone resulting from vitamin D deficiency, which is associated with a higher fracture risk. Osteoarthritis of the spine or improper positioning on the bone density table can result in falsely elevated BMD results.

If the Z-score is more than one SD below that expected for age, the cause of low bone mass should be determined. Modifiable risk factors should be corrected, such as ongoing tobacco use or alcohol abuse. If a patient is on medications associated with bone loss, alternatives should be considered. If a patient is on glucocorticoids, the lowest possible dose should be prescribed. It may be necessary to do a laboratory evaluation to look for an etiology of low bone mass. Tests to consider include TSH, ESR, SIEP/UIEP, intact PTH, 25 Vitamin D, celiac antibodies, urine calcium, phosphorus, and bone alkaline phosphatase. If a cause of low bone mass is identified, it is evaluated and treated.

The urine N-telopeptide (NTX) is a test that measures bone breakdown products. The second urine sample of the morning is the most useful. A value of 40 to 50 bone collagen equivalent/millimoles (BCE/mmol) suggests ongoing bone loss and predicts loss of BMD and fracture. A value less than 10 BCE/mmol suggests a low bone turnover state and perhaps an increased risk of microdamage and a tendency toward stress fractures.

Treatments

All patients with low bone mass should be advised to take 1,200 to 1,500 milligrams (mg) calcium per day, divided into two to three servings, by diet or supplements. Calcium carbonate is associated with a small risk of kidney stones. When this concern exists, calcium citrate may decrease this risk. The recommended vitamin D intake is being reevaluated. Patients should get 800 to 1,000 international units (IU) per day. The level can be measured and dose adjusted when necessary. Patients should strive to participate daily in a weight-bearing exercise program with emphasis on balance and falls prevention.

The National Osteoporosis Foundation (NOF) recommends treating postmenopausal women with a T-score of -2.0 or greater or -1.5 or greater if other risk factors for osteoporosis are present. Care must be based on a patient's bone density results and other comorbid medical conditions.

Surgical procedures are being explored to attempt correction of vertebral deformities. These procedures include vertebroplasty and kyphoplasty. In vertebroplasty, cement is injected into the compressed vertebral body. In kyphoplasty, a balloon is inserted into the compressed vertebra, and polymethyl methacrylate is injected. Both procedures are indicated for pain relief. Long-term studies to evaluate benefit and safety are needed. Primary risks include neurological impairment as a result of extrusion of cement near the spinal cord and increased risk of vertebral fractures above and below the surgical site. Early treatment of hip fractures reduces morbidity and mortality associated with hip fractures. Ideally, repair is within 24 hours.

Pharmacological treatments are either antiresorptive (they inhibit bone loss caused by the activity of osteoclasts—cells associated with bone removal) or anabolic (they increase production of osteoblasts—cells associated with production of bone). Antiresorptive therapies reduce osteoclast resorption. Anabolic therapies increase osteoblast function. The FDA mandates that new therapies demonstrate reduction in fracture risk.

There has been recent concern of a small risk of avascular necrosis of the jaw with bisphosphonate therapy. It appears most commonly in patients treated with monthly intravenous zoledronic acid for metastatic cancer, in patients with poor dental hygiene, and in patients with low bone turnover. All of these agents appear to be associated with increased bone density and a reduction in vertebral and nonvertebral fractures.

Hormone replacement therapy (HRT) has come in disfavor for the treatment of osteoporosis due to the associated risk of stroke, myocardial infarction, and breast cancer. The Women's Health Initiative (WHI) study was the first randomized double-blind study to

---

KEY FACTS

Description

A systemic disorder characterized by skeletal fragility and an increased risk of insufficiency fractures.

Causes

Bone density declines with age. Certain medical conditions predispose to bone loss.

Risk factors

Include female gender, postmenopausal state, Caucasian and Asian race, low adult weight, family history of osteoporosis, and personal history of a fracture as an adult.

Symptoms

Include loss of height and thoracic kyphosis.

Diagnosis

Dual energy X-ray absorbtiometry (DEXA) and evaluation by experienced medical personnel.

Treatments

Calcium and vitamin D supplementation, weight-bearing exercise program, and medications to preserve or improve BMD.

Pathogenesis

Without treatment, there is a progressive decline in bone density associated with increased fracture risk.

Prevention

Appropriate intake of calcium, vitamin D and weight-bearing exercises throughout a lifetime.

Epidemiology

In the United States, there are 700,000 vertebral fractures, 300,000 hip fractures, and 250,000 wrist fractures annually. As the population ages, the incidence is expected to increase.

demonstrate a reduction in hip fracture with the use of HRT. If a woman chooses to take HRT, it may well prevent postmenopausal bone loss. Generally, the bisphosphonates are more potent in the prevention of osteoclast resorption than HRT.

The selective estrogen receptor modulator (SERM) FDA-approved for the treatment of osteoporosis is raloxifene. This agent has been shown to reduce the risk of vertebral fractures but not of hip fractures. Side effects include hot flashes, leg cramps, and an increased risk of thrombosis.

Teriparatide is the only anabolic agent FDA-approved for the treatment of osteoporosis. It is a self-injection given daily for two years. It improves BMD and reduces the risk of vertebral and hip fractures. Early on, it may be associated with orthostatic hypotension. There has been an increased risk of osteosarcoma in rats treated with this agent. This has not been seen in humans, dogs, or monkeys. It is useful in patients with severe osteoporosis, patients not responding to bisphosphonate therapy, and in patients with a low bone turnover state.

Calcitonin is of questionable efficacy in bone density improvement and fracture reduction and therefore is not considered a mainstay of osteoporosis treatment.

Pathogenesis and prevention

Bone is composed of matrix and mineral. The matrix consists of type I collagen and a cellular component called osteoblasts, which form bone and osteoclasts, which resorb bone. Bone remodeling is a dynamic process. Peak bone mass is achieved by age thirty. Thereafter, osteoclast function outweighs osteoblast function, and there is a 0.5 to 1 percent loss of bone each year. In women, for the two years before menopause and up to five years after menopause, there can be a 5 percent loss every year. Most Caucasian women become osteoporotic at age 70.

Mineral is composed of hydroxapatite containing calcium and phosphorus. If a patient does not consume or absorb enough calcium, secondary hyperparathyroidism occurs. Calcium is then removed from the skeleton to maintain appropriate serum levels. As a result, bone loss occurs. Both primary and secondary hyperparathyroidism is a cause of osteoporosis.

It is critical that children, teens, and young adults get regular exercise and have adequate calcium and vitamin D intake so that they reach a maximal peak bone mass. Patients should avoid behaviors known to contribute to osteoporosis such as tobacco use and alcohol excess. Falls prevention should be a goal for all

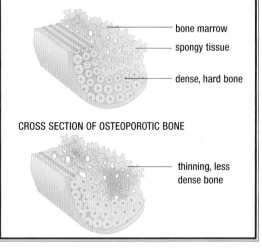

OSTEOPOROSIS

Osteoporosis is a decrease in the density of bone, as a result of the loss of collagen, and thus of calcium. Osteoporosis affects both hard and spongy tissue.

CROSS SECTION OF NORMAL BONE

— bone marrow
— spongy tissue
— dense, hard bone

CROSS SECTION OF OSTEOPOROTIC BONE

— thinning, less dense bone

patients. Physicians must screen all patients at risk for osteoporosis and treat those with indications for pharmacological therapy.

Epidemiology

Osteoporosis is an increasingly prevalent condition that accounts for more than 700,000 vertebral fractures, 300,000 hip fractures, and 250,000 wrist fractures annually in the United States. This results in significant morbidity and mortality and a large economic burden on society due to the costs of caring for these individuals, who often fail to regain their pre-fracture functioning state. Many patients must live in nursing homes either temporarily or permanently after a hip fracture. Osteoporotic fractures are more common in women, but the mortality rate after hip fracture is higher in men. The risk of mortality within the first year after a hip fracture is up to 20 percent.

Severe osteoporosis is associated with a loss of confidence, a fear of falling, and often social isolation, as patients go out less. As a result, depression becomes common. Once a patient becomes severely kyphotic, little can be done to correct the deformity.

Linda A. Russell

See also
- Bone and joint disorders • Fracture
- Hormonal disorders

Pancreatic disorders

The pancreas can be affected by several diseases; they include congenital malformations, tumor formation, and inflammatory or metabolic conditions.

The pancreas is a major digestive gland, embedded below and behind the stomach between the duodenum and the spleen. It consists of two major components, the glandular (acinar) part and the endocrine part (islets). The acinar or exocrine tissue is responsible for producing the digestive juices with active enzymes and represents 90 percent of the pancreas. Enzymes are secreted from acinar cells when the pancreas is stimulated by ingestion of food. Pancreatic juice collects in a system of ducts that join to form the main pancreatic duct, which, with the bile duct, enters the duodenum. The activated enzymes mix with the food and chemically break it into fragments that can be absorbed into the bloodstream. Only a relatively small portion of the pancreas volume comes from the pancreatic islets, which nestle between the acinar tissue and produce several hormones. The most important hormones are insulin and glucagon, which regulate the blood sugar in a very narrow range.

Pancreatitis

Acute pancreatitis is a sudden inflammation. It is most commonly related to gallstones or alcohol consumption, but other triggers, such as medications and viruses, have been identified. Pancreatic enzymes are highly potent agents that can quickly digest food. Several security mechanisms are built in to prevent these enzymes from attacking and autodigesting the pancreas itself. For example, the enzymes are stored in separated cellular compartments as inactive pre-enzymes, which only become activated once they are secreted and have traveled through the duct system to the small bowel. Under pathological conditions, these mechanisms fail, and enzyme activation accidentally occurs within the pancreas. Trypsin, an enzyme that cleaves proteins and peptides, plays a key role, as it is not only able to activate itself but also all other enzyme precursors. The smallest amount of accidentally activated trypsin may initiate a rapid and uncontrolled amplification of active enzymes. These events lead to an acute inflammatory reaction of the pancreas (acute pancreatitis). Symptoms depend on the extent of tissue injury or destruction. The spectrum ranges from a mild and self-limited disease with some acute abdominal pain to a very severe, life-threatening condition (necrotizing pancreatitis). The diagnosis is confirmed with detection of elevated pancreatic enzymes (amylase, lipase) in the blood and imaging studies such as computed tomography (CT). Treatment in most cases is food restriction, and the patient is given fluids; in severe cases, intensive care monitoring and surgery may be needed. After resolution of the gallstone pancreatitis, the gallbladder should be removed (cholecystectomy).

Chronic pancreatitis is a more subtle disease process that leads to a loss of glandular tissue and ultimately to a lack of digestive enzymes in the intestinal tract. Long-standing excessive alcohol consumption is the most common etiology, but the exact pathophysiology is still poorly understood. It has been speculated, however, that the chronic toxic effects injure both the acinar and duct cells. In an initial attempt at repair, fibrillary proteins are deposited to these damaged areas. As more damage occurs, however, these proteins continue to

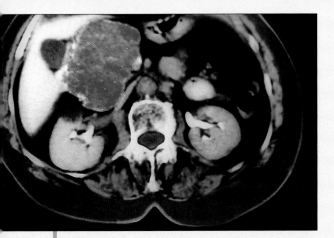

This CT scan of a patient's abdomen shows a cystic pancreatic tumor (in red). The liver is yellow, the kidneys are pale red, and the spine is pink.

precipitate in the pancreatic duct system. The channels become increasingly plugged, and the enzyme-producing acinar cells eventually turn off. The organ slowly transforms into scar tissue that may contain calcifications, which may be seen on an X-ray. More commonly, however, the diagnosis of chronic pancreatitis is suspected from the lack of pancreatic enzymes, which leads to poorly digested food (fatty stools), weight loss, anemia, and sometimes secondary diabetes mellitus. The disease may develop silently or cause various degrees of chronic or recurrent pain attacks in the upper abdomen. It is important to keep in mind that all symptoms are nonspecific and can be mimicked by or coexist with pancreatic cancer. Treatment for chronic pancreatitis usually is conservative. It should include discontinuation of alcohol consumption, oral supplementation of digestive enzymes in capsules with each meal, pain control, and possibly monitoring of the diabetes. Surgical decompression of the clogged duct system has become a rare approach.

Tumors

The pancreas can be affected by several diseases that range from congenital malformations to inflammatory or metabolic conditions to tumor formation. Both the glandular (acinar) part and the pancreatic islets can form tumors. The most common type of exocrine tumor is pancreatic cancer, which is highly malignant and carries a poor prognosis. Rarer forms of glandular tumors include cystadenomas. The islets consist of several cell types, each of which produces a different hormone. Each of these cell types may develop an uncontrolled growth and form a tumor, such as insulinoma, glucagonoma, or gastrinoma. Some islet cell tumors metastasize (are malignant), while others do not. About 80 percent of these endocrine tumors continue to excessively secrete their original hormone and cause respective symptoms. For example, the loss of feedback control in an insulin-producing tumor (insulinoma) results in dangerously low blood sugar levels (hypoglycemia). Islet cell tumors can occasionally be found in conjunction with tumors in other endocrine organs.

Congenital malfunctions and malformations

The most common congenital pancreatic malfunction is found in the context of cystic fibrosis. While the lung disease eventually determines survival, the lack of pancreatic secretory enzymes together with the dry mucus membranes results in a very thick bowel content, which can clog the bowels and cause a bowel obstruction. Apart from pulmonary care and potential lung transplantation, these patients need a rigid bowel program with enzyme supplements and laxatives. Anatomical malformations of the pancreas, which are relatively rare, result from faulty organ development in utero. The most common of these is pancreas anulare, in which the pancreas forms a ring around the duodenum.

Acquired malformations

Pancreatic pseudocysts are fluid-filled cavities in the pancreas that may result from pancreatitis or trauma. They may reach several centimeters in size and cause compressive symptoms to other organs. Surgical or other interventions are needed for treatment.

Diagnosis

The pancreas is not easily accessible. Ultrasound or CT are the most important imaging tools. Endoscopic retrograde choledocho-pancreatography (ERCP) is an endoscopic procedure to cannulate (to insert a tube into) the bile and pancreatic duct to obtain images and perform interventions (stone retrieval, sphincterotomy, and stent placement). MRCP (magnetic resonance cholangio-pancreatography) achieves the same images without surgery.

Andreas Kaiser

Paralysis

Paralysis is a general term used to describe an inability to move one or several parts of the body. A lesser degree of weakness is termed *paresis*. Paralysis can be congenital or acquired and has many causes, including cerebral palsy, trauma, tumor, or stroke; or autoimmune, toxic, infectious, musculoskeletal, or metabolic compromise of the motor pathways in the nervous system.

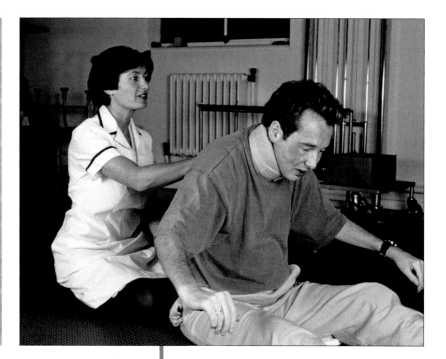

A physiotherapist assists a man with paralysis of all four limbs (quadriplegia) to balance in a supported "long sit position." The patient has a broken neck and has to relearn how to balance in this particular position.

Paralysis can occur at any level of the nervous system and may also be due to psychiatric conditions. Paralysis may be partial (paresis) or complete (plegia), mild or life threatening. It may involve one side of the body (hemiparesis or hemiplegia); all four limbs (quadriparesis or quadriplegia); the lower limbs (paraparesis or paraplegia); a single limb (monoparesis or monoplegia); or an isolated muscle group supplied by a single motor nerve (mononeuropathy). Paralysis can develop suddenly or slowly over time. Paralysis is an important cause of disability in the United States because the limitation in movement prevents individuals from carrying out activities of daily living. The diagnosis, prevention, and treatment of paralysis are determined by its etiology (cause).

Causes and risk factors

Some common causes of paralysis include stroke, cerebral palsy, multiple sclerosis, Guillain-Barré syndrome, spinal cord injuries, central nervous system tumors, and various neuropathies (for example, Bell's palsy). Risk factors are variable and are based on the causative disease process. For example, the risk factors in stroke include heredity, high blood pressure, sex, diabetes mellitus, and age. In multiple sclerosis, the risk factors relate to geographical location in that the farther an individual lives from the equator in the first fifteen years of life, the greater his or her chance of developing the disease. Women are also at a higher risk. The etiology is presumed to be autoimmune, but the precise cause is unknown.

In some parts of Asia and Africa, the polio virus remains endemic and continues to be an important cause of paralysis due to one of its complications, poliomyelitis. However, it has been eradicated in most industrialized parts of the world through vaccination.

Symptoms, signs, and diagnosis

Paralyzed individuals will usually complain of loss of movement or weakness in the affected part of the body. The loss of strength may also sometimes be associated with numbness or paresthesias (abnormal touch sensation, such as burning or prickling). The symptom of weakness is verified on neurological examination, which focuses on isolated testing of the major muscle groups. When paralysis is caused by damage to the central nervous system, there may be associated symptoms, such as trouble producing speech (aphasia) or numbness. In many cases, these associations can aid in determining the anatomical location of the disease process.

In stroke or in certain infectious or metabolic conditions, an individual may not be able to describe weakness, but an examiner may find decreased muscle tone, absent reflexes, pathological reflexes, muscle atrophy, increased muscle tone, or spasticity.

Alternatively, if paralysis is caused by damage to the peripheral nervous system, there may be associated pain. Metabolic abnormalities such as electrolyte imbalances tend to cause more widespread weakness. An infectious cause may be suggested if there is fever, diarrhea, vomiting, mental status changes, neck stiffness, insect bites, or another affected person who ate the same food.

Diagnostic testing is guided by a physician's assessment of the pattern and chronological development of the paralysis and associated symptoms. If these factors lead to suspicion of a disease process in the brain or spinal cord, computed tomography (CT) or magnetic resonance imaging (MRI) of the brain, spinal cord, or brachial plexus is used to examine the tissue in detail and to look for evidence of stroke, tumor, infection, or demyelination. If the lesion is suspected in the peripheral nervous system, such as the peripheral nerves, neuromuscular junction or muscle, electromyography (EMG) is used. Diseases of the muscle that cause paralysis are sometimes diagnosed using a muscle biopsy. When the cause of paralysis is thought to be a metabolic disorder or to be systemic in nature (autoimmune), then blood tests are used to aid in diagnosis. These tests may include investigation for antibodies known to be associated with certain conditions, such as acetylcholine receptor antibodies found in myasthenia gravis, or genetic mutations associated with specific conditions (amyotrophic lateral sclerosis and superoxide dismutase) or metabolic disturbances (hypocalcemia, hypokalemia).

Treatments and prevention

Dynamic preventive treatments such as widespread vaccination for polio virus have essentially eradicated poliomyelitis as a cause of paralysis in industrialized parts of the world, although it remains an important cause of paralysis in parts of Africa and India.

In the United States and most of Europe, stroke is treated in the first three hours of onset with drugs designed to break up the clot obstructing an artery. Close monitoring and control of blood pressure, glucose

---

KEY FACTS

Description

Paralysis is a general term used to describe an inability to move a part, or parts, of the body. Weakness, as distinct from paralysis, is designated *paresis*, and has the same causal factors as paralysis.

Causes

There are multiple causes of paralysis that originate from different levels of the nervous system; some more common examples are: stroke, tumor, neuropathy, amyotrophic lateral sclerosis, trauma, and Guillain-Barré syndrome.

Risk factors

Reduction of modifiable risk factors is based on the specific disease process causing paralysis. In stroke, these include lowering blood pressure, smoking cessation, lowering cholesterol, tight glycemic control in diabetes mellitus, and treatment of obstructive sleep apnea.

Symptoms

The pattern of weakness, associated symptoms, and time course of onset are essential features that aid in characterizing the type of paralysis, its cause, and treatment.

Diagnosis

Aimed at the suspected part of the body affected, it may include MRI, CT, EMG, X-rays, or blood tests in conjunction with a detailed medical history and physical examination.

Pathogenesis

Mechanisms of paralysis vary based on the underlying disease process. In stroke, the process is vascular due to inadequate blood supply or bleeding into the brain. Tumors cause mass effect and compression of important anatomical structures. Demyelinating diseases, such as multiple sclerosis, are caused by disruption or loss of the myelin sheaths in the central nervous system. The result is impaired signal transmission.

Prevention

Strategies are aimed at the disease process responsible for paralysis. In stroke, prevention consists of medical and dietary modifications that will lower blood pressure and cholesterol and will optimize glucose control. A healthy diet, exercise, and smoking cessation are also important preventive factors for stroke. In polio, vaccinations are powerful prevention strategies. In diseases such as primary central nervous system tumors or multiple sclerosis, there are no known prevention strategies.

Epidemiology

Strokes are one of the leading causes of paralysis; in 2000, around 1 million people had some form of paralysis after a stroke.

TYPES OF PARALYSIS

Depending on where the damage occurs in the nervous system, paralysis can affect one side of the body, the lower half of the body, or the trunk and all four limbs.

spinal cord

spinal nerves

paralyzed area (dark)

hemiplegia

paraplegia

quadriplegia

level, and temperature are also important treatments in the acute setting of stroke. However, most of the treatment is aimed at primary and secondary prevention of stroke, which entails reducing modifiable risk factors such as high blood pressure, high cholesterol, poor glucose control in diabetes, and obstructive sleep apnea.

In demyelinating diseases, such as multiple sclerosis, immunomodulating agents or immunosuppressant agents are used, as well as filtering of blood to remove pathogenic antibodies (plasma exchange).

Although treatment is usually directed at the specific disease process causing paralysis, paralysis of any etiology is treated with aggressive physical therapy and rehabilitation because immobility, in and of itself, can lead to atrophy, deconditioning, contractures, and other morbidity. There are some new therapies, such as constraint-based therapy, which is aimed at restricting the functional parts of the body so that an individual is made to use the dysfunctional limb, rehabilitating it into function.

Pathogenesis

Mechanisms of paralysis vary depending on the cause. There are two broad types of stroke, hemorrhagic (bleeding) and ischemic (blocked vessel). Paralysis in ischemic stroke occurs as a result of rupture of a cholesterol plaque or embolization of clot material from the heart that clogs a cerebral artery. The blocked artery leads to inadequate perfusion of brain tissue and subsequent cell death and edema. Often, the tissue that dies involves the motor fibers of the nervous system, which control strength and movement. If these areas of the brain are affected, the appropriate signals required for coordinated muscle movements are not transmitted to the spinal cord, nerves, and muscles. As a result, the patient experiences paralysis.

Paralysis can be reversible or permanent, depending on the cause. In general, paralysis from stroke and multiple sclerosis is permanent, with rehabilitation potential occurring over a period of months after the initial event. Other causes of paralysis, such as amyotrophic lateral sclerosis or tumors, are progressive in nature. Paralysis from an electrolyte or endocrine abnormality can be completely reversible.

Epidemiology

The incidence of cerebral palsy is 2 in 1,000 in developed countries; in 30 percent of cases, the spastic form is found. In 2005, polio, another cause of paralysis, was endemic in six countries; worldwide, there were around 2,000 cases of polio.

Meredith Roderick and Robert Daroff

See also
• Diabetes • Metabolic disorders • Multiple sclerosis • Sleep disorders • Stroke and related disorders

Parathyroid disorders

The parathyroid glands are located in the neck near the thyroid. The parathyroid glands make parathyroid hormone (PTH), which regulates blood calcium levels by a feedback mechanism. PTH is critical to calcium, phosphorus, and vitamin D metabolism. Parathyroid disease results from over- or underproduction of PTH or from resistance to parathyroid hormone.

Eighty percent of adults have four small parathyroid glands, although between one and twelve glands have been observed. In the United States, about 100,000 people develop hyperparathyroidism (a condition in which excess PTH is produced) each year. Risk increases with age, and in women over 60 years, 2 in 1,000 will develop the condition. In around 85 percent of cases it is the result of a noncancerous tumor—an adenoma, in which case it is called primary hyperparathyroidism, which leads to elevated blood calcium and PTH levels. In less than 1 percent of cases, primary hyperparathyroidism is caused by parathyroid cancer.

If all glands are overactive, which occurs in 15 percent of patients, or if there are extremely low levels of calcium, the condition is called secondary hyperparathyroidism, which is associated with chronic kidney failure.

Symptoms and diagnosis

Hypercalcemia is an abnormally high level of calcium in the blood as a result of excess parathyroid hormone. Symptoms are fatigue, nausea, abdominal pain, mental confusion, heart arrhythmias, or seizures. Patients may suffer from kidney stones and osteoporosis. Because calcium is being removed from the bones, the calcium is excreted in large amounts in the urine to try to restore a normal blood level; this has the effect of developing stones in the kidneys. Hyperparathyroidism may be the result of another disease that lowers blood calcium levels. In these cases, the output of PTH is increased in order to raise the blood calcium. This is secondary hyperparathyroidism, and it is the body's response to low calcium levels. Common causes of secondary hyperparathyroidism are kidney disease and vitamin D deficiency. Patients may have bone pain and muscle aches.

A deficit of PTH is called hypoparathyroidism; this can be caused by abnormal development, destruction, or decreased function of the glands. In adults, the most common cause of hypoparathyroidism is destruction of the glands in the neck during surgery. Patients have low calcium levels, and symptoms include numbness, tingling around the mouth, and muscle cramps.

Very rarely, patients have resistance to PTH and do not respond to the hormone. This group of diseases is called pseudohypoparathyroidism. Patients will have symptoms due to the low calcium. Bone X-rays of the skull and hands help diagnose the condition. Laboratory blood tests are used to measure calcium levels and parathyroid hormone. The causes of most parathyroid diseases are poorly understood, so there are no known ways to reduce the risk of developing them.

Treatments

If hyperparathyroidism is mild, usually no treatment is needed, although the patient's calcium levels and kidney function will be checked regularly. Drugs may be given if calcium levels are very high. In hypoparathyroidism, PTH is given to replace the hormone. Tumors of the parathyroid are removed surgically.

Mary Ruppe

KEY FACTS

Causes
Hyperfunction of the parathyroid gland.

Risk factors
Mostly unknown. Genetic mutations in rare cases.

Symptoms
Fatigue, nausea, abdominal pain, mental confusion, heart arrhythmias, or seizures.

Diagnosis
History, physical examination, and lab testing.

Treatments
Surgery; or, if mild, periodic laboratory testing.

Pathogenesis
Loss of feedback control of PTH production.

Prevention
Most cases are not preventable.

Epidemiology
In the United States, about 100,000 people develop hyperparathyroidism each year.

See also
- Bone and joint disorders • Cancer
- Hormonal disorders • Kidney disorders

Parkinson's disease

Parkinson's disease (PD) is a chronic, slowly progressing neurodegenerative movement disorder. Its main pathological hallmark is the death of nerve cells (neurons) in a specific region of the brain (substantia nigra pars compacta).

The neurons that are lost in PD are nerve cells that produce dopamine. Dopamine is a chemical neurotransmitter that transmits nerve signals between the substantia nigra and a brain region called the corpus striatum. These signals typically produce normal muscle activity. The loss of dopamine allows striatal neurons to discharge action potentials (fire) without regulation and leaves the afflicted person unable to control his or her muscle movements. It is apparent that 50 to 80 percent of neurons in the substantia nigra may be lost before disease symptoms appear. The symptoms of PD have been known for centuries. It was not until 1817, however, that the disorder became a recognized disease entity.

Causes and risk factors

Parkinson's disease is the most common form of a disease cluster, called parkinsonism, all forms of which share the primary symptoms. Parkinson's disease is classified in two general categories: familial and sporadic. The familial forms of the disorder are caused by gene mutations in any one of about eight identifiable genes. The causes of sporadic or idiopathic Parkinson's disease are unknown but are most likely the result of environmental risk factors acting on genetically susceptible individuals when aging.

Many environmental risk factors have been identified. Decreased risk appears to be associated with such factors as diet (vitamin E, multivitamins), smoking, alcohol, and caffeine. Increased risk appears to be related to such factors as aging, gender (men are at higher risk than women), race (whites are at higher risk than others), family history, life experiences (trauma, stress, and depression), infectious agents (encephalitis and herpes), environmental exposures (heavy metals, well water, farming, and pesticides). A compound that was produced in an attempt to synthesize street heroin called MPTP (1-methyl 4 phenyl 1, 2, 3, 6-tetrahydropyridine) also causes PD-like symptoms and is used, in fact, to study possible mechanisms of neuronal destruction in various disease models.

Aging is a risk factor for Parkinson's disease. It usually affects people over fifty, and the average age of onset is around sixty years. Some people, however, especially those with familial PD, manifest an "early onset" form of the disease before their fortieth year.

Symptoms

The loss of striatal neurons and decreased striatal dopamine concentrations lead to the typical characteristics of PD. These include altered muscle function that negatively impacts many bodily activities that involve movement. Altered muscle function results in the cardinal symptoms of resting tremor in the limbs, hands, and face, including the jaw; muscle (cogwheel) rigidity; slow voluntary movement (bradykinesia); and postural instability, with impaired balance and coordination. As the disease progresses, patients usually have difficulty with speech and with walking, and in advanced cases there may be loss of movement. These collective symptoms are caused by excess muscle contraction due to decreased dopamine production. More subtle, non-motor consequences include cognitive impairment, mood disorders, sleep disturbances, sensation disturbances, altered autonomic function, changes in sensation, and minor problems with language.

Resting tremor is usually one of the earliest symptoms. It presents on one side, is most severe in the resting state, and decreases in intensity with movement. It is estimated, however, that perhaps as many as 30 percent of patients have barely detectable tremor (akinetic tremor). Cogwheel muscle rigidity, or jerky, alternating resistant or nonresistant movements, or both, is observed when a limb is moved passively by the examiner. Bradykinesia and postural instability also result from poor muscle control, owing to the lack of adequate dopamine production and the loss of dopaminergic neurons. This leads to impaired balance and altered postural reflexes that often result in loss of balance and subsequent falls.

PD patients often experience other motor symptoms, such as changes in gait, especially in more advanced cases. The patient may be observed "shuffling," using short steps with minimal foot elevation, accompanied by a shuffling sound as the footwear scuffs along the floor. These patients often fall, especially on a cluttered walking surface. They will often have a decreased arm swing due to the short steps and bradykinesia. Even turning is difficult and is done in a series of small steps without flexing the trunk and neck. Another motor symptom of the advanced patient is a stooped posture, which can become so severe that the upper torso may be at right angles with the rest of the trunk. Eventually, the patient may experience festination, an increasing gait that, when combined with postural changes and poor balance, results in a fall. Akinesia, or "freezing," is also experienced by the advanced PD patient. The patient cannot move his or her feet, especially in confined or obstructed places or when first initiating a step from a standing position.

Other motor effects include alterations in speech and swallowing. Problems with speech include hypophnia, a soft, hoarse, and monotonal speech; and festinating speech, an excessively rapid, usually soft and unintelligible style of speaking. Weak swallowing (dysphagia) and a stooped posture often lead to drooling. In these patients, salivary or food aspiration can lead to poor lung clearing and pneumonia. About 50 percent of patients experience fatigue. Often, patients blink infrequently and can acquire a masklike facial appearance (hypomimia) with a blank expression. Decreased motor activity also impairs the patient's ability to shift positions in bed and to rise from a sitting position. It impairs fine motor coordination and causes an overall loss or severe decrease in movements such as the walking arm swing. These more advanced patients tend to make small letters when handwriting (micrographia).

As the diseases progresses, most patients develop motor symptoms even though they have been treated successfully for symptoms over many years. Motor symptoms begin to manifest with the normal treatment regimen. This is known as "wearing off." Initially it is treated by more frequent administration of levodopa (a drug that increases dopamine levels). "On-off" is another complication that arises over time. The effectiveness of levodopa suddenly disappears and the patient becomes rigid and may have tremors and slow movement. An additional dose of medication can usually, with a little time, overcome this effect. Apomorphine injection also can be used, and it is effective in just a few minutes after administration.

Patients can develop mild to severe uncontrolled movements (dyskinesia) with spasms, writhing, twitching or contraction of muscles, and chorea (involuntary jerky movements) that may often occur as a side effect at the peak of levodopa effect. As the disease progresses, it becomes more difficult to control. Many PD pa-

tients also experience nonmotor effects. Cognitive impairment includes executive dysfunction, memory loss, and ultimately dementia in a significant number of cases. Executive dysfunction implies that the patient has problems with planning, abstract thinking, mental agility, initiating appropriate actions within a framework of rules including determining appropriate and inappropriate reactions to environmental circumstances, and appropriately processing sensory input information. These symptoms may be the early stages of dementia, which affects 20 to 40 percent of patients. Dementia often manifests with difficulty in abstract thinking, memory deficits, and behavioral abnormalities.

Depression is a notable mood disorder in PD patients. Because there are no tools to assess depression specifically in PD, it is difficult to determine the degree to which this disorder permeates the afflicted population. It is felt, however, that it is very common and may affect 50 percent or more of people with the disorder. Depression often goes undetected in this population because it is assumed the behavior may be an unavoidable consequence of the disease. A skilled professional can distinguish depression from the effects of PD since people without PD present with a different profile.

KEY FACTS

Description
A chronic, progressive neurodegenerative disorder.

Causes
Gene mutations and environmental factors.

Risk factors
Aging, diet, race, ethnicity, gender, exposure to chemicals, and infectious agents.

Symptoms
Tremor in the hands, limbs, and face. Poor balance and coordination. Depression, memory loss, and dementia.

Diagnosis
Based on the symptoms. PET can help diagnosis.

Treatments
Increasing dopamine levels.

Pathogenesis
Cognitive impairment, dementia in some cases.

Prevention
None as yet.

Epidemiology
Statistics are variable; best estimates are that around 1 million people in the United States have been diagnosed, and three times that number are believed to be undiagnosed.

During the course of PD and the related parkinsonian disorders, sleep disturbances affect most patients. Altered sleep patterns can profoundly influence the patient's quality of life, affecting performance at work and activities such as driving. Sleep can also be altered by the medications prescribed for PD, especially those that act on dopamine systems. Studies of sleep in this population have found disrupted night sleep, greater leg movements, sleep apnea, drug-independent sleepiness, and REM sleep behavior disorder. In REM sleep behavior disorder, the normal muscle paralysis (atonia) that occurs during REM sleep is disturbed in a way that allows the patient to retain muscle tone. Thus, the patient can respond to dreams in an often violent manner, potentially causing severe injury to himself or herself or another person in the same bed. PD patients also frequently experience restless leg syndrome, a neurological consequence characterized by strange, unpleasant sensations in the legs. Significant disruption in normal sleep patterns can lead to exhaustion.

The senses can be affected in this neurological disorder. Visual function, such as detecting differences in contrast, spatial orientation, color discrimination, binocular vision, and oculomotor control may be impaired. Other disturbances include a decreased ability to properly modulate blood pressure changes in response to changes in body position; dizziness; altered proprioception (awareness of movement and spatial orientation of body parts to each other), reduction (microsmia) or loss (anosmia) of smell acuity, and pain related to the demands placed on the musculature.

Seborrheic dermatitis (oily skin) is fairly common in PD. Later in the course of the disease, urinary incontinence, constipation, altered sexual function, and weight loss can occur.

Diagnosis and treatments

There is not a definitive diagnostic test or combination of tests for PD. The diagnosis of the disease is based mainly on the hallmark symptoms discussed above and the unified PD rating scale. In combination with these, positron emission tomography (PET), an instrumental test that is useful in observing organ function, greatly increases diagnostic accuracy. Good specificity for the test is provided because radioactive test substances that mimic dopamine can show that dopamine uptake is decreased.

Treatment of symptoms with medications is often the first approach to managing the disorder. Usually, the type of medications, the dose and frequency of administration, and the combinations of medications must be adjusted over time during the course of the disorder. Many of the medications have significant side effects; the patient's physical well-being and mental health must be closely monitored. Most of the medications primarily control symptoms by increasing available dopamine levels. The most widely used drug for the treatment of PD tremor is levodopa. However, only a small portion, probably not more than 5 percent, of the levodopa gets into the brain. The remaining material is metabolized in other tissues and eventually causes significant side effects. Also, the administered levodopa inhibits the normal production of levodopa, so doses must be increased over time. In addition to levodopa, inhibitors (carbidopa and benserazide) of the nonbrain enzymes that convert levodopa to dopamine can be administered in "combination therapy" with levodopa to decrease the amount of levodopa that is metabolized before it reaches the brain. These inhibitors also decrease the side effects experienced by the extraneural metabolism of levodopa.

When symptoms are not controlled by medication, surgery, such as deep brain stimulation, pallidotomy, and thalamotomy, may be tried. Speech therapy and exercise may improve quality of life for the PD patient.

Pathogenesis and epidemiology

There is no cure for PD, but medications or surgical procedures give significant symptomatic relief for extended periods. Because the disease follows a chronic course, long-term management is important. Adjustments in medications, family and patient education, the use of support personnel and groups, maintenance of well-being, exercise, and nutrition all help.

An estimated 0.37 percent, or 1 million people, in the United States suffer from PD, and an estimated 3 to 4 million people with PD remain undiagnosed. Around 15,000 per year in the United States die from PD. Some data has associated increased PD mortality with countries using agricultural pesticides. The incidence of PD may depend on gender, age, and ethnicity. Men have a higher incidence of PD than women; the incidence in both genders increases over the age of 60; and Hispanics have the highest rate of the disease, followed by non-Hispanic whites, Asians, and blacks.

David Ullman

See also
- Aging, disorders of • Dementia
- Disabilities • Muscle system disorders
- Paralysis

Pelvic inflammatory disease

Pelvic inflammatory disease (PID) is an infection of the female reproductive tract, which causes sickness and infertility worldwide.

PID is caused by infections, usually chlamydia and gonorrhea, and these bacteria are the targets for treating the disease. If left untreated, 18 percent of women will have chronic pelvic pain, 9 percent will have an ectopic pregnancy, and 20 percent will be infertile. The organisms causing PID usually spread up the female reproductive tract from the vagina, through the cervix, and can infect the uterus, fallopian tubes, and peritoneum. PID is complex because there are many ways it can present in women. In the United States more than 1 million women develop PID yearly.

Causes and risk factors

Common organisms that cause PID are chlamydia and gonorrhea, and possibly bacteria that lead to bacterial vaginosis. Many women do not have any symptoms, but most experience pelvic pain and may also have vaginal discharge or bleeding. Women at increased risk for PID are those with STDs (sexually transmitted diseases), PID in the past, early age sexual activity, those not using good barrier contraception, and those with many sexual partners. Other risk factors include vaginal douching or using an intrauterine contraceptive device. Using oral contraceptive pills may reduce the risk of PID.

Diagnosis and treatments

It is recommended that all women with abdominal pain be examined and tested for STDs. Tests that are helpful in diagnosing infection are the presence of white blood cells (WBC) in a vaginal swab or increased blood WBC counts. Ultrasound scans of the reproductive tract are also useful and can show thickening of the fallopian tubes in women with PID. Other changes related to inflammation may be seen with magnetic resonance imaging or computed tomography scans. Biopsy samples taken from the uterus can show inflammation changes under the microscope, and laparoscopy may be needed to confirm the diagnosis.

Tests include radiological examinations and exploratory surgery to look for the disease, if treatment with medications are not effective. The most effective way to reduce the incidence of PID is to prevent it from developing. Screening women for chlamydia and gonorrhea who do not have symptoms and treating those women with antibiotics that can act against chlamydia and gonorrhea and possibly bacterial vaginosis are effective measures in preventing PID. There are different patterns of drug resistance of these organisms in different parts of the world, so regional variations may decide which antibiotic is chosen. Early treatment of those with PID will also prevent the development of complications. Whether the treatment is given in the hospital or at home depends on the severity of the PID.

PID is a serious condition and causes medical issues for women worldwide. Early screening and treatment can prevent many long-term complications.

Moeen Panni

KEY FACTS

Description
An infection of the female reproductive tract.

Causes
Caused by chlamydia and gonorrhea.

Risk factors
Sexual activity at an early age, many sexual partners, IUCDs, previous PID, and an STD.

Symptoms
Pelvic pain, vaginal discharge, and bleeding.

Diagnosis
Examination, blood tests, ultrasound, radiological examinations, and exploratory surgery.

Treatments
Early screening and treatment can prevent many of the long-term complications. Antibiotics.

Pathogenesis
If left untreated, the disease can lead to chronic pelvic pain, ectopic pregnancy, and infertility.

Prevention
Regular checkups, prompt treatment of infection.

Epidemiology
Around 1 million cases of PID yearly in the U.S.

See also
- Chlamydial infections • Ectopic pregnancy
- Female reproductive system disorders
- Gonorrhea • Infections, bacterial
- Infertility •Sexually transmitted diseases

Peritonitis

Infection of the peritoneum may be primary (without evident cause), secondary (related to an intra-abdominal process), or a complication of peritoneal dialysis.

Primary or spontaneous bacterial peritonitis (SBP) occurs in adults with cirrhosis and ascites and children with kidney damage or cirrhotic livers with large nodules. Risk factors for SBP include advanced cirrhosis, prior episode of SBP, coexisting gastrointestinal bleed, and low protein concentration in the fluid in the peritoneal cavity. The microorganisms causing SBP include E. coli, Klebsiella, *Streptococcus pneumoniae*, and *Streptococcus* species (19 percent). Fever, abdominal pain, nausea, vomiting, diarrhea, and altered mental status are common symptoms, but many patients are asymptomatic. Diagnosis of SBP requires paracentesis, in which a needle is used to puncture the body cavity, to take fluid for culture, to relieve the pressure of excess fluid, or to inject medication. Treatment of suspected SBP should be started as soon as cultures are obtained. Empiric antibiotics should be given—that is, without definite knowledge of the disorder but based on the fact that they were effective in similar cases. Clinical improvement occurs within 48 hours. Treatment for five days is as efficacious as longer courses. Mortality has declined from 95 percent to 40 percent since 1924. In high risk patients, antibiotic prophylaxis decreases the recurrence rate of SBP.

Secondary peritonitis

Perforation of the gastrointestinal or urogenital tract caused by infection, trauma, or surgery leads to secondary peritonitis. A large number of microorganisms spill into the peritoneal cavity, leading to polymicrobial infection with anaerobes (especially *Bacteriodes fragilis*), enterobacteraceae, streptococci, enterococci, and clostridia. *Neisseria gonorrhoeae* may be present in female genital tract infection. Activation of the immune system by the protein cytokine can cause inflammation, toxins can be released when bacteria die, and anaerobic and aerobic bacteria can cause sepsis and abscesses. Abdominal pain aggravated by motion is a predominant symptom. Anorexia, nausea, vomiting, fever, and abdominal distension are seen. Marked abdominal tenderness with rebound tenderness, rigidity, and hyperresonant or absent bowel sounds are other signs. High heart rate, fast breathing, and low blood pressure signify septic shock. An increase in white cells and elevated serum amylase levels are frequent. Dilated bowel loops or free air may be seen on radiographs. Ultrasonography or computed tomography scans of the abdomen detect lesions and guide drainage of fluid or abscess. Surgery to control the contamination, remove necrotic tissue, and drain abscesses is essential. Antibiotics should be started immediately after obtaining blood cultures. Supportive measures to maintain circulation, oxygenation, and nutrition are critical. Survival depends on the age of the patient, co-morbid conditions, duration of peritoneal contamination, and the microorganisms involved. Peritoneal dialysis carries a risk of peritonitis.

Nigar Kirmani

KEY FACTS

Description

Infection of the peritoneum may be primary, secondary, or related to peritoneal dialysis.

Causes

Primary: enteric gram negatives and streptococci. Secondary: bowel anaerobes and gram negatives. Peritoneal dialysis: gram positive bacteria.

Symptoms

Fever, abdominal pain, nausea, vomiting and diarrhea. Abdominal tenderness, rebound tenderness, and hypoactive bowel sounds.

Diagnosis

Elevated cell count in fluid in peritoneal cavity and positive culture are diagnostic.

Treatment

Broad spectrum antibiotics are needed. Surgical drainage and anaerobic coverage are essential for secondary peritonitis.

Pathogenesis

Translocation of intestinal bacteria, spillage of bowel contents and infection of catheter exit site.

Prevention

Antibiotic prophylaxis prevents recurrences of SBP.

Epidemiology

SBP occurs in cirrhotics with ascites and children with nephrotic syndrome. Secondary peritonitis occurs after bowel perforation, trauma, or surgery.

See also
- Cirrhosis of the liver • Infections, bacterial
- Kidney disorders

Personality disorders

Personality disorders are a group of disorders described by the *Diagnostic and Statistical Manual of Mental Disorders,* fourth edition (DSM-IV), as "an enduring pattern of inner experience and behavior that deviates markedly from the expectations of the individual's culture, is pervasive and inflexible, has an onset in adolescence or early adulthood, is stable over time, and leads to distress and impairment." Personality disorders are notoriously difficult to treat.

Although personality disorders have their onset in adolescence or early adulthood, they are considered adult disorders. Personality disorders are pervasive and maladaptive patterns of human behavior. These enduring patterns of inflexible and aberrant behavior are not a consequence of another psychiatric disorder, medical condition, or substance abuse.

Causes and risk factors

Numerous factors may contribute to the development of personality disorders. Some of these factors are biological, while others are environmental. The interactions between biological and environmental factors are complex. For instance, Cluster A personality disorders are more common in the biological relatives of patients with schizophrenia. Depressive disorders are common in the family backgrounds of patients with borderline personality disorders.

A strong association has been demonstrated between individuals with histrionic personality disorders and patients with somatization disorder, in which people think they have a physical illness, but no cause can be discovered for the symptoms. Parental alcoholism and antisocial behavior are prevalent in the families of individuals who have antisocial personality disorder.

Since children's behavior is shaped by their family environment, personality disorders are often viewed as direct results of these interactions, or they may serve as adaptation strategies to their specific families. For example, very active children may be restrained in their activities by overly protective and controlling parents. Consequently, those children might develop coping strategies that predispose them toward avoidant behavior.

Individuals at high risk for the development of personality disorders are often abused children, children raised in chaotic family environments, children with close relatives diagnosed with personality disorders and major psychiatric illnesses, and children whose parents are alcohol and substance abusers.

Diagnosis

The assessment of the symptoms and patterns of behavior should be based on as many sources of information as possible. From the diagnostic point of view, it is also advisable to conduct more than one clinical interview with an individual prior to a diagnosis being given. In addition to the fact that the ethnic, cultural, and social background of the individual must be taken into account, it is important to assess the stability of symptoms in a variety of contexts. With the exception of one type of personality disorder, antisocial personality disorder, the diagnosis of personality disorders can be applied to adolescence and young adults; however, in order to diagnose a personality disorder in an individual prior to age eighteen, the symptoms must be present for at least one year. When individuals meet the criteria for more than one personality disorder, each of them should be diagnosed separately. Personality disorders are coded on Axis II of DSM-IV, as opposed to any other psychiatric disorders, which are coded on Axis I.

Based on the DSM-IV, a diagnosis of personality disorder requires that an individual must experience significant problems in two or more of the following general areas in addition to the number of specific symptoms. These general diagnostic criteria are cognition, affectivity, interpersonal functioning, and impulse control. It has previously been noted that the general concept of the category of personality disorders is mostly based on Western understanding of personality and the definition of "normalcy."

Symptoms

The personality disorders are grouped into three clusters in the DSM-IV, based on their symptom similarities. Cluster A covers the paranoid, schizoid, and schizotypical personality disorders. Individuals from this cluster often appear to be odd or eccentric. Cluster B is made up of the antisocial, borderline, histrionic, and narcissistic personality disorders. Individuals from this cluster are often described as emotional, dramatic, and unpredictable. Cluster C includes the avoidant, dependent, and obsessive-compulsive personality disorders. Individuals from this cluster are often described as anxious. There is an additional DSM-IV category of personality disorder: not otherwise specified (NOS). This category is usually applied in the clinical cases in which an individual is considered to have a personality disorder that is not included in the DSM-IV (for example, passive-aggressive personality) or an individual exhibits symptoms of more than one type of personality disorder.

Cautionary note

Although the cluster system has proved helpful for research and educational purposes, the DSM-IV adds a warning note that there are limitations to the system, not least because some people have co-occurring personality disorders from different clusters.

Cluster A personality disorders

Paranoid individuals with paranoid personality disorder are often suspicious of others and preoccupied with doubts regarding the motives of other people. Those individuals have major difficulties in establishing close relationships because of their fear that the information they share can be used against them. Such people are also prone to bear grudges and have difficulty forgiving insults or other real or perceived injuries. Because they lack trust in other people, these individuals have an excessive need to be self-sufficient and have a strong desire to control their environment.

Schizoid individuals with schizoid personality disorder often demonstrate a lack of desire for intimacy. They often have a restricted affect in emotional situations and appear to be disinterested in developing close relationship with others. They rarely experience or display emotions such as anger or excitement.

Schizotypical individuals with this disorder are characterized by a marked discomfort concerning close relationships as well as cognitive and perceptual distortions. It is not uncommon for these individuals to have ideas out of reference or even have some paranoid ideations. Their affect is usually restricted. Under stressors, these individuals may experience transient psychotic episodes with a duration from a few minutes to hours.

Cluster B personality disorders

Antisocial individuals with this disorder are characterized by a pervasive pattern of disregard for, and viola-

---

KEY FACTS

Description

Pervasive and maladaptive patterns of behavior that lead to the significant impairment of functioning in major areas, in the clear absence of other psychiatric or medical conditions or changes in personality related to alcohol or substance use.

Causes and risk factors

Personality disorders may be the result of multiple interactions between the individual's characteristics, such as temperament, and environmental factors, for example cultural and social norms and family upbringing.

Diagnosis

The diagnosis of personality disorder is usually made by a clinician based on the results from clinical evaluations. There are no laboratory tests or other procedures available that can provide a definitive diagnosis.

Symptoms

Based on the similarity of symptoms, personality disorders are grouped into three clusters in the DSM-IV. Cluster A covers the paranoid, schizoid, and schizotypical personality disorders. Cluster B is made up of the antisocial, borderline, histrionic, and narcissistic personality disorders. Cluster C includes the avoidant, dependent, and obsessive-compulsive personality disorders. There is also a DSM-IV category of "personality disorder not otherwise specified" (NOS) for those individuals who do not clearly fit into any of the described personality disorders.

Treatments

The types of treatments depend on the particular subtype of personality disorder, severity of symptomatology, and comorbid conditions (that is, substance use disorders, eating disorders, and anxiety disorders). Treatment is typically successful when it is individualized and may include both psychotherapy and pharmacotherapy.

Pathogenesis

The outlook varies. Some personality disorders diminish during middle age without any treatment, while others persist throughout life despite treatment.

Prevention

Early identification and treatment of individuals at high risk.

Epidemiology

Varies across different personality disorders.

tion of, the rights of others, which begins in childhood or early adolescence and continues into adulthood. For this diagnosis to be given, the individuals must be at least 18 years of age and must have been diagnosed with conduct disorder prior to the age of 15. Lack of empathy, arrogance, superficial charm, and self-assurance are hallmarks of this disorder.

Borderline individuals with this disorder are characterized by a pattern of instability in their personal relationships, self-image, marked fluctuation of affect, and impulsivity at least in two areas (for example, unsafe sexual practices, gambling, binge eating, or substance abuse). Their dysphoric mood is often disrupted by episodes of anger or extreme anxiety and despair. Under stress, some of these individuals are prone to psychotic-like symptoms, such as ideas out of reference, body-image distortions, and hallucinations. Histrionic individuals with this disorder are characterized by excessive emotionality and attention-seeking behavior. These individuals often become depressed and upset if they are not the center of attention. They are novelty driven and become easily bored with their usual routine. Their appearance and behavior can be inappropriately sexual and seductive.

Narcissistic individuals with this disorder are characterized by a need for admiration, a lack of empathy, a sense of self-importance, and exploitative attitudes toward others. They often believe that they are superior and expect others to recognize it as well. These individuals are very sensitive to criticism and may become extremely agitated or angry because of it.

Cluster C personality disorders

Avoidant individuals with this disorder are usually preoccupied with feelings of inadequacy and hypersensitivity to rejection or negative evaluation in social situations. They prefer to have minimal social interactions because of their fears of criticism or humiliation. There are often shy, quiet, and isolated. In many cases, individuals with this disorder also fit the criteria for social phobia.

Dependent individuals with this disorder are characterized by marked difficulties with the decision-making processes of everyday life. These individuals often lack the initiative to take control of major areas in their lives. They tend to form a close relationship in order to obtain the care and support they need. They rarely question authorities and usually display compliant behaviors to avoid displeasing other people.

Obsessive-compulsive individuals with this disorder are preoccupied with orderliness, perfectionism, and a

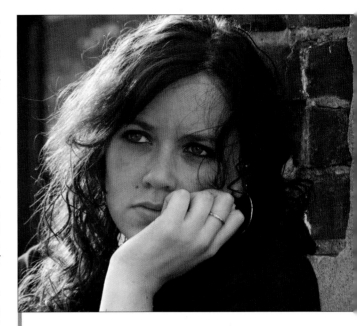

For someone who has a personality disorder, poor social functioning and an inability to adapt to changing circumstances can cause distress in everyday life. It can impinge on all relationships and cause occupational problems.

need for mental and interpersonal control. Their everyday relationships have a formal and serious quality, and their interpersonal style is often described as stiff or rigid. They are preoccupied with concerns that things have to be done a specific, "correct" way; subsequently, they have difficulties accepting ideas or suggestions from other people.

Treatments

The treatment of personality disorders is complicated by the fact that affected individuals rarely seek help on their own. Most of the patients view their problems as part of their self-image, which explains their reluctance to participate in treatment. Subsequently, the type of treatment depends on the willingness of the affected individuals to accept a need for change, the severity of the symptoms associated with specific personality disorders, and comorbid conditions. A growing body of evidence supports the notion that a biopsychosocial approach to the treatment of personality disorders provides a foundation for integrating diagnosis and treatment modalities. Based on this approach, psychotherapy and pharmacotherapy can be matched to meet the individual needs of patients. A variety of psychotherapeutic methods have been tried for personality disorders. Each of them provides interventions based on the theoretical understandings of the development of personality disorders. On a practical level, different schools of psychotherapy are not mutually exclusive, but rather overlap and complement each other. The psychotherapeutic modalities are often aimed at examining the psychodynamic aspects of the patient's relationships, enhancing problem-solving skills and the ability to tolerate frustrations, stressors, and the uncertainty of daily life, and improvement of cognitive skills.

Each personality disorder subtype requires specific modifications of therapeutic goals, and objectives and must be based on realistic expectations of how much character change can be achieved by the particular patient.

The pharmacotherapy of personality disorders is not organized around different subtypes, but rather targets symptom domains such as physical aggression, hyperactivity, impulsiveness, transitory psychotic symptoms, anxiety, and mood reactivity. For example, it is not uncommon to prescribe antipsychotic medications to patients with paranoid and schizotypal personality disorders during a brief psychotic episode.

Patients with borderline personality disorder can be also given antipsychotics during episodes of transient paranoid ideations or dissociative symptoms. Mood stabilizers such as lithium, carbamazepine, lamotrigine, and valproate can be used to improve impulsiveness, anger outbursts, and sudden mood changes. Antidepressants and anti-anxiety medications are also clinically effective therapeutic agents in the manage-

If a person has a narcissistic personality disorder, he or she feels an unrealistic sense of self-importance. The person needs a lot of praise but cannot accept criticism and so tends to have unsatisfactory relations with other people.

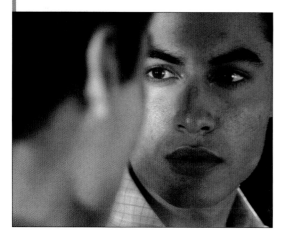

ment of depressive symptoms, episodic dysphoria (feeling sick or unhappy), irritability, sleep problems, and anxiety.

Pathogenesis

Although personality disorders are lifelong patterns of maladaptive behavior with an onset in adolescence or early adulthood, most of the individuals experience periods of remissions and exacerbations. Positive life experiences and major life events, such as the death of a parent or spouse, marriage, birth of a child, and retirement can modify the course of personality disorders and the age of diagnosis.

Prevention

The preventive strategy involves the early identification of children and young adolescents who are at high risk based on family histories and significant environmental variables, such as chaotic family upbringing. Once an at-risk individual is identified, therapeutic measures aimed at the prevention of the development of full-blown disorder are implemented.

Epidemiology

The prevalence of personality disorders varies in different population samples. It is estimated that 0.5 to 2.5 percent of the general population meet the criteria for paranoid personality disorder, about 2 percent for schizoid, and about 3 percent for schizotypical. The prevalence of antisocial personality disorder is about 3 percent in men and 1 percent in females in community settings, but the prevalence of this disorder is 10 times higher in prisons or other forensic settings. About 2 percent of the general population carry a diagnosis of borderline personality disorder; about 75 percent of those patients are women. It is estimated that histrionic personality disorder occurs in about 2 percent of the general population. Fewer than 1 percent of the population have narcissistic personality disorder, and 75 percent of them are men. About 1 percent of the population have avoidant or obsessive-compulsive personality disorders, and between 0.5 and 1 percent have dependent personality disorder.

Oleg Tcheremissine

See also

• Alcohol-related disorders • Anxiety disorders • Asperger's disorder • Autism • Bipolar disorder • Depressive disorders • Mental disorders • Mood disorders • Psychotic disorders • Schizophrenia • Substance abuse and addiction

Phenylketonuria

Phenylketonuria (PKU) is an autosomal recessive disorder in which the absence of the enzyme phenylalanine hydroxylase (PAH) results in the buildup of phenylalanine in the blood and urine. This buildup leads to mental retardation and neurological problems if not treated early in life with dietary modification.

Phenylketonuria (PKU) is an inborn error of metabolism in which affected individuals lack the enzyme phenylalanine hydroxylase (PAH). Without this enzyme, these individuals cannot metabolize the amino acid phenylalanine. The inability to metabolize phenylalanine leads to a buildup in the bloodstream, which results in cognitive impairment and a "mousy" odor of the body and urine. Other findings include neurological manifestations as well as lighter skin pigmentation and occasionally an eczematous rash.

PKU is a result of an abnormal gene that is inherited in an autosomal recessive fashion. There is no single mutation that predominates in PKU, and a person must inherit an affected gene from each parent. With such a low incidence of this disorder, newborn screening programs have been instrumental in identifying affected individuals. Testing should also be performed to rule out lack of tetrahydrobiopterin, an essential cofactor.

Treatments

Treatment of this disorder involves restriction of phenylalanine intake within one month after birth. Well-established phenylalanine-free diets have been in use since the 1930s. Some patients with PKU will also require tyrosine supplementation. Infants who are not appropriately treated with diet restriction can develop severe mental retardation within six months of birth, as well as asthma and hyperactivity. Optimal outcomes require continuation of the diet throughout life, as some sequelae (complications) can manifest after childhood. Individuals must also avoid aspartame because one of the breakdown products of this artificial sweetener is phenylalanine.

As a result of an effective newborn screening program, pregnant mothers who have PKU have become a concern. Pregnant women with poor diet adherence have a much higher incidence of having offspring with mental retardation, microcephaly, or congenital heart defects than the general population. These risks are increased with elevated phenylalanine levels during pregnancy with microcephaly and mental retardation occurring in 73 to 92 percent of offspring. These risks are independent of the PKU status of the fetus.

Wade Schwendemann and Brian Brost

KEY FACTS

Description

An inborn error of metabolism leading to impaired cognitive development and neurophysiological function if not appropriately treated.

Causes

Phenylketonuria (PKU) is inherited in an autosomal recessive fashion when a pair of abnormal genes is inherited. The gene for phenylalanine hydroxylase (PAH) is faulty and unable break to down phenylalanine. More than 400 mutations in this region can result in PKU.

Risk factors

There are no known risk factors.

Symptoms

Presenting symptoms include mild to severe mental retardation, developmental delay, seizures, and abnormalities of gait, sitting posture, or stance. There can be a "mousy" odor of the body or urine.

Diagnosis

Elevated levels of phenylalanine in the blood. Those with classic PKU have levels over 20 mg/dL without treatment.

Treatments

Treatment of this disorder consists of a phenylalanine-restricted diet. With proper and early dietary modification, nearly all effects of the disorder can be avoided.

Pathogenesis

Lack of the PAH enzyme leads to a buildup of phenylalanine; the exact mechanism of the mental retardation is unknown.

Prevention

No known method of preventing the inheritance of this disorder, although the sequelae can be prevented by aggressive treatment.

See also
- Genetic disorders • Mental retardation
- Metabolic disorders

Plague

Plague is an ancient disease that has killed hundreds of millions of people. It is one of the most deadly diseases humans have ever known. The disease never completely disappears, and the world has experienced three major outbreaks, or pandemics, of plague.

The first pandemic of plague was in 541 C.E. The outbreak began in Egypt and then moved across Europe, killing over 100 million people. Seven hundred years later, a second outbreak killed one in three people in Europe. During this time, people began calling plague the Black Death or the great pestilence. A third pandemic swept around the world in 1855. It eventually spread to every inhabited continent and killed more than 12 million people in China and India alone. There are still approximately 1,000 to 3,000 cases in the world each year. Now, however, the chances of a pandemic are very low. Plague used to kill about 90 percent of the people who got sick, but thanks to antibiotics, now only one out of seven cases of plague is fatal.

Causes

Plague is a zoonosis, that is, a disease that can spread naturally from animals to humans. Plague is caused by an infection with the bacterium *Yersinia pestis*. The bacteria live in animals such as rats, prairie dogs, marmots, and other rodents. Fleas bite these animals and pick up the bacteria. The fleas then jump onto humans and bite them, giving them the infection.

Plague has two main forms. One is bubonic plague, which results from fleabites. It gets its name from the large, swollen, and tender lymph nodes, called buboes, which it causes. These swollen lymph nodes are usually in the neck, under the arms, or at the top of the legs. The other main form of the disease is pneumonic plague. This occurs when the infection is in the lungs.

Bioterrorism

Naturally occurring plague is not the only form of the disease; several countries have found ways to turn plague into a biological weapon. Many countries conducted research with plague, and a few actually created weapons. The Japanese army used plague as a weapon against the Chinese in 1940. In this particular

KEY FACTS

Description
A disease of animals that can infect humans. Bacteria called *Yersinia pestis* cause plague. It occur in two forms: bubonic plague and pneumonic plague.

Causes
A bite from an infected flea causes bubonic plague. Pneumonic plague occurs in some people with bubonic plague when the bacteria travel to the lungs. Other people get pneumonic plague when exposed to airborne droplets from a person with pneumonic plague. Some biological weapons can also cause plague.

Risk factors
Yersinia pestis lives on every continent except Australia. The infected fleas usually come from rats, prairie dogs, marmots, and other rodents.

Symptoms
A patient with plague feels very ill. People with bubonic plague will develop large painful masses of lymph nodes, called buboes, usually in the armpit or at the top of the leg. Those with pneumonic plague may have chest pain, trouble breathing, and a cough that brings up bloody material from the lungs.

Diagnosis
Doctors will make their initial diagnosis based on the patient's symptoms. Special laboratories can perform tests to verify the diagnosis.

Treatments
Health care providers treat plague with intravenous or oral antibiotics.

Pathogenesis
In bubonic plague, bacteria grow in the lymph nodes and release toxins that make the patient very ill.

Prevention
Anyone exposed to plague should begin taking antibiotics as soon as possible to reduce the chance of becoming infected. People with pneumonic plague can spread the disease to others not infected. They should be isolated and health care workers must use protective equipment when caring for these patients.

Epidemiology
If untreated, bubonic plague kills 30 percent of its victims in around four days. Untreated pneumonic plague kills 95 percent of its victims in three days. In rural areas of the United States, 10 to 15 cases occur annually. Worldwide, 1,000 to 3,000 cases occur annually, in countries such as Africa, Asia, and South America.

case, the attackers dropped plague-infected fleas from an aircraft. This attack caused 120 deaths. After World War II, both the United States and the Soviet Union were able to create a weapon system that spread the bacteria directly, without the need for fleas. The United States never took this project very far, but it is believed that the Soviet Union did a substantial amount of work in this area.

Plague is a problem only in extremely unsanitary conditions in poorer areas of the world where there are regular small outbreaks; there are only occasional outbreaks in developed countries. As living conditions improve around the world, the number of people who develop plague continues to fall. However, because plague is well-established in wild rodents, it probably will never be totally eradicated. Rat extermination should be carried out in both developed and undeveloped countries.

Diagnosis

Plague is not very difficult to diagnose in the laboratory. It has a distinct appearance under a microscope. A scientist in a laboratory can use several tests to examine samples of blood or other body substances from a patient to make certain the disease is plague. A patient with plague also produces antibodies to the bacteria. Laboratory tests that show elevated antibody levels would also confirm that a person was infected.

Treatments

Doctors can treat plague with antibiotics. For quite some time, the antibiotic of choice was streptomycin. This particular medication is not always widely available, and pregnant women should not use it, so doctors may use another medication, such as gentamicin. Health care providers will usually give these medications as an injection, either into the muscle or into a vein. If there are many people who develop the disease at one time, it may not be possible to start intravenous lines on everyone. Doctors may treat patients with oral medications. In this case, the preferred medications are doxycycline or ciprofloxacin, which are acceptable for both adults and children. Plague can be prevented if an exposed person is treated with antibiotics. A vaccine can prevent plague but may not be available in sufficient quantities if plague were used as a biological weapon.

Prevention

Pneumonic plague causes special problems because it spreads from person to person, in droplets that spray

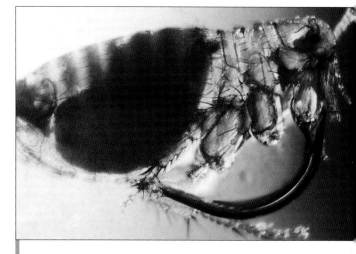

*This greatly magnified picture shows a plague-infected oriental rat flea (*Xenopsylla cheopsis*) after feeding on an inoculated mouse. This flea is known to transmit the bacterium* Yersinia pestis, *the causative agent of plague.*

with each sneeze. Because of this, doctors and nurses must isolate individuals with pneumonic plague so that they do not infect others. People who take care of those with plague must wear personal protective equipment, including a face mask.

In areas where plague is enzootic (known to exist in a locality), preventive measures should be taken. These include eliminating any sources of food or shelter for rodents near homes; ensuring that rodents do not have any means of access to homes; treating pets, such as dogs and cats, with insecticides; avoiding touching dead or sick rodents; and taking care not to handle sick domestic animals, especially cats. Hunters in affected localities should wear gloves before touching dead animals. Hikers and campers must use an appropriate insecticide on clothing and avoid rodent nests. Any pets accompanying hunters, hikers, or campers should also be sprayed with an appropriate insecticide.

Epidemiology

In 2003 the World Health Organization reported 2,118 cases of plague in nine countries. Of these cases, 182 of the victims died.

Richard Bradley

See also

• Anthrax • Avian influenza • Filariasis
• Infections, animal-to-human • Infections, bacterial • Malaria • Rabies • Rickettsial infections • West Nile encephalitis

Pleurisy

Pleurisy is an inflammation of the lining of the lungs that causes pain on breathing or coughing. Pleurisy most commonly results from an infection (pneumonia, viruses, or TB), but can also be caused by chest trauma, rheumatic diseases, lung cancer, and other disorders.

The lungs and inner chest wall are lined by a thin, smooth, self-lubricating tissue called pleura. When a person has pleurisy, this lining becomes inflamed and roughened, such that each breath can produce a grating sound called a "friction rub," which can be heard with a stethoscope. Pleurisy is usually caused by lung infections, but other conditions can also cause pleural inflammation. In some cases, the inflammation causes the accumulation of pleural fluid in the potential space between the pleural surfaces just outside the lung.

Symptoms and diagnosis

The main symptom of pleurisy is sudden pain in the chest, made worse with deep breathing, coughing, and chest movement. Pain may be referred to areas away from the site of origin, such as the shoulder, lower chest, neck, or abdomen, which can be confused with intra-abdominal disease. If sufficient pleural fluid accumulates, it can compress the underlying lung, causing rapid or difficult breathing.

Pleurisy is easily diagnosed when the characteristic pleuritic pain occurs. A pleural friction rub is diagnostic but may be transient in nature. Chest radiographs are useful to demonstrate pleural fluid. Analysis of the pleural fluid when present is the most helpful diagnostic test in establishing a diagnosis in most cases of pleurisy. This is done using a procedure called thoracentesis, in which a fine needle is inserted into the chest to reach the pleural space and extract fluid.

Treatments

The pain of pleurisy is controlled with acetaminophen, nonsteroidal anti-inflammatory drugs, or occasionally with narcotics, depending on the severity of the pain. Treatment of the underlying cause of pleurisy is essential. Bacterial pneumonia is treated with antibiotics. Viral infections are usually self-limiting and do not require medication other than symptomatic relief.

Alternative treatments can be used along with traditional therapy to heal pleurisy. Acupuncture and botanical medications may alleviate pleuritic pain and breathing problems. Contrast hydrotherapy and homeopathic treatment can also be efffective in relieving the pain.

Pleurisy can be prevented depending upon the cause. Early treatment of pneumonia can prevent the accumulation of fluid (pleural effusion).

Isaac Grate

KEY FACTS

Description

Inflammation of the lining of the lungs that causes roughening of the lining and acute pain with breathing and coughing.

Causes

Pleurisy is caused by a number of conditions, including bacterial and viral infections, tuberculosis, cancer, trauma, certain systemic diseases, and other conditions.

Symptoms

Sudden pain in the chest, made worse with deep breathing, coughing, and chest movements.

Diagnosis

A diagnosis of pleurisy is made when a patient is experiencing the characteristic pleuritic pain, or the pleural friction rub can be heard through a stethoscope, or both. Chest radiographs may show accumulated fluid.

Treatments

Depends on the cause of the pleurisy. Bacterial infections are treated with antibiotics; viral infections are self-limiting and run their course without medications.

Epidemiology

None available.

Risk factors

None known.

Prevention

Early treatment of pneumonia with antibiotics, or treatment of the underlying disease.

See also

Pneumonia

Pneumonia is a common respiratory illness, affecting millions of people annually. It ranges in severity from mild to serious and can even be fatal, depending upon the type of infecting organism, the victim's age, and underlying health status. People at higher risk for pneumonia include the elderly, smokers, young children, and people with anatomic problems, chronic conditions, or compromised immune systems.

Pneumonia is caused most often by bacteria and viruses and less often by fungi and parasites. Pneumonia may also occur because of various lung injuries or other medical issues. More than one hundred strains of microorganisms can cause pneumonia, yet only a few are responsible for most cases. The smallest airways of the lungs are surrounded by alveoli (air-filled sacs), which are vital to oxygen and carbon dioxide exchange. Destructive, invading microorganisms trigger an immune system response, causing inflammation and interruption in gas exchange. The symptoms of infectious pneumonia are caused by both destructive, invading microorganisms and the immune system's response. Lobar pneumonias involve only a single lobe or lung section; multilobar pneumonias involve more than one lobe and are often more serious.

Bacterial pneumonia

In adults and children over five years of age, bacterial pneumonias are typically the most common and most serious. The term *atypical pneumonia* refers to pneumonia caused by certain bacteria: *Legionella pneumophila*, *Mycoplasma pneumonia*, and *Chlamydophila pneumoniae*. Atypical bacteria and viruses are the most common causes of interstitial pneumonia, which involves the areas between the alveoli (interstitial pneumonitis). The word *atypical* is used because healthier people are commonly affected and the pneumonia is generally less severe and responds to different antibiotics from other bacteria. An exception is *Legionella pneumonia*, which can be severe, with high mortality rates. Although bacteria are typically inhaled, they can also reach the lungs through the bloodstream, if there is an infection elsewhere in the body. Many of the types of bacteria that cause pneumonia can be found in the nose or mouth of healthy people. *Streptococcus pneumoniae* (pneumococcus) is the most common pneumonia-causing bacterium in all age groups except newborn infants and is the most common cause of lobar pneumonia. Another important cause of pneumonia is *Staphylococcus aureus*. Less common bacterial causes include *Hemophilus influenzae* and *Pseudomonas aeruginosa*. Many of the less common causes of bacterial pneumonia live in the gastrointestinal tract and may enter the lungs if vomit is inhaled.

Viral pneumonia

Besides damaging lung tissue, viral pneumonias can affect other organs and disrupt many body functions. Although respiratory syncytial virus (RSV) is the major pathogen in viral pneumonias, these types of pneumonias can also be caused by other viruses, including influenza, parainfluenza, adenovirus, cytomegalovirus (CMV), and herpes simplex virus. Herpes simplex virus is a rare cause of pneumonia, except in newborns. People who have compromised immune systems are at risk for CMV pneumonia. Viral pneumonias are the most common types of pneumonias in children less than five years of age.

Community-acquired pneumonia

Community-acquired pneumonia is infectious pneumonia in a person who has not recently been hospitalized. It is the most common type of pneumonia; its most common causes, which differ by age group, include *S. pneumoniae* (the most common cause worldwide), the atypical bacteria, *H. influenzae*, and viruses. The term *walking pneumonia* has been used to describe a type of community-acquired pneumonia of less severity, usually caused by an atypical bacterium or virus.

Hospital-acquired pneumonia

The more serious hospital-acquired pneumonia (nosocomial pneumonia) is acquired during or after hospitalization for another illness or procedure. Its causes, microbiology, treatment, and prognosis, are different from those of community-acquired pneumonia. Up to 5 percent of patients hospitalized for other causes subsequently develop pneumonia. Many have risk factors for pneumonia, like mechanical ventilation, prolonged malnutrition, underlying heart and lung diseases, decreased amounts of stomach acid, and compromised immune systems. The microorganisms a person is exposed to in a hospital are often different from those at home and they are more dangerous; they include resistant bacteria such as methicillin-resistant *S. aureus* (MRSA) and *P. aeruginosa*.

Aspiration pneumonia

Aspiration pneumonia (aspiration pneumonitis) is caused by inhaling oral or gastric contents while eating or as a result of reflux or vomiting. The resultant lung inflammation can contribute to infection, since the material aspirated may contain anaerobic bacteria. Aspiration is a leading cause of death among hospital and nursing home patients.

Less common pneumonia classifications include fungal pneumonia, which can occur in people with compromised immune systems; parasitic pneumonia, in which parasites typically enter the body through the skin or by swallowing, then travel to the lungs through the blood; and chemical pneumonia, which is caused by chemical toxins that enter the body through inhalation or skin contact. Often, pneumonias are classified as acute (less than three weeks duration) or chronic. Chronic pneumonias tend to be either noninfectious or mycobacterial, fungal, or mixed bacterial (caused by airway obstruction). Acute pneumonias are further divided into classic bacterial pneumonias (*S. pneumoniae*), atypical pneumonias (*M. pneumoniae* or *C. pneumoniae*), and aspiration pneumonias.

Symptoms of pneumonia

The symptoms of pneumonia include cough (dry or productive), chest pain, respiratory distress, and fever. Increased respiratory rate is the most consistent clinical manifestation. Headache, stiff and aching muscles and joints, loss of appetite, fatigue, sore throat, and gastrointestinal complaints (nausea, vomiting, diarrhea, abdominal distention) may also be present. Infectious pneumonias are often preceded for several days by symptoms of an upper respiratory infection. Less common forms of pneumonia can also cause anemia, rashes, and neurological syndromes. In the elderly, pneumonia may manifest itself atypically, with new or worsening confusion or unsteadiness leading to falls. Infants with pneumonia may experience the above symptoms but may also have a decreased appetite and be increasingly sleepy.

Diagnosis

People with suspected pneumonia should undergo a medical evaluation that includes a thorough physical examination and a chest X-ray, since pneumonia shares symptoms with other conditions and can be difficult to diagnose in people with other illnesses.

A physical examination may reveal the above symptoms, as well as low blood pressure, increased heart rate, or low blood oxygen. People with respiratory distress, confusion, or low blood oxygen need immediate medical attention. Listening to the lungs with a stethoscope reveals diminished breath sounds and crackling sounds or wheezing. Feeling the way the chest expands, tapping the chest wall, and palpating for increased chest vibration can also help to identify affected lung areas. Chest X-rays can reveal affected lung areas, confirm the pneumonia diagnosis, and in-

---

KEY FACTS

Description

Infection of human respiratory tract.

Causes

Infection by either bacteria or viruses, less commonly by fungi and parasites. Can also be caused by lung injury.

Risk factors

African Americans, newborns, elderly, people who smoke, and people whose immune system is compromised are at more risk. People who are hospitalized and on mechanical ventilators, those suffering from malnutrition, or those who have underlying heart or lung diseases are also at risk.

Symptoms

Dry or productive cough, fatigue, loss of appetite, chest pain, sore throat, fever, nausea, vomiting, diarrhea, aching muscles and joints.

Diagnosis

Physical examination and chest X-ray. Examination of blood and sputum for microorganisms.

Treatments

Antibiotics and supportive care.

Pathogenesis

Sepsis or septic shock can occur, leading to liver, kidney, brain, and heart damage.

Prevention

Treating underlying illnesses; quitting smoking; vaccination of vulnerable groups.

Epidemology

In the United States, around 5 million cases occur each year; about 1 million will need hospitalization. Pneumonia is the fifth leading cause of death in people older than 65 in the United States. In 2000 around 8 percent of patient deaths were a result of pneumonia.

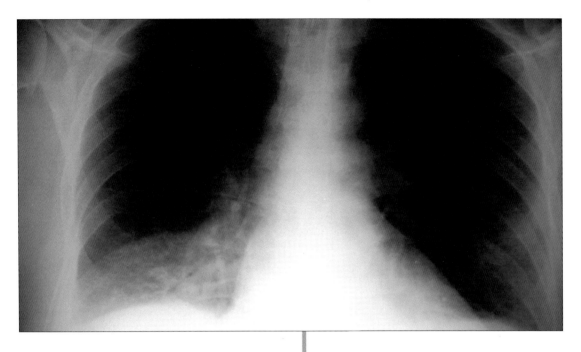

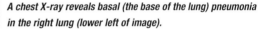

A chest X-ray reveals basal (the base of the lung) pneumonia in the right lung (lower left of image).

dicate certain complications. They are not diagnostic alone and must be considered in combination with other clinical features. By evaluating the location, distribution, and appearance of affected areas, chest X-rays can distinguish between pneumonia types and help predict the course of illness, though they cannot determine the microbiological cause. A chest computed tomography (CT) scan or other tests may be useful.

The diagnostic evaluation and microbiological classification may include a sputum culture, blood tests (blood cultures, a complete blood count, and blood tests for antibodies to specific viruses), bronchoscopy, urine tests, throat swab, and even an open lung biopsy, if the case is particularly serious and the diagnosis evasive. The definitive diagnosis of a bacterial infection requires isolation of an organism from the blood, pleural fluid, or lungs. The sample can then be cultured to look for infection and test for antibiotic sensitivities. Since cultures typically take a few days, they are mainly used to confirm sensitivities to an antibiotic already in use or as an epidemiological tool to define incidence and prevalence. A white blood cell count may be useful in differentiating viral pneumonia from bacterial pneumonia. The definitive diagnosis of a viral infection rests on the isolation of a virus or detection of viral antigens in a sputum sample.

Treatments

Treatment of suspected bacterial pneumonia is based on the presumptive cause and on the patient's clinical appearance. Antibiotics are the mainstay of treatment. Antibiotics are not effective in the treatment of viral pneumonias, though they are often used to prevent or treat the secondary bacterial infections that can occur in lungs damaged by viral pneumonia. The more serious forms of viral pneumonia can be treated with antiviral medications, although these treatments are often beneficial only if started within 48 hours of symptom onset. Supportive care for pneumonia may include treatment for the relief of associated symptoms, increased fluids, incentive spirometry (to show if the airways are narrowed), oxygen supplementation, and chest clearance therapy. Most cases of pneumonia can be resolved within one to three weeks without hospitalization using oral antibiotics, rest, fluids, and home care. However, the elderly and those with respiratory distress or other medical problems may need more intensive treatment. If the pneumonia does not improve, symptoms worsen, or complications occur, hospitalization and intensive care may be needed. Serious infections can result in respiratory failure requiring noninvasive or invasive mechanical ventilation.

The antibiotic choice depends on the nature of the pneumonia, the area's most common pneumonia-causing microorganisms and their sensitivities, and the age and underlying health of the victim. Pneumonia treatment is ideally based on the causative microorganism and its antibiotic sensitivities, but specific causes are identified in only 50 percent of cases, even after extensive evaluation.

The duration of treatment is traditionally seven to ten days, but shorter courses may be sufficient. A combination of antibiotics may be administered in an attempt to treat all possible causes.

Complications

Complications of pneumonia are usually the result of the spread of infection within the body. Occasionally, the microorganisms infecting the lungs will cause fluid (effusion) to build up in the pleural cavity (the area between the lungs and chest wall). If the microorganisms themselves are present, the fluid collection is called an empyema. When pleural fluid is present in a person with pneumonia, the fluid can often be collected with a needle and examined. Depending on the examination results, complete drainage of the fluid may be necessary, often requiring a chest tube. In severe cases, surgery may be required because, if the fluid is not drained, the infection may persist, since antibiotics do not penetrate well into the pleural cavity. The treatment for empyema is based on its stage, which can be ascertained by imaging studies.

Sepsis or septic shock most often occurs with bacterial pneumonia when microorganisms enter the bloodstream and the immune system responds. Individuals with sepsis or septic shock need hospitalization and intensive care; intravenous fluids and medications help keep their blood pressure from dropping. Sepsis can cause liver, kidney, brain, and heart damage, among other problems, and often causes death.

Rarely, bacteria in the lung will form a pocket of infected fluid called an abscess that can usually be seen on a chest X-ray or chest CT. They typically occur in aspiration pneumonia and often contain several types of bacteria. Antibiotics are usually adequate to treat a lung abscess, but the abscess may have to be drained.

In the United States, about 1 in 20 people with pneumococcal pneumonia will die. In cases where the pneumonia progresses to a bacterial blood infection, 1 in 5 will die. Pneumonia caused by *M. pneumoniae* is associated with few deaths; however, about half of those who develop MRSA pneumonia while on a ventilator will die. In regions of the world without advanced health care systems, pneumonia is much more deadly. Limited access to health care, X-rays, antibiotics, and the inability to treat underlying conditions contribute to higher death rates. Ultimately, an individual's prognosis depends on the type of pneumonia, symptom severity, appropriate treatment, complications, their age, and underlying health.

Prevention

Appropriately treating underlying illnesses can decrease a person's risk for pneumonia. Smoking cessation is important, not only because it limits lung damage but because cigarette smoke interferes with the body's natural defenses. Testing pregnant women for Group B *Streptococcus* and *Chlamydia trachomatis* and then giving antibiotic treatment, if needed, reduces pneumonia in infants. Suctioning the mouth and throat of infants with meconium-stained amniotic fluid decreases the rate of aspiration pneumonia.

Vaccination of infants against *H. influenzae* type B has led to a dramatic decline in cases. Vaccinations against *H. influenzae* and *S. pneumoniae* in the first year of life have greatly reduced their role in pneumonia in children. Vaccinating children against *S. pneumoniae* has led to a decreased incidence in adults, since many adults acquire infections from children. For adults in the United States, the vaccine against *S. pneumoniae* is currently recommended for all healthy individuals older than sixty-five and any adults with chronic conditions or compromised immune systems. A repeat vaccination may be required. Vaccines against RSV are available for high-risk populations. Influenza vaccines should be given yearly to health care workers, nursing home residents, and pregnant women.

Epidemiology

Pneumonia is a major cause of death among all age groups. In children, the majority of deaths occur in the vulnerable newborn period, with over 2 million deaths each year worldwide (1 in every 3 deaths). Mortality from pneumonia generally decreases with age until late adulthood, though it is a leading cause of death among the elderly and chronically ill. More cases of pneumonia occur during the winter months than at other times of the year; it occurs more commonly in males than females and more often in African Americans than Caucasians. Hospitalized people are at higher risk for pneumonia, and those with chronic health conditions or compromised immune systems are at risk for repeated episodes.

Julie A. McDougal

See also
• Aging, disorders of • Antibiotic-resistant infections • Infections, bacterial • Infections, viral • Respiratory system disorders

Poliomyelitis

There is evidence suggesting that poliomyelitis existed since ancient times. Although its contagiousness was established in the nineteenth century, the viral etiology of poliomyelitis was confirmed in the early twentieth century. Since the discovery of the virus, tremendous efforts led to a successful vaccine development. Such urgent need was dictated by continued increase of worldwide polio epidemics that peaked in the mid-twentieth century. It was important to prevent an illness that could cause significant disability and death.

In the United States the effort to create an effective vaccine began with the support of President Franklin D. Roosevelt and the establishment in 1938 of the National Foundation for Infantile Paralysis (now the March of Dimes), which supported both scientists conducting research on this disease and patients affected by this illness. Polio has been eradicated from the Western Hemisphere. In the rest of the world, the majority of cases are reported from several countries in Africa and the Indian subcontinent (such as Nigeria, Somalia, Afghanistan, Pakistan, and India). The Global Polio Eradication Initiative was launched in 1988, when poliomyelitis crippled an estimated 1,000 children per day. The initiative aims for global polio eradication in the first decade of the twenty-first century. The initiative uses several strategies involving surveillance of paralytic polio cases, supplemental immunizations on national immunization days, and ensuring universal vaccine coverage with oral poliovirus vaccine (OPV) for children in the first year of life.

Poliomyelitis is caused by serotypes 1, 2, and 3, polioviruses that are members of the enterovirus group. Type 1 poliovirus was responsible for most of the paralytic polio cases in the pre-immunization era. Since the introduction of the first polio vaccine in 1957, the number of cases steeply declined in the developed world; in the United States the last naturally occurring case of poliomyelitis was in 1979. In the rest of the world, the incidence of polio has reduced by 99 percent from 350,000 cases in 1988 to 1,918 cases reported in 2002 as polio vaccines became more widely available.

Pathogenesis

Poliomyelitis is transmitted from human to human through the fecal-oral route via contaminated hands, food, or water. People with subclinical forms of polio can shed the virus with feces for several weeks, thus becoming a source of the infection for others. Incubation period for poliomyelitis is 7 to 14 days

KEY FACTS

Description
Poliomyelitis (or polio) is a highly contagious viral infection that is known to invade the nervous system and cause paralysis.

Causes
By poliovirus, which is a virus that includes 3 distinct groups called serotypes (serotypes 1, 2, and 3).

Risk factors
It is a contagious disease; anyone who has no prior specific immunity (antibodies) is susceptible. Children younger than 5 years are at risk for contracting polio. Male and female genders are equally at risk for the infection.

Symptoms
Polio can present with several different clinical symptoms, including fever, headache, and stiff neck; the most serious one is paralytic polio.

Diagnosis
Diagnosis is made by recovering the virus from the body fluids or by the measurement of specific antibodies against polioviruses.

Treatment
As for many viral illnesses, there is no antiviral medication active against poliovirus.

Pathogenesis
The disease spreads through direct contact with infected body fluids; the virus invades nerve cells.

Prevention
The best way to prevent polio is to maintain specific antibody protection against the virus. This is commonly achieved by vaccination.

Epidemiology
Due to aggressive immunization campaigns and the Global Polio Eradication Initiative led by the World Health Organization, poliomyelitis has been eliminated in most of the world, apart from parts of Asia and several countries in Africa, where there is a high burden of endemic cases.

(range 5 to 35). The virus enters through the nose or mouth into the digestive system, where it multiplies and spreads to the lymphatic system and blood. Polioviruses have a specific preference for invading and destroying nerve cells (neurons) in the brain and spinal cord. The nerve cells regulate the function of various muscles; as a result of the destruction of nerve cells by polioviruses, muscles cannot function.

Symptoms and complications

The spectrum of clinical manifestations of polio ranges from subclinical (unapparent polio) to paralytic polio. In 90 to 95 percent of cases the infection with polioviruses results in subclinical or unapparent polio with minimal or no symptoms. Abortive poliomyelitis, which is another clinical presentation of this infection, has nonspecific features typical for many viral illnesses (fever, headache, sore throat, and abdominal pain) and no evidence of nervous system invasion. Nonparalytic poliomyelitis has typical features of any enteroviral infection, with symptoms such as fever, headache, and meningeal irritation. Both nonparalytic polio and abortive polio typically resolve without any residual complications. Around 0.1 percent of polio infections result in paralytic poliomyelitis distinguished into spinal and bulbar forms. In very rare cases, paralytic polio can evolve in a matter of hours. Spinal paralytic polio originally presents with the same symptoms as abortive polio, followed by a symptom-free interval of several days. Afterward, the fever recurs along with meningeal irritation causing headache, vomiting, and stiff neck, as well as muscle pains. A characteristic feature of paralytic polio is development of asymmetric paralysis with involvement of different muscle groups. Legs are usually more affected than arms. A paralysis or loss of muscle control in polio is described as flaccid (floppy) and can range from the involvement of some muscle groups to the involvement of trunk and both arms and legs (quadriplegia). Involvement of the chest wall muscles and diaphragm results in compromised breathing, which frequently necessitates mechanical support. Additional symptoms include muscle twitching and muscle spasms. The development of paralysis usually stops when the fever resolves. Some factors were found to be associated with a higher chance of paralysis, such as pregnancy, strenuous exercise, tonsillectomy, and intramuscular injection. Up to one-third of paralytic polio cases could evolve into a form called bulbar polio, in which the virus invades the brain stem and involves cranial nerves that control muscles responsible for swallowing and breathing.

Bulbar polio is associated with the highest mortality compared to the other forms of polio. Overall mortality from paralytic polio is 5 to 10 percent and is commonly a result of respiratory suppression.

Encephalitis is a rare and uncommon form of poliomyelitis that presents with confusion, altered consciousness, and seizures.

Subclinical and abortive polio resolve without any sequelae. Up to two-thirds of patients with paralytic polio continue to have residual weakness for the rest of their lives, resulting in disability. Infection with poliovirus results in a serotype-specific antibody development. This is not necessarily protective against infection with other polioviruses.

A condition called postpoliomyelitis syndrome is described in up to 40 percent of survivors of paralytic polio; it develops 20 to 30 years after the original infection. This condition is not well understood, but it is believed that new onset muscle weakness is a result of a premature death of the nerve cells.

Diagnosis and treatments

Polioviruses can be commonly recovered by viral culture from throat secretions or feces, and on some occasions from the cerebrospinal fluid. Virus isolation is important when the differentiation of the wild (found in nature) type virus from the vaccine-associated virus is necessary. Cerebrospinal fluid is often analyzed to check the number of cells and the protein content. A blood test detecting the antibody response to this virus is also available; for confirmation, the blood tests are performed in the acute and recovery phase. The diagnosis of poliomyelitis is confirmed if there is a fourfold increase in two antibody measurements.

There is no specific treatment for poliomyelitis. Treatment is typically aimed toward relief of symptoms. Bed rest is especially important in paralytic illness. In cases in which muscles of respiration are involved, mechanical ventilation is sometimes necessary.

Prevention

The best way to prevent poliomyelitis is vaccination, which induces antibody production and subsequent protection from the infection. Two vaccines have been widely used in the world. The first licensed vaccine was the inactivated poliovirus vaccine (IPV) developed by Jonas Salk. IPV is an injectable vaccine and is given at 2, 4, and 6 to 18 months, and at the age of 4 to 6 years. After improving the vaccine's ability to induce antibody responses, it is now exclusively used in the United States. IPV does not induce local immuni-

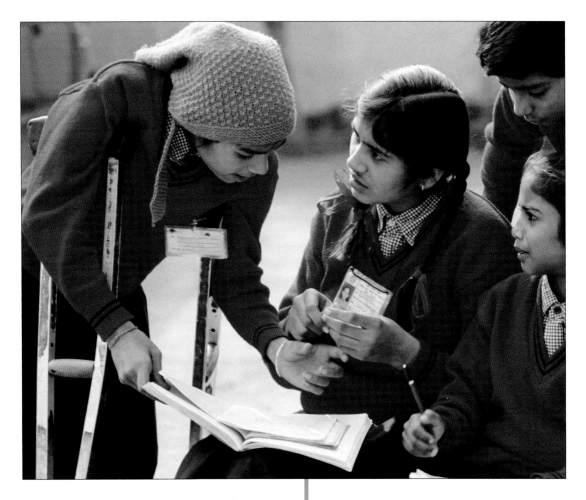

ty (antibody production) in the gastrointestinal tract; therefore IPV vaccinated individuals could theoretically shed the virus with feces and become a source of the infection.

Another vaccine that was introduced in the 1960s is a live oral poliovirus vaccine (OPV) developed by Albert Sabin. Due to ease of administration and cost effectiveness, it is widely used in most of the developing world. The advantage of this vaccine is development of local antibody response in the gastrointestinal tract and shedding of the vaccine-associated virus in the stool. In this situation the virus could be passively spread to nonimmune individuals and result in the development of protective antibody.

The oral vaccine is given at two, four, and six months of age with a booster dose at the age of four. The use of this vaccine is responsible for a significant worldwide decrease in cases of poliomyelitis. OPV is also available in a monovalent serotype specific formulation (mOPV). As part of the Global Polio Eradication Initiative, mOPV1 is now being increasingly used.

An Indian schoolgirl disabled by polio confers with her classmates. Although a global initiative to eradicate the disease is underway, setbacks in parts of India have been encountered. Overall the number of cases has decreased worldwide.

In contrast to the inactivated poliovirus vaccination, on rare occasions OPV is a cause of vaccine-associated paralytic poliomyelitis (VAPP). Around 93 cases of VAPP were reported per 291.4 million doses of vaccine that were distributed in 1969 to 1980 in the United States. The disorder occurs in recipients of the vaccine, in a close family member, or in caregivers. Clinical features of the VAPP are similar to naturally occurring paralytic polio.

Diana Nurutdinova

See also
- Immune system disorders • Infections
- Infections, viral • Muscle system disorders
- Nervous system disorders • Paralysis

Post-traumatic stress disorder

Post-traumatic stress disorder (PTSD) is an anxiety disorder in which psychological and physiological symptoms follow an exposure or confrontation with life-threatening traumatic experiences. These may be military combat, hostage situations, rape, torture, or natural and man-made disasters. The intensity of this trauma relates to the severity of symptoms of PTSD. PTSD patients can be effectively treated with different pharmacological agents and psychotherapy.

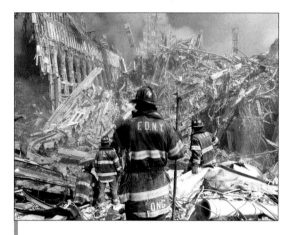

Firefighters clear debris after the devastation of the twin towers tragedy in 2001 in New York. Many people, including rescue workers, suffered from PTSD following the attack.

PTSD is a psychiatric disorder that historically has been studied in the context of combat experience. However, it has been recognized that other types of trauma, such as child abuse, torture, hostage situations, or violent crimes can also be associated with the development of PTSD. *The Diagnostic and Statistical Manual of Mental Disorders,* fourth edition (DSM-IV), specifies that a life-threatening traumatic event must be witnessed or experienced by the individual, and the response to this event must involve intense fear or horror. Based on currently available data, it is evident that the proximity to and the intensity of the traumatic event are related to the probability of developing the disorder and the severity of its symptoms.

Causes and risk factors

The development of PTSD reflects an interaction of constitutional and environmental factors. Research indicates that a smaller hippocampus, a part of the brain that is actively involved in the processes of fear and memory, may be associated in PTSD patients with specific risk and resilience factors. Experiencing a traumatic event increases plasma and brain concentrations of corticosteroids and neuroactive steroids, which increases responsiveness to glucocorticoids or other neuroendocrine measures, or both, that have been observed in combat-related PTSD. It has been also shown that a person's coping strategies could play a critical role in the development of the disorder. Specifically, avoidant coping strategies have been associated with greater PTSD symptoms, while more problem-focused cognitive style applied to reinterpretation and adaptation to the traumatic experience has been associated with fewer symptoms.

A growing body of evidence indicates that individuals who have a history of childhood trauma are more likely to develop PTSD later in life. The severity and duration of this initial traumatic experience are associated with increased severity of PTSD symptoms later in life. Also, a history of depression in first-degree relatives increases someone's vulnerability to PTSD.

Diagnosis and symptoms

In PTSD, people primarily develop three domains of symptoms: reexperiencing the traumatic event, avoiding stimuli associated with the trauma, and experiencing an increase in autonomic arousal. Symptoms of reexperiencing the trauma include recurrent and intrusive recollections of events, distressing dreams, acting or feeling as if the traumatic events are recurring, and physiological and psychological distress following exposure to the internal or external cues related to the trauma. Symptoms of avoidance include an effort to avoid recurrent thoughts or activities associated with the trauma, inability to recall an important aspect of the traumatic event, decreased interest and participation in significant activities, feelings of being numb or detached from reality, restricted affect, and a sense of a foreshortened future. Symptoms of increased arousal include irritability, insomnia, hypervigilance, difficulty concentrating, and enhanced startle response. The diagnosis of PTSD is only made when symptoms persist for at least one month. According to the DSM-IV, there are three subtypes of PTSD, based on the time course. Acute PTSD refers to an episode that lasts less than three months. Chronic PTSD refers to an episode lasting three months or longer. Delayed-onset PTSD refers to an episode that develops six months or more after exposure to the trauma.

Treatments

Pharmacotherapy is effective in the treatment of PTSD, acting to reduce its core symptoms and commonly associated symptoms of depression. Selective serotonin reuptake inhibitors, or SSRIs (citalopram, escitalopram, fluvoxamine, fluvoxetine, paroxetine, and sertraline), along with venlafaxine, a serotonin-norepinephrine reuptake inhibitor, have become first-line treatments of PTSD based on their overall efficacy and tolerability. Sexual dysfunction, weight gain, and sleep disturbance are common adverse effects associated with SSRI treatment. In the case of PTSD, benzodiazepines, such as alprazolam, diazepam, and clonazepam, have been also shown to be effective, well tolerated, and safe, in the absence of comorbid substance- and alcohol-abuse disorders. However, in the long term, antidepressants may may help target depressive symptoms. In addition, discontinuing long-term therapy with benzodiazepines can be difficult because, in some patients, anxiety symptoms could be exacerbated. Side effects of benzodiazepines include general sedation, slurred speech, memory impairment, and ataxia.

There is a growing body of data that indicates that a course of propranolol started shortly after an acute traumatic event helps reduce PTSD symptoms one month later. However, larger studies are needed for propranolol. Psychotherapeutic interventions include supportive techniques, cognitive-behavioral therapy, psychodynamic therapy, and group therapy. The most common therapeutic targets include dealing with intense emotional content, recovering a sense of self, new coping strategies, and reestablishing connections with the outside world. A combination of psychotherapy and medications is the most effective therapeutic option for PTSD.

Prevention

Individuals whose professional responsibilities expose them to possibilities of experiencing or witnessing traumatic events may benefit from additional education about the signs and features of PTSD. Treatment such as a critical incident stress debriefing is a proven therapeutic modality intended to prevent the development of full-blown PTSD following trauma. In addition, administration of propranolol shortly after traumatic exposure may be useful to mitigate PTSD symptoms or perhaps even prevent its development.

Epidemiology

In the United States, lifetime prevalence of PTSD in the adult community population is around 8 percent. However, in specific populations, such as military personnel, firefighters, police officers, search-and-rescue personnel, refugees, and victims of natural and man-made disasters, prevalence of PTSD is higher.

Oleg Tcheremissine and Lori Lieving

KEY FACTS

Description

An anxiety disorder with psychological and physiological symptoms after experiencing or witnessing a life-threatening trauma.

Causes

Changes in neural system in response to a life-threatening traumatic event.

Risk factors

Childhood trauma and family history of depression.

Symptoms

Reexperiencing the trauma; avoiding emotional experiences related to the trauma; sleep disturbances, and feeling increased arousal.

Diagnosis

If the symptoms last at least one month.

Treatments

Antidepressants, anxiolytics, adrenergic agents, and psychotherapy.

Pathogenesis

PTSD can occur at any age, including childhood.

Prevention

Educating people whose professions expose them to traumatic experiences.

Epidemiology

The lifetime prevalence among adults in the U.S. is around 8 percent. Women are twice as likely as men to be diagnosed with PTSD; in specific populations of patients, these figures are higher.

See also

• Anxiety disorders • Depressive disorders •
Mental disorders • Occupational disorders

Preeclampsia

Preeclampsia, which is life threatening, is a common condition that can affect pregnant women.

Preeclampsia occurs more often in the very young and very old pregnant patient, and in the first rather than later pregnancies. Once the condition has been diagnosed, the only treatment is to deliver the baby as soon as can be arranged. Preeclampsia is considered more a syndrome than a disease, with different problems that may have different causes. The root of the problem probably comes from abnormalities with the process of attachment of the placenta. This leads to a number of changes affecting most organs in the body.

Eclampsia is more common in patients with associated diseases of high blood pressure, diabetes, and kidney disease. The symptoms of preeclampsia are contracted blood vessels, swelling and damage to the liver, changes in blood clotting, and poor function of the kidneys. These changes lead to high blood pressure, blood clotting problems, and protein in the urine. Further progression of the disease leads to brain swelling, headache, visual problems, and then seizures, along with very severe blood clotting problems.

Preeclampsia is defined by a blood pressure more than 140/90 (mmHG) and more than 300 milligrams of protein in the urine over a 24-hour period. Severe forms of the syndrome include higher blood pressures (more than 160/110), larger amounts of protein in the urine (5 grams in 24 hours), seizures or signs of liver damage with low blood platelets (HELLP syndrome: hemolysis, elevated liver enzymes, and low platelets).

Early diagnosis of the condition has reduced deaths in pregnant patients in developed countries; however, up to 11 percent of pregnancies are still affected. In developing countries, 50,000 mothers die of eclampsia every year. In the United Kingdom and United States it is one of the leading causes of maternal death. Preeclampsia is a very serious condition; even when diagnosed, there is a risk for mother and baby. A patient has to be 20 weeks pregnant for the diagnosis to be made. There may be swelling, but this is no longer considered a definitive symptom. Some patients have seizures; then it is called eclampsia.

The main treatment of preeclampsia is to deliver the baby, either vaginally or by a cesarean section. The medical issues dictate which method is used and can be done fastest. Seizures can occur before or even up to a week after delivery of the baby. Magnesium sulfate helps prevent seizures, although when they are happening, antiseizure medicines are used. High blood pressure must be controlled as well as the clotting problems that occur from reduced platelet counts or low blood clotting factors. This may be done by transfusion of platelets or fresh frozen plasma to prevent bleeding.

After delivery, treatment may continue for a week, depending on the severity of the preeclampsia. With early detection and treatment, many lives can be saved. If left untreated, women may die. There is a high risk of the baby dying or having medical problems such as lung and nervous system diseases as a result of its prematurity. Early diagnosis is the only preventive measure. In the United States, each year around 150,000 women suffer from preeclampsia, about 3 to 4 percent of pregnancies. About 70 percent of these are first pregnancies. Around 18 percent of maternal deaths are due to preeclampsia.

Moeen Panni

KEY FACTS

Description
A common condition of pregnancy.

Causes
Probably abnormalities of the placenta.

Risk factors
Hypertension, diabetes, and kidney disease.

Symptoms
Liver swelling, dysfunction of kidneys, high blood pressure, and protein in urine.

Diagnosis
Made when there is hypertension, edema, and protein in the urine.

Treatments
Delivery of the baby as soon as possible.

Pathogenesis
Left untreated, women die of organ failure, often liver rupture, seizures, and bleeding in the brain.

Prevention
Early diagnosis reduces deaths.

Epidemiology
Around 3–4 percent of pregnancies are affected.

See also
• Pregnancy and childbirth disorders

Pregnancy and childbirth

Pregnancy is a complex process that lasts about 38 weeks between conception and labor. In the regular course of events, normal women give birth to normal children with few problems. However, many problems can occur. Irregularities in pregnancy and disorders of childbirth may present complications to the birth process and the newborn.

Pregnancy and childbirth disorders may be classified as: risks before pregnancy; pregnancy complications, such as miscarriage, placental and amnion disorders; labor problems; and disorders of both mother and baby after birth.

The female reproductive organs are all located within the body and comprise the following: ovaries, fallopian tubes, uterus, cervix, and vagina. The ovaries are located at about hip level on each side of the body; these primary female reproductive organs contain a solid mass of cells, or ova. The ova, or eggs, form in the female at about the third month of fetal development. Under the influence of hormones, eventually about 300 to 400 eggs reach maturity at the time when the female matures sexually. Each month an egg is released from the ovary. From the ovary the egg passes into the fallopian tube. The fallopian tubes are located near the ovaries but not connected to them. The fallopian tubes or oviducts, which are the passageway from the ovary to the

uterus, are about 5 inches (12 cm) long. The end of the tube near the ovary is called fimbriated because fingerlike projections create waves that cause the mature egg to move into the fallopian tube. If sperm are present in the tube, it is there that fertilization takes place. Rarely, the fertilized egg will try to implant in the tube, causing a tubal or ectopic pregnancy.

The uterus is a hollow, muscular organ, shaped like an upside-down pear, in which the fertilized egg implants and develops. The lining of the uterus is covered with ciliated cells and numerous glands, the uterine glands.

The cervix is at the lower end of the uterus that opens to a wider channel called the vagina, which is the passageway through which the baby passes during the birth process. At puberty, ovarian function begins when the menstrual cycle and ovulation are linked to complex hormonal action of the hypothalamus at the base of the brain, the pituitary, and the ovaries.

A pregnancy is divided into three trimesters. The first trimester is from week one through 14. For about the first three days after fertilization in the fallopian tubes, the egg, which is now called a zygote or morula, begins to divide. As it divides, it becomes a blastocyst and moves along the tubes to implant in the endometrium, the lining of the uterus. At the end of the second week, blood cells begin to form. During week three, hormonal changes cause the endometrium to thicken, and its blood nourishes

RELATED ARTICLES

the blastocyst. In week four the amniotic sac develops around the embryo (as it is now called) to buffer shocks. The embryo's heart is already beating. The sac immediately begins to fill with water from the mother about 12 days after conception; after about 12 weeks, fetal urine makes up most of the fluid. The spine and nervous system start to form. During week five, the first organs form; arms and legs are little buds, and the digestive system is developing. In week six the head and inner parts of the ear begin to enlarge. Now called a fetus, the young offspring receives nourishment from the placenta through the mother's umbilical cord. By the end of weeks eight through fourteen, all internal organs are formed. During these critical weeks of formation, it is imperative that the mother avoids any substances that could cause fetal malformation.

The second trimester is from weeks 14 to 28. As muscles and systems are growing, the mother begins to feel movement. At the end of week 24, the fetus is still not able to live independently of the mother, although in rare cases, nursing and support care may help the offspring survive. As the pregnancy advances, it is normal for the mother to suffer from indigestion, heartburn, and constipation. Weight pressure on internal organs can cause hemorrhoids and varicose veins in the legs.

The third trimester is from weeks 29 to 40. The fetus now looks like a baby. However, the baby is thin because the subcutaneous fat has not developed. Although babies may survive if born during these early weeks, the longer the term in the uterus, the better the chances for a normal birth. At birth the average baby weighs around 7½ pounds (3.4 kg).

Risk factors before pregnancy

A high-risk pregnancy is one in which the woman or baby are more likely to become ill or die or have complications before, during, or after delivery.

Certain conditions or characteristics may place a woman at high risk before pregnancy. These factors include physical and social characteristics, problems during previous pregnancies, or preexisting health conditions.

Physical characteristics such as age, weight, and height often affect pregnancy. For example, girls aged 15 and younger are at risk for preeclampsia,

ECTOPIC PREGNANCIES: MISPLACED EMBRYOS

In a normal pregnancy, the egg is fertilized in the fallopian tube and implants in the uterus; however, in an ectopic pregnancy the egg may not reach the uterus but begins to grow someplace else. Although on rare occasions the fertilized egg may begin to grow in the ovaries, cervix, or abdominal cavity, the most common site is in the fallopian tubes. Risk factors include narrow or blocked tube, pelvic inflammatory disease (PID), previous ectopic pregnancy, exposure to diethylstilbestrol as a fetus, or a tubal ligation that was unsuccessful.

In an ectopic pregnancy, the fetus cannot survive, and the pregnancy must be terminated as soon as possible to save the woman's life. Surgery is performed with a laparoscope or the drug methotrexate may be used to shrink the embryo and its placenta. Ectopic pregnancies occur one in one hundred to two hundred pregnancies; the number is rising, especially among nonwhites.

a condition in which blood pressure is raised and the woman may have edema and proteinuria, and underweight or undernourished infants. Women over 35 are at risk for high blood pressure, gestational diabetes, or labor complications. Women who weigh less than 100 pounds are likely to have small underweight babies; obese women may develop diabetes and have large babies that are difficult to deliver.

Women who are short in stature may have small pelvises that create a difficult passage through the birth canal. The baby may lodge against the pelvis, a condition called shoulder dystocia. Other maternal structural abnormalities may include a double uterus or weak cervix that opens as the fetus grows.

Social characteristics can also affect risk. People of low socioeconomic status (SES) or unmarried mothers have increased risk in pregnancy. The reason for this correlation is unclear but may involve a lower level of prenatal care. Women who have had premature delivery, miscarriage, or Rh compatibility tend to repeat the same problems in later pregnancies.

Disorders before pregnancy

A previous disorder can increase problems of pregnancy. Pregnancy puts a great deal of stress on the body. For example, the heart must work harder, and women with the following preexisting conditions must be especially cautious.

Heart disease. Women with previous heart defects can safely give birth to healthy children; however, these women need careful monitoring.

High blood pressure. Women with high blood pressure before pregnancy are likely to have serious problems during pregnancy.

The tendency for preeclampsia, a blood pressure condition that may develop in normal pregnancies, increases if there is a preexisting history.

Anemia. Hereditary anemias, such as sickle-cell anemia, hemoglobin S-C disease, and some thalassemias may cause pneumonia, urinary tract infections, and uterine infections.

Kidney diseases. Women with kidney disorders may find their condition worsens with pregnancy, and high blood pressure and preeclampsia may develop. Many women who undergo dialysis can give birth to a healthy baby.

Seizure disorders. Anticonvulsants, which are medications to control seizures, may cause birth defects. Some women may be able to discontinue the medications during pregnancy; however, seizures may harm the woman and fetus.

Sexually transmitted diseases. Diseases such as chlamydia and gonorrhea may cause premature labor and eye infections in the newborn.

Syphilis can be transmitted through the placenta and cause severe birth defects. Women with HIV infections transmit the virus as the baby passes through the birth canal; retroviral drugs may be given, and a cesarean section may reduce transmittance. Genital herpes is passed to the baby as it passes through the birth canal; this virus can produce a life-threatening condition called herpes encephalitis.

Diabetes. Having diabetes before pregnancy can produce complications such as high blood pressure and kidney damage.

Liver and gall bladder disorders. Women with these disorders tend to have miscarriages.

Asthma. Preexisting asthma conditions are unpredictable. In about one-fourth of women with asthma, the condition improves with pregnancy; in about one-fourth of the women, asthma worsens; and the other half remain the same as before pregnancy. Women with severe asthma who are treated with prednisone risk premature birth to the infant.

Autoimmune disorders. Abnormal antibodies can cross the placenta and damage the fetus. Systemic lupus erythematosus (SLE) or lupus may worsen, get better, or appear for the first time. Flare-ups are most common immediately after birth.

Fibroids. Noncancerous slow-growing tumors in the uterus may enlarge during pregnancy, causing premature labor, difficult birth positions, and repeated miscarriages. There may be more than one, and they can be pea-sized or as large as a grapefruit.

An obstetrician measures a pregnant woman's abdomen to ensure that she is the correct size for the stage of pregnancy. In a small percentage of pregnancies, the uterus is larger than expected because there is too much amniotic fluid.

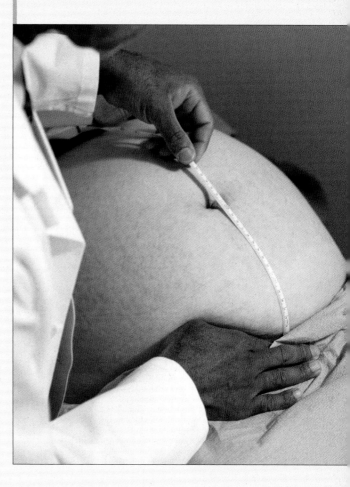

Pregnancy complications

Complications can develop during pregnancy that are independent of preexisting conditions. They include miscarriage, gestational diabetes, preeclampsia and eclampsia, and several other pregnancy problems.

Miscarriage. The medical term for miscarriage, or the loss of a fetus before 24 weeks of pregnancy due to natural causes, is spontaneous abortion. About 15 percent of pregnancies that end in miscarriage are the result of high-risk pregnancies; 85 percent of these occur during the first 12 weeks. The general consensus is that a birth defect or genetic defect caused the early miscarriage. The remaining 15 percent occur during weeks 13 to 24 and usually have no identified cause. Spotting or bleeding from the vagina and uterine cramps indicate a miscarriage. The physician will advise the woman to stay off her feet and to get bed rest.

Gestational diabetes mellitus (GDM). This is a type of diabetes that affects only pregnant women. As the fetus grows, hormones that are normal in most women work against the body, and as a result, the woman is unable to make sufficient insulin, which causes blood sugar to build up. If not treated, this can cause problems for both the mother and the fetus. Gestational diabetes mellitus occurs in about 7 percent of pregnancies but can usually be controlled by diet and exercise.

Preeclampsia and eclampsia. Associated with swelling of the face and hands (not feet, which is normal in pregnancy), preeclampsia is a complication that involves high blood pressure that develops late in pregancy (after the twentieth week). This dangerous condition, one of the most common complications of pregnancy and one of the leading causes of death of mother and fetus in the United States, occurs in about 3 to 4 percent of pregnancies. Preeclampsia can lead to eclampsia, which can lead to coma, seizures, and death. High blood pressure and high levels of protein in the urine are signs of eclampsia; delivering the fetus is usually the only definite cure.

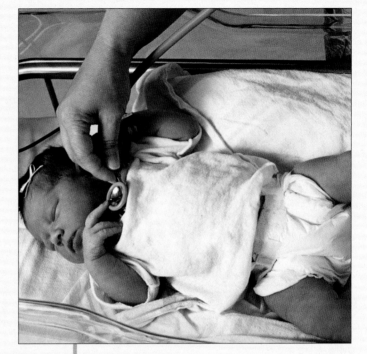

A newborn baby has its breathing checked. After birth a series of checks are done, including examination of hips, spine, posture, cries, behavior, and reflexes.

Hypermesis gravidarum. Although morning sickness is common in preganacy, hypermesis gravidarum results in extremely severe nausea and excessive vomiting during pregnancy. This leads to weight loss, dehydration, and liver damage. Patients should be evaluated for unsuspected liver disease, kidney infection, pancreatitis, intestinal blockages, or head lesions, all of which can cause excessive vomiting. Termination of the pregnancy may be essential for those who do not respond to therapy.

Placental and amnion problems. The placenta, the inner lining of the uterus during pregnancy, becomes the lifeline between the mother and fetus. Inside the uterus is the amnion, a membrane containing fluid that cushions the fetus. The umbilical cord connects with the placenta and provides nourishment and oxygen to the fetus and removes waste products. Potential problems with the placenta, amniotic fluid, or umbilical cord are many. The placenta may separate from the uterus (from a few millimeters to complete detachment). This condition is known as abruptio placentae. The cause is unknown, but it is associated with cardiovascular diseases, rheumatoid diseases, and the use of cocaine.

Unknown bleeding may be hidden behind the placenta, causing serious blood loss and more serious complications, such as shock. Another condition occurs when the placenta is located over or near the cervix, in the lower part of the uterus. It may cause painless but profuse bleeding, and the baby must be delivered surgically by cesarean section.

Too much or too little amniotic fluid may cause disorders. Normally, the amniotic fluid increases until about 28 to 32 weeks of pregnancy, when it measures about 1 quart (945 ml). The volume remains the same, then decreases when the baby is full-term. Some pregnancies have too little fluid, which is a condition called oligohydramnios, or too much amniotic fluid, which is called polyhydramnios. Whether these become serious conditions depends on the stage of pregnancy. Birth defects of the kidneys and urinary tract are more likely if there is too little amniotic fluid. Too much fluid may put stress on the diaphragm and result in breathing problems for the mother or cause problems of early delivery.

Labor complications

Labor begins with contractions of the uterus and normally proceeds with 50 percent of women delivering within one week and 90 percent within two weeks of the date due. No more than 10 percent deliver on their specified due date. Timing may become a problem. If labor starts before the 37th week of pregnancy or after the 42nd week, the health of the fetus may be endangered. Even in about 10 percent of normal pregnancies, the amnion ruptures before labor begins. If labor does not begin soon after, the risk of infection increases, so labor will be induced. Sometimes both labor and delivery need help. Induction of labor is the artificial starting of labor, which is usually brought about by giving the drug oxytocin, a hormone that induces contractions. The drug, identical to the hormone produced in the pituitary gland, may also hasten a labor that is proceeding too slowly. When the opposite happens and labor is moving too forcefully, the woman may be given painkillers or drugs such as terbuline or ritodrine that may stop or slow contractions.

If labor is prolonged or the fetus is abnormally positioned, forceps or metal tongs that fit around the head may be used to help delivery. A vacuum extractor that fits on the baby's head may also be used.

During a normal birth, the umbilical cord and placenta follow as the afterbirth. In about one in 1,000 deliveries, the umbilical cord precedes the baby and may prolapse or rupture prematurely, preventing blood supply to the fetus. A nuchal cord (when the umbilical cord is wrapped around the fetus's neck) occurs in about one-fourth of deliveries. Normally, it causes no problems, but if the doctor finds this, he or she will slip the cord over the baby's head.

Cesarean section. When the doctor determines that it is safer to surgically remove the baby, he or she may deliver the baby through an incision in the mother's abdomen and uterus. About one-fourth of deliveries in the United States are by cesarean section. This is major surgery with an obstetrician, anesthesiologist, nurses, and sometimes a pediatrician involved in the

POSITION OF FETUS

Toward the end of the pregnancy, the fetus gets ready for birth. The normal birth position is head-first, facing the mother's back and face, with body angled to one side and neck bent. However, abnormal positions may occur. If a fetus faces forward or has the face or brow facing down, the neck is in an abnormal position and the head requires more space to pass through the vagina. The baby may have to be repositioned by forceps or vacuum extractor. When a baby presents itself as feet, shoulder, or buttocks first, it is called a breech position. Such births are dangerous because the feet are delivered first but the head is caught inside the mother, resulting in possible damage to the brain and spinal cord. Shoulder dystocia is a condition that occurs when one shoulder lodges against the mother's pubic bone and the baby is caught in the birth canal. The head may come out, but the baby cannot breathe because of pressure on the chest. If the baby cannot be repositioned, the baby may be pushed back into the vagina to be delivered by a cesarean section.

procedure. A horizontal incision is usually made in the lower part of the uterus. The mother is encouraged to walk around as soon as possible after delivery to prevent pulmonary embolism, a blood clot that may form in the legs and then move to the lungs. Compared with vaginal delivery, the mother has more overall pain afterward and a longer recovery time.

Mother and baby after birth

Several conditions that require emergency care may develop after delivery. During a difficult labor, the amniotic fluid enters the mother's bloodstream and travels to her lungs, causing the arteries to constrict. The heart may begin to beat rapidly, and the woman may go into shock and even cardiac arrest and death. Uterine bleeding or excessive hemorrhage from the uterus is a major concern. In a normal delivery, about 1 pint (470 ml) of blood is lost, primarily because some blood vessels are opened as the placenta detaches from the uterus. More than 1 pint (470 ml) is considered excessive. After delivery the woman is monitored carefully for one hour to make sure the uterus has contracted. Another rare condition is an inverted uterus, when the uterus is turned inside out and protrudes through the cervix. This serious medical condition must be corrected by surgery.

Newborn problems

If labor does not proceed normally and the fetus has not been receiving enough oxygen, there may be a complication of fetal distress. Rarely, a baby does not start to breathe at birth and requires resuscitation. Both these conditions affect the baby's well-being.

A problem may occur during pregnancy that can damage the fetus. Fevers with temperature of 103°F (39.4°C) or more during the first trimester risk miscarriage or birth defects to the fetus. Some infections can cause serious birth defects, for example German measles (rubella), which can cause defects of the heart and inner ear; and toxoplasmosis (cat scratch fever), which can cause damage to the eyes and liver. Other conditions such as chicken pox, herpes simplex, or listerosis can also harm the fetus.

Erythroblastosis fetalis. This condition is Rhesus (Rh) incompatibility, that is, a mismatch between the blood of the fetus and the blood of the mother. When an Rh negative mother is carrying an Rh positive fetus,

---

ABORTION AND TERMINATION

A spontaneous abortion is one that is brought about by natural causes and that occurs up to 24 weeks of pregnancy; if the baby dies after 24 weeks, it is called stillborn. A therapeutic abortion is induced by medical means—either by drugs or surgery. In the United States therapeutic abortions for voluntarily ending pregnancy are legal only in the first trimester.

A threatened abortion is when there is bleeding or cramping during the first 24 weeks, indicating that the fetus may be lost. An inevitable abortion occurs when pain or bleeding leads to dilation of the cervix, meaning the fetus will be lost.

A complete abortion is the expulsion of all the fetus and placenta in the uterus; an incomplete abortion means only part of the contents is expelled. This may lead to a septic abortion, which means there is an infection that can occur before, during, or after the abortion.

A missed abortion is when the dead fetus is retained in the uterus for four weeks or longer. A habitual abortion means the woman has had three or four miscarriages.

---

the mother can develop antibodies against the fetus. The Rh factor is a molecule on the surface of red blood cells. A person who has the factor is Rh positive; a person who does not is Rh negative. If a mother is sensitized during a first pregnancy, she may build up antibodies that cross the placenta to the fetus and destroy the red blood cells faster than the fetus can produce new ones. If untreated, the baby may be born with the condition erythroblatosis fetalis. Depending on the degree, the child may develop serious conditions and brain damage. Mothers are monitored to take steps to prevent the condition. If the level of the antibody is too high, the fetus is given a transfusion, and labor is induced. Women with Rh negative blood are given an injection of Rh antibodies at 28 weeks of pregnancy and within 72 hours after a delivery of a baby with Rh positive blood. The treatment destroys any of the blood cells that have entered across the placenta, and later pregnancies are not at risk.

Evelyn B. Kelly

Prevention

The primary causes of mortality (illness) and morbidity (death) are not natural disaster, old age, or even wars. Rather, modifiable behaviors are the leading causes of mortality in the United States and, arguably, worldwide.

The exact percentage of morbidity and mortality that could be prevented or delayed by making fairly simple behavioral changes is not known. However, a study has reported that the leading causes of death in the United States in the year 2000 were tobacco use (18.1 percent of total U.S. deaths), poor diet and physical inactivity (16.6 percent), and alcohol consumption (3.5 percent). These are all modifiable behaviors—behaviors that can be changed through prevention efforts.

A limited number of behaviors contribute markedly to diseases that are major killers. These behaviors are often established during adolescence, and include unhealthy dietary behaviors; inadequate physical activity; tobacco use; alcohol and other drug use; unsafe sexual behaviors that may result in HIV infection or unintended pregnancies, or both; behaviors that can lead to violence, such as drinking too much; behaviors that can lead to unintentional injuries, for example, driving a motor vehicle after drinking too much alcohol; inadequate handling of stressful conditions; use of firearms; and inadequate hygiene. The 2002 world report on violence and health published by the World Health Organization (WHO,

Geneva) lists these top ten causes of death for all its member states. However, data gathering is inadequate or poor in many countries of the world, and many countries are either not members or have not filed a report, so these statistics must be evaluated in view of these limitations.

Among both children and adults, the leading causes of death today are closely related to modifiable behaviors. Only some of them will be addressed here because the list of modifiable behaviors that lead to disease or death is long and complex. Among adults, chronic diseases such as cardiovascular disease, cancer, and diabetes are the nation's leading killers. Eating low-fat foods and fruit and vegetables, getting regular physical activity, and refraining from tobacco use would prevent many premature deaths. These health-related behaviors are usually established in youth and track into adulthood.

Many prevention researchers believe that positive health behavior choices need to be promoted during childhood and adolescence through targeted health promotion and disease prevention efforts before unhealthy behaviors are initiated and become ingrained. Some have characterized prevention as "the creation of conditions, opportunities and experiences that encourage and develop healthy, self-sufficient children and that occur before the onset of problems." However, this definition does not cover the scope of prevention science, in particular because prevention efforts can target people of any age, in any situation, in any country, and for many different behaviors.

RELATED ARTICLES

What is prevention?

Prevention is different from treatment because it is aimed at general population groups with various levels of risk for any health problem. The goal of prevention is to reduce health risk factors and enhance health protective factors. Prevention efforts use specific theories and frameworks to match interventions to the needs of a particular (targeted) population. Prevention has been defined in many ways, and definitions continue to evolve. In 1948 the World Health Organization (WHO) identified three successive stages of prevention. These stages were criticized later as being too focused on disease. They were therefore modified to include behaviors that affect the overall quality of life, and to reflect the fact that prevention can involve medical intervention, behavioral intervention, or changes in public policy. Below are modified definitions of the three stages of prevention originally presented by the WHO.

Primary prevention. This stage targets initial prevention and includes all activities designed to prevent the onset of the initial episode of any disease, adverse health episode, or condition. Primary prevention efforts are designed to protect individuals and to avoid problems prior to signs or symptoms of problems. This includes activities, programs, and practices that change opportunities, risks, and expectations surrounding individuals.

Secondary prevention. This stage of prevention targets mitigation and control and covers all activities aimed at the prevention of further episodes of disease, adverse health episode, or condition. Secondary prevention identifies persons in the early stages of problem behaviors or disease and attempts to avert the ensuing negative consequences by inducing people to change behavior through counseling or treatment. It is often referred to as early intervention.

Tertiary prevention. This stage concentrates on the reduction of complications or relapse. In terms of disease, this stage includes all prevention activities aimed at the reduction of the incidence of chronic incapacity or complications in a population and thus aims to reduce the functional consequences of an illness. In more general terms, tertiary prevention strives to end problem behaviors or to ameliorate their negative effects, or both, through treatment and rehabilitation. This is most often referred to as treatment but also includes rehabilitation and relapse prevention.

Health disparities

The top ten causes of death in the United States and in the world have already been discussed. Heart disease (cardiovascular disease, or CVD) is the most deadly worldwide, regardless of gender, race, or location. Poor diet, physical inactivity, smoking, alcohol use, stress, obesity, and overweight are all major contributors to heart disease. Cancer and stroke follow close behind. One of the main causes of stroke is atherosclerosis, when fatty deposits build up on the walls of the blood vessels that supply blood (arteries) to the brain. Atherosclerosis is in turn caused by high cholesterol. Other behavioral causes of stroke include smoking, high cholesterol, and drug and alcohol use. In youth, major causes of death are accidents, suicide, and homicide. These are related to alcohol and drug use, poverty, depression, and stress.

Hispanic and African American populations in the United States are more likely to die from unintentional injury and diabetes than the general population. This is in part a result of lower overall socioeconomic status (SES), which is related to poorer workplace safety, lack of time to prepare healthy meals or exercise, lack of access to healthy foods including fresh fruits and vegetables, and lack of safe places (for example, parks, trails, and gyms) in which to be physically active. The comparatively high incidence of suicide and assault in these populations and the prevalence of HIV/AIDS in African Americans further attest to the health disparities in the United States. Health disparities between the developed and developing countries are masked in worldwide statistics, which group all people together to show the overall top ten causes of death at the global level. Globally, in 2002, HIV/AIDS was the fourth leading cause of death.

Prevention approaches

The stage of prevention appropriate to the problem that is to be addressed, as well as any health disparities and other population characteristics, such as reading level or SES, need to be taken into account when developing prevention programs. Public health researchers frequently divide prevention approaches into three subsets: universal, targeted, and indicated.

Universal. This approach addresses the entire population with messages and programs aimed at

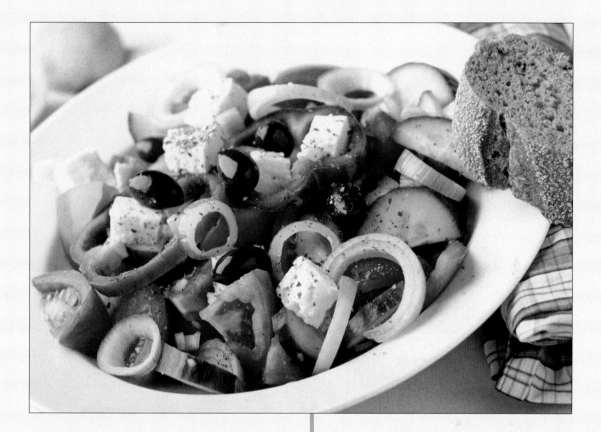

Vegetables and fruit are a vital part of a healthy diet; they help prevent disease and they are an excellent source of essential vitamins and minerals, which are needed to fight infection.

preventing or delaying problem behaviors. An example of the universal approach is the President's Council on Physical Fitness and Sports (PCPFS), which strives to make the health and fitness of all Americans a top priority. The Council dates back to 1956, when President Dwight D. Eisenhower signed the council into existence.

Targeted. This approach selects subsets of the total population that are assessed to be at risk for problem behaviors by virtue of their membership to a particular population segment. An example of the targeted approach would be Body and Soul, which is a dietary intervention conducted through African American churches. Body and Soul was tailored specifically to the needs of African American families and thoroughly researched in African American churches. The intervention is based on food choices, activity preferences, language usage, and motivating factors that emerged in extensive research within the African American community.

Indicated. This approach identifies individuals who are exhibiting early signs of problem behavior(s), and targets them with special programs to prevent further onset of difficulties. An example of the indicated

approach might be a needle exchange program designed to prevent drug users from becoming HIV positive.

These common categories in prevention might lead to misunderstandings because of the terminology that is used to differentiate tailoring from targeting. Tailored interventions adapt prevention programs and materials to the characteristics, needs, and interests of individuals. Targeted interventions adapt prevention programs and materials to the characteristics of a particular audience based on age, gender, ethnicity, or other factors but that do not provide information unique to the individual. A tailored intervention to increase mammography in women provided personalized letters to each participant. Each letter included a drawing of a woman matched to the age and race of the recipient and messages tailored to the recipient's personal barriers and beliefs about mammography and breast cancer. A targeted

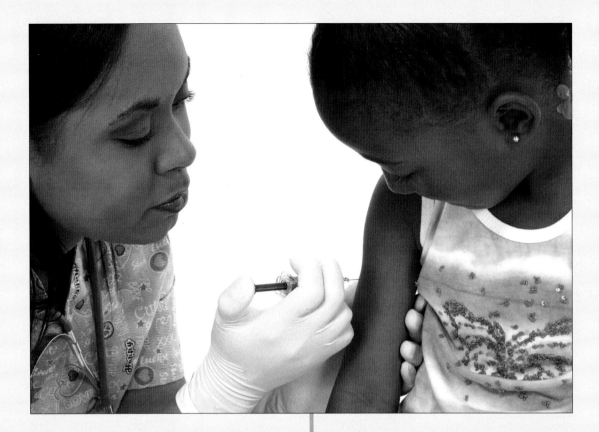

intervention to increase mammography in Latina women used a large-scale population-based survey in Latina women to understand their screening behavior, knowledge, and attitudes about cancer, as well as their reading levels and other preferences. This information was used to develop a culturally appropriate booklet that included testimonials from Latinas, based on the general characteristics of this population, and it was sent to all participants in the intervention.

Public health and specific health-related behaviors

Sanitation is a part of daily life. However, this has not always been the case. During the nineteenth century, 25 percent of women who delivered babies in hospitals were dying of puerperal sepsis, or childbed fever. Dr. Ignaz Semmelweis observed in the late 1840s that medical students were coming from their autopsy lectures to deliver babies without washing their hands, causing many women to die. This observation caused him to postulate that the students were carrying diseases into the operating room and infecting the mothers. His solution was simple: hands should be washed with a chlorinated solution before

Vaccination is used to confer immunity against disease; vaccination programs also are implemented to prevent disease from spreading through a population.

all medical procedures. He was met with ridicule and skepticism, and it was not until the 1870s that Louis Pasteur made the same observation and became a proponent of hand washing before operations.

Today, hand washing is thought of as the beginning of modern sanitation efforts. The CDC estimates that 5 percent to 15 percent of hospitalized patients die of nosocomial infections (infections that originate or occur in a hospital setting). Hospital personnel can also catch the diseases of the patients they treat, causing many hospitals to institute a hand washing policy between each patient. Hand washing is also an important way to prevent the spread of disease in schools and offices and can reduce health care costs.

Sun safety

Exposure to ultraviolet (UV) light is the most modifiable risk factor for skin cancer. Behavior largely determines how much UV light a person is exposed to, making it ideal for a behavior-modification approach. Sun safety includes many actions, including wearing sunscreen (at least SPF 15), avoiding exposure to the sun during the middle of the day, avoiding artificial UV light (such as tanning beds), and wearing clothing that covers the skin (including hats that shield the back of the neck and face). While sunscreen is one aspect of sun safety, it does offer protection against UVB and UVA rays and has been shown to significantly decrease the incidence of squamous cell carcinoma, a common form of skin cancer. Protective clothing (for example, long-sleeve shirts, pants, and wide-brimmed hats) also plays a significant role in sun safety by protecting the skin from harmful rays, especially during the critical hours between 10 AM and 2 PM when the angle of the sun's rays is almost vertical. It is also important to avoid the strongest rays, seek out natural shade, and wear protective covering during this time, thereby reducing the amount of sun exposure. Sun safety has many implications for preventing diseases such as cancer in the majority of the population.

Treatment compliance

Noncompliance to prescribed treatment regimens include not taking the full dose of a medication, not having prescriptions filled, saving expired medications for use in the future, using others' medications, and taking alternative therapies not prescribed by a physician, all of which may cause increased health care costs for consumers and insurance companies. This presents a problem for the United States; because the general population is aging, health care costs and the prescribing of drugs are rapidly increasing. Compliance has important health benefits, such as preventing the progression of disease in the individual and the spread of infectious disease in the general population. Furthermore, with chronic lifestyle-related diseases such as diabetes mellitus on the rise, compliance with treatment regimens goes beyond the health effects and becomes a factor in sustaining the economy by promoting productive years of life. Another "treatment" is vaccination or immunization, particularly in childhood. Immunization has been called the most important public health intervention in history, after safe drinking water. It has saved millions of lives over the years and has

prevented hundreds of millions of cases of disease. Much effort is made in the United States and worldwide to ensure that parents vaccinate their children when vaccinations are available, and to provide them when they are not. Thus, prevention has wide-reaching effects on several aspects of the general population.

Screening behavior

Screening behavior is necessary for the prevention of several chronic diseases, including many cancers (for example, lung, colorectal, breast, prostate, and skin cancer), hypertension, and diabetes mellitus. Screenings include yearly checkups and are an important way to prevent the development of chronic disease; however, many people are not regularly screened. In fact, one of the first theories of health behavior to be developed, the health belief model, was introduced in the early 1950s to explain widespread failure of the asymptomatic U.S. population to undergo screening tests for conditions such as lung cancer. Interventions to increase screening behavior have focused on mobile clinics, stations in grocery stores, and mass media campaigns (such as the CDC's Screen for Life: National Colorectal Cancer Action Campaign). More recently, community-based centers are being targeted as places to screen a large proportion of the population. Screening is important in prevention because it usually catches diseases when they are in the early stages, enabling health professionals to focus on primary or secondary prevention when health outcomes are more likely and treatment less expensive.

Sexually transmitted diseases

There are several sexually transmitted diseases (STDs) that threaten health, such as herpes, but none is as life threatening as AIDS. In the United States alone, more than 900,000 cases of AIDS have been reported since 1981. HIV is human immunodeficiency virus; AIDS is acquired immune deficiency syndrome. "Acquired" means that it is contagious or that people can get infected through others. Immune deficiency is a weakness in the body's system that fights diseases. The syndrome refers to a group of health problems that make up a disease. AIDS is caused by the HIV. By killing or damaging cells of the body's immune system, HIV progressively destroys the body's ability to fight infections and certain cancers. HIV is spread by sexual contact with an infected person, by sharing needles or syringes, or both (primarily for drug injection) with someone who is infected, or through transfusions of infected blood. Babies born to HIV-infected women may become infected before or during birth or through breast-feeding after birth.

Safe sexual practices are the most important key to HIV/AIDS prevention. However, there are many cultural, religious, and moral obstacles involved in the promotion of safe sex. In some cases, depending on culture, funding issues, and age of the audience, abstinence is promoted in lieu of safe sex. Careful research has shown that latex or polyurethane condoms provide a highly effective mechanical barrier to HIV. However, for condoms to provide maximum protection, they must be used consistently (every time) and correctly.

Stress, mental health, and coping

The single behaviors or clusters of behaviors discussed above are related to health and can prevent disease. However, healthy living often involves a complex web of behaviors and interactions between mind, body, and environment. For instance, stress occurs when a challenging situation arises for which an individual does not have the resources to cope. It is thought that the relationship between stress and disease may be, in part, due to a weakened immune system as a result of stress. For example, it has been suggested that there may be impairment of healing and delay in recovery as a result of stress-induced neuroendocrine activation. Another hypothesis is that high stress levels can lead to other behaviors that increase risk for disease, such as alcohol, tobacco, and drug use. Disease may also occur as a result of the body's inability to adapt and maintain homeostasis in the face of stress. Homeostasis is the principle of self-regulating information feedback by which constant conditions are maintained in the human body. Stress has been implicated in the onset of several diseases, including cardiovascular disease and some cancers. Stress, if left unchecked, also has the potential to affect general mental health, leading to increased vulnerability to anxiety and depression and even suicide. Therefore, stress management and effective

coping are key factors in disease prevention.

Stress monitoring is one viable coping strategy, since tracking stress levels can provide information for appropriate intervention. Supplying a health care provider with information about real time stress levels allows the provider to assess stress exposure and tailor stress-reduction strategies accordingly. Patterns or particular triggers may be identified that in turn allow for the development of strategies to deal with specific precursors. When used as a coping resource, stress monitoring has been found to be a significant predictor of life satisfaction.

Effective coping strategies are needed to deal successfully with stress and mental health issues. Identifying appropriate coping techniques depends on the situation and the person. Traditionally, coping has been categorized into two broad categories: emotion-focused and problem-focused activities. In recent years these have been extended to include other categories, such as withdrawal or seeking support. Strategies considered to be "adaptive" coping strategies focus on activities that will help to reduce or remove the source of stress. Therefore, problem-focused strategies are seen as more adaptive than emotion-focused strategies. However, when personal control cannot be exercised to remove or reduce stressors, emotion-focused strategies, including avoidance and seeking support, are useful to maintain psychological well-being.

Problem-focused strategies include seeking information to help solve the issue; evaluation and development of solutions; rethinking to help reduce the threat and thus allow for a broader view to identify possible solutions; seeking information from others on how they have solved similar situations; and setting goals to deal with different aspects of the stressor. Some examples of emotion-focused strategies are relaxation, physical activity, meditation, avoidance, creative expression, emotional eating, and seeking support. When choosing a coping strategy, effectiveness is key. The person should not focus solely on one strategy; a combination of different techniques may be needed and should deal with stress in the short term as well as the long term. It may be useful to avoid stressful situations as necessary, but it will be more adaptive and healthful if activities to reduce or eliminate the source of stress within the

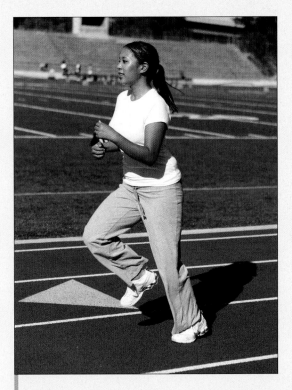

Getting regular exercise is an important factor in preventing illness. Just 20 to 30 minutes of vigorous or moderate activity three or five times a week are enough to ensure that bones, joints, and muscles remain healthy.

situation are undertaken and if they are tailored to the individual and to the specific setting.

A healthy lifestyle

As mentioned above, the leading causes of morbidity and mortality in the United States and worldwide are behavioral. Therefore, leading a healthy lifestyle is probably the most efficient and well-rounded strategy to prevent disease. The key term is *lifestyle*; it is important that these healthy behaviors are integrated and become part of everyday living. They should not be regimens or prescriptive behaviors but a normal part of a daily routine. This requires making changes that are realistic and that can be gradually incorporated into a normal life.

A healthy diet that, at minimum, meets the recommended standards can greatly reduce risk for a whole host of diseases. Proper diet ensures that the dietary needs of the body are met and that unhealthy foods do not detract from proper bodily function.

National health agencies recommend five to nine servings of fruit and vegetables per day, with an emphasis on vegetables, and limiting fat intake to 30 percent of calories, with an emphasis on reducing saturated and trans fats. Plenty of water and less salt and sugar are also recommended. Choosing low-calorie foods that are rich in nutrients will help ensure that the body gets enough energy without adding unnecessary empty calories, such as sugar. Variety and balance are important in order to maintain dietary health as well as to keep people happy about their dietary choices. Food not only affects physical health but can also have an impact on mood, so eating healthily helps to keep both the body and mind in good condition.

Regular exercise is another important lifestyle behavior that can reduce disease risk; it is recommended that adults engage in at least 30 minutes of moderate activity at least five days per week or 20 minutes of vigorous activity on at least three days per week. For children and adolescents, the guidelines vary somewhat, but there is general agreement that pediatric populations should engage in at least 60 minutes of physical activity on most days of the week. Lifestyle physical activity behaviors, such as taking the stairs and parking farther from one's destination, can be easily incorporated to achieve some of this recommended activity. Physical activity helps to maintain good health by building healthy bones, muscles, and joints. It reduces risk for heart disease, diabetes, and high blood pressure. Exercise may improve these ailments, control weight, and reduce stress, depression, and anxiety.

Proper nutrition and regular exercise will help someone maintain a healthful weight. Overweight and obesity put people at increased risk for the leading causes of illness and death in the United States, heart disease and some cancers, as well as other serious health conditions, including metabolic syndrome, sleep apnea, diabetes, stroke, and osteoarthritis. Maintaining or obtaining a healthy weight is dependent upon the right balance of diet and exercise. People must eat enough to provide the body with enough energy to keep going and should exercise enough to burn off excess incoming energy.

Tobacco, alcohol, and drug use also have a significant impact on health and disease prevention. Tobacco use is the leading preventable risk factor for asthma, heart disease, stroke, and various cancers. No amount of smoking or oral tobacco use is healthy. Alcohol use is the third leading preventable cause of death in the United States. Prolonged abuse can lead to liver disease, cancer, cardiovascular disease, and poor psychological health. If people want to drink alcohol, they should drink it in moderation, following medical guidelines. Drug use, aside from its direct consequences, has also been linked to unintentional injury, physical confrontations, unsafe sexual practices, and other high-risk behaviors. In particular, sharing needles for drug use is a significant contributor to the HIV epidemic. Drug use can upset the homeostatic balance of the body, and addiction can lead to serious physical, mental, and social consequences. Further, use of any of these substances can impact health.

It is clear that numerous health behaviors interact to produce a healthy or unhealthy lifestyle. To maintain good health, the individual must engage in behaviors that will promote health and must be aware of how all of these behaviors are interrelated. A healthy lifestyle includes—but is not limited to—good nutrition, regular exercise, not smoking, and proper stress management. Together, these behaviors as well as others promote health and help to prevent disease.

Environmental factors

The state of the environment affects the entire world population, as is evidenced by recent effects of global warming. Although environmental hazards vary by location, one influential aspect of the environment is air quality. Air quality can have detrimental effects on respiratory health by exacerbating asthma and slowing growth in children. Both indoor and outdoor pollutants can cause asthma, and since asthma is linked to physical inactivity, more children are at risk for other health problems. It is very difficult to reduce overall air pollution. However, exposure to pollutants such as secondhand smoking and auto exhaust can be managed. Reducing exposure to air pollutants can stop lung growth retardation, reduce asthma symptoms, and improve general health status.

Another important environmental health issue is access to safe places for children to play and for adults to use for exercise. Researchers have suggested that lack of access to places for safe recreation in combination with easy access to fast foods that are

cheap and energy dense are major contributory factors in the epidemic of obesity that is a problem worldwide.

War, politics, and policy

Health promotion and disease prevention are always a matter of priority. War is one obvious major behavioral cause of preventable death that is a product of choices made and priorities that are set as part of politics and policy. The poverty of some in the face of the plenty of others is, at some level, a policy decision—a choice that is made by people, politicians, and policy makers. Public policy that allows for poor hygiene, lack of safe drinking water, and open sewer systems in some nations contributes to open areas of stagnant water that allow free mosquito breeding and hence endemic strains of malaria and widespread diarrheal diseases.

Blaming the victim occurs when people are held to be responsible for their illness and for physical or psychological problems, and health thus may become a valued asset with moral overtones. The evolution of victim blaming has been ascribed to the rising collective costs of medical treatment and to the notion of reciprocal rights. Personal irresponsibility in health-related behaviors is seen by many as antisocial because it raises health costs for the entire community and has a negative influence on the just distribution of relatively scarce commodities.

However, prevention efforts that are limited to information on individual behavior modification contribute to an exclusive and erroneous focus on personal control. An emphasis on changing individual factors to the exclusion of systemic factors can lead to absolving management from responsibility for work conditions and job demands. It can lead people to absolve governments from responsibility to support social programs and research into the social and environmental causes of ill health. It can deceive people into overlooking opportunities to deal with significant environmental determinants of disease. Everyone has a responsibility to guard his or her health through preventive behaviors. However, the political and policy impact on personal and public health show that responsible government and world leadership are central to health promotion and disease prevention.

Donna Spruijt-Metz, Britni Belcher,
and Selena T. Michel

Prostate disorders

Several disorders may affect the prostate, including benign prostatic hyperplasia (enlarged prostate), prostatitis (inflammation of prostate), and prostate cancer.

The prostate is part of the male reproductive system. It is a walnut-sized gland that produces fluid that mixes with sperm to form semen. The prostate lies below the bladder and surrounds the upper part of the urethra, the tube that carries urine from the bladder through the penis to the exterior. Because of this proximity to the urinary system, prostate disorders often affect urination.

Benign prostatic hyperplasia

Benign prostatic hyperplasia (BPH) is a noncancerous enlargement of the prostate gland. Because the prostate continues to grow during a man's lifetime, BPH becomes increasingly common with older age, affecting around half of men aged 50 years and 90 percent of men aged 80 years. BPH is not linked to prostate cancer. Other terms for BPH include benign prostatic hypertrophy, lower urinary tract symptoms (LUTS), prostatism, or bladder outflow obstruction.

Causes and risk factors

The precise cause of BPH is not known. Some studies suggest that BPH is associated with hormones that regulate prostate growth, such as testosterone, estrogen, and dihydrotestosterone. Other evidence suggests BPH is linked with aging and the testes, since the disorder is more common in older men and does not develop in men whose testes were removed before puberty. The major risk factors for BPH are older age and a family history of BPH.

Symptoms, signs, and diagnosis

As the prostate enlarges, it compresses the urethra, obstructing the passage of urine; the bladder cannot produce enough force to empty itself, hence urine is left in the bladder. The symptoms of BPH vary from person to person and do not necessarily indicate the size of the prostate or the severity of disease. It is also possible to have BPH without suffering any symptoms.

Common symptoms include difficulty or pain when passing urine, frequent or urgent need to urinate (especially at night), a weak stream of urine, inability to

KEY FACTS: BPH

Description

Benign prostatic hyperplasia (BPH) is a non-cancerous enlargement of the prostate gland. The prostate gland is part of the male reproductive system and produces fluid that mixes with sperm during ejaculation.

Causes

The cause of BPH is not known. Contributing factors are likely to include advancing age and male hormones. Prostate enlargement is a normal part of aging, and most men have enlarged prostates by the age of 80 years.

Risk factors

The main risk factors for BPH are older age and a family history of the disorder. The only men not at risk of developing BPH are those whose testes were removed before puberty.

Symptoms

BPH puts pressure on the urethra, causing problems with urination. Common symptoms are pain or difficulty urinating; a frequent or urgent need to urinate, or both; difficulty starting to urinate; a weak urine stream; leaking or dribbling; and feeling that the bladder is still full despite urinating.

Diagnosis

BPH is diagnosed from symptoms, examination of the prostate, and the results of blood, urine, and imaging tests. The symptoms of BPH are similar to other prostate disorders, so tests may be done to exclude prostatitis and prostate cancer.

Treatments

Some cases improve without treatment. Mild BPH may simply require regular monitoring. Severe or persistent BPH is treated with drugs or surgery to remove excess prostatic tissue that is compressing the urethra, or shrink the prostate.

Pathogenesis

Without treatment, symptoms may improve, stay the same, or increase in frequency or severity, or both. BPH may also recur after successful treatment. Long-standing BPH can cause serious complications, such as inability to urinate, urinary tract infections, and kidney damage.

Prevention

BPH cannot be prevented.

Epidemiology

BPH becomes more common after the age of 40 and affects most men after 80, although not all will have symptoms. After adjusting for age, there is very little geographic or racial variation in the prevalence of BPH around the world.

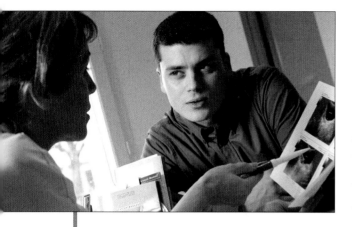

A consultant discusses the findings on a prostate ultrasound scan with a patient. Ultrasound scanning may be done to confirm that there is prostate enlargement.

begin urinating, leaking or dribbling, and the feeling of incomplete bladder emptying.

BPH is diagnosed on the basis of symptoms and investigations. The main test is a digital rectal examination (DRE), during which the doctor inserts a gloved and lubricated finger into the rectum to feel the size and condition of the prostate. A blood test called prostate-specific antigen (PSA) may be performed to help rule out prostate cancer, which has similar symptoms to BPH. Other tests include analysis of urine samples for glucose, blood, or signs of infection; urinary flow studies to measure the strength and volume of urine flow; imaging tests or cystoscopy to view the prostate; and urodynamic studies to determine bladder function.

Treatments and prevention

Many cases of BPH do not require treatment. If the prostate is only slightly enlarged or the symptoms are mild, the patient may simply be monitored with regular checkups. This is known as "watchful waiting."

For more severe or persistent symptoms, several treatments are used. Drugs can help relax the muscles around the prostate or shrink the prostate gland itself; ultrasound waves, microwaves, or radiofrequency energy may be used to destroy excess prostate tissue; or part of the prostate may be removed surgically. Surgery for BPH is usually performed via the urethra so that no external incision is needed. At present there is no way of preventing BPH.

Prostatitis

Prostatitis means inflammation of the prostate gland. It is the most common prostate disorder in men under 50 years of age. There are different types of prostatitis. It may develop suddenly (acute prostatitis) or gradually (chronic prostatitis) and may be caused by infection (bacterial prostatitis) or have no known cause (nonbacterial prostatitis). Other terms for prostatitis include *prostatodynia* and *pelvic pain syndrome*.

Bacterial prostatitis is an infection of the prostate gland caused by bacteria spreading from the urethra, bladder, large intestine, or other part of the body. Nonbacterial prostatitis is not due to bacteria, but the precise cause is unknown. Potential causes include other infectious agents, structural abnormalities of the urinary tract, or pelvic muscle spasm.

Risk factors for prostatitis include urinary tract infection, a urinary catheter, rectal or perineal injury, structural abnormalities of the urinary tract, and occupations or activities that subject the prostate to vibration.

In acute prostatitis the symptoms typically arise suddenly and are severe, whereas chronic prostatitis may be asymptomatic or cause symptoms that are mild or variable in severity.

All forms of prostatitis can cause problems with urination similar to those for BPH. Additionally, prostatitis can cause symptoms of infection, such as fever, chills, nausea, and vomiting; pain in the lower back, pelvis, and genital area; pain when urinating; blood in the urine; pain with ejaculation; painful bowel movements; and blood in the semen or urine.

Prostatitis is diagnosed based on symptoms, physical examination (often including DRE), and analysis of urine for bacteria and white blood cells. Samples of prostatic fluid and semen may also be tested for bacteria.

Treatments and prevention

Bacterial prostatitis is treated with antibiotics, sometimes with muscle-relaxant, analgesic, and anti-inflammatory drugs. If treatment is not successful, part of the prostate may be removed surgically via the urethra. Nonbacterial prostatitis may also be treated with antibiotics. Other treatments include exercises, relaxation techniques, and lifestyle changes to relieve symptoms. Some cases of prostatitis can be prevented by avoiding infection of the urinary and reproductive tracts.

Joanna Lyford

See also
- Aging, disorders of • Bladder disorders
- Cancer, bladder • Cancer, prostate
- Hormonal disorders • Infections • Male reproductive system disorders • Urinary tract disorders

Psoriasis

Psoriasis is a chronic inflammatory disease that results from a genetic predisposition to the disease and from environmental factors. The genetic basis is evident because it is seen more often in some families and there is a high rate of concordance among twins. Triggering factors include skin trauma, infection, psychological stress, certain medications, alcohol consumption, and pregnancy. Patients with a family history of psoriasis are at increased risk for developing the disease.

Psoriasis is typically diagnosed by its characteristic clinical appearance. Classically patients develop sharply demarcated red plaques (raised plateaulike lesions) with silvery white scale distributed about the scalp, trunk, and limbs, with a predilection for extensor surfaces such as the elbows and knees.

The second most common form of psoriasis is called guttate psoriasis and is typified by red droplike lesions that classically appear on younger patients after streptococcal sore throat.

Other forms include pustular (small blisters containing sterile pus on a red base) and erythrodermic (redness of more than 90 percent of the body surface area due to persistent and severe inflammation). Psoriasis frequently affects the nails, causing small pits, discoloration, and lifting of the nail plate. Of particular importance, up to one-third of patients with psoriasis can have an associated arthritis called psoriatic arthritis.

Treatments and prevention

There are many topical and systemic therapies for psoriasis. Management of this chronic disease requires recognizing the extent of the disease, as well as the possible side effects of treatment. In general, limited skin disease can be managed with topical corticosteroids in combination with other steroid-free agents such as vitamin D_3 analogues, retinoids (vitamin A–type molecules), salicylic acid, and coal tar.

More widespread disease may be treated by exposure to ultraviolet light (phototherapy), without additional medications (psoralens) to increase light sensitivity. Additional therapies include oral vitamin A–type drugs (retinoids), chemotherapy agents such as methotrexate, or immunosuppressive agents such as cyclosporine. A group of medications known as biologics has become available for the treatment of extensive psoriasis. Biologics are proteins produced by molecular biology techniques and include antibodies that bind molecules involved in causing psoriasis. Often topical therapies are combined with light therapy or nontopical medications for adequate relief. There are no known preventive measures at this time.

Adam Korzenko and Richard Kalish

KEY FACTS

Description
Psoriasis is a chronic inflammatory disease of the skin.

Causes
Both genetic and environmental factors contribute to psoriasis.

Risk factors
The most important risk factor is a family history of psoriasis.

Symptoms
Red patches and plaques with silvery white scale over extensor surfaces. Psoriasis may also affect scalp, nails, palms and soles, and joints.

Diagnosis
Clinical grounds and skin biopsy.

Treatment
Topical corticosteroids, vitamin D_3 analogues, coal tar, salicylic acid, topical and oral retinoids, phototherapy without additional psoralens, methotrexate, cyclosporine, and biologics.

Pathogenesis
The exact mechanism remains unclear. Several lines of evidence suggest that psoriasis is an autoimmune disease mediated by T-lymphocytes.

Prevention
There are no known preventive measures at this time.

Epidemiology
The prevalence of psoriasis has been estimated at 2 percent of the world's population. There is a bimodal incidence with peaks at 20 to 30 years and 50 to 60 years. Psoriasis affects males and females equally.

See also
- Arthritis • Genetic disorders
- Immune system disorders • Skin disorders

Psychotic disorders

Psychosis is a general term that refers to distortions or alteration in a person's thoughts or perceptions. The person loses touch with reality and has frightening thoughts, for example that someone is trying to kill him or her. The person's thoughts and perceptions have changed or distorted. This is one of many examples of the symptoms that may be experienced by someone with a psychotic disorder.

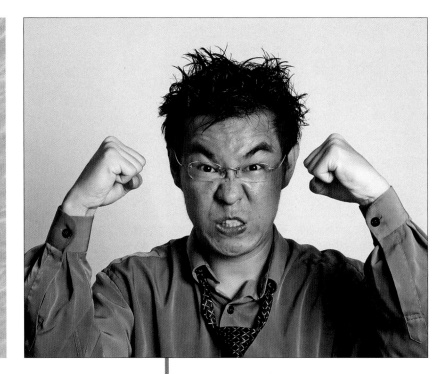

Auditory hallucinations, in which the individual hears one or two voices talking, can be distressing for the person involved. Usually, but not in every case, these voices make very negative comments about the person.

Everyone continually takes in information from their environment, information that is received through the senses, including visual (sight), auditory (sound), gustatory (taste), olfactory (smell), and tactile (touch). Each of these five important sensory functions, functions that are taken for granted each day, become distorted in psychosis and result in people viewing things or people around them that are not present. Individuals with psychosis may also experience delusions, which are fixed beliefs that are not based in reality, or they have difficulties in organizing or generating their thoughts.

Psychotic disorders are illnesses in which psychosis is the primary symptom. It is important to keep in mind that many disorders, including nonpsychiatric medical illnesses, may have psychosis as a symptom. For example, individuals with epilepsy, brain tumors, or those who have suffered a severe head injury may develop psychosis.

Another common cause of psychosis is drugs of abuse, such as amphetamines, PCP, or cocaine. In addition, drugs such as LSD are in a class of drugs called hallucinogens, which bring about changes in beliefs and perceptions. Although these drugs of abuse can induce psychosis, drug abuse and dependence are not considered psychotic disorders. Psychotic disorders include several psychiatric illnesses that are associated with psychosis (see box, page 704). Since how people perceive the world around them is essential to ground them in reality, it can easily be seen how psychotic disorders, which alter the perception of reality, can be such devastating illnesses.

Causes

More is known about the cause of psychosis than the cause of psychotic disorders. The symptom of psychosis is nonspecific, being present not only in psychotic disorders but also in a number of nonpsychiatric medical disorders and substance abuse disorders.

Psychosis is a symptom, whereas psychotic disorders are illnesses. The development of psychosis appears to be related to an overabundance of the neurochemical dopamine. Drugs that increase dopamine, such as amphetamines or cocaine, or medications used to treat Parkinson's disease, can result in psychosis.

Both genetic and environmental factors are associated with psychotic disorders. For example, if an identical twin develops schizophrenia, the other twin has a 50 percent chance of also developing the illness. This decreases to a 15 percent chance in fraternal twins. Since identical twins have identical genes, but fraternal twins, like siblings, share only 50 percent of their genes, genetic factors play a large role in the development of schizophrenia. However, 50 percent of identical twins who have a co-twin with schizophrenia do not develop the illness.

Thus it can be reasoned that environmental factors also play a role in the development of schizophrenia, as well as the other psychotic disorders.

Environmental factors

There have been numerous environmental factors that have been implicated in psychotic disorders. Many of the factors that have been investigated include events that occur very early in life, such as an infection during pregnancy or complications during birth. The current thinking about the cause of psychotic disorders is that there are individuals born who are genetically predisposed toward illness but only develop the illness in the context of specific environmental stressors.

Symptoms

Psychotic disorders have psychosis as their common feature. Psychosis can come in a number of different forms, but the characteristic features include hallucinations, delusions, or disordered thought. Auditory hallucinations are the most common type of hallucination and can vary from indistinct noises (for example, mumblings, people shouting in the distance, or the wind blowing) to one or more distinct voices. The voices most often make negative and degrading comments about or directed toward the person, and at times two voices may converse among themselves. Command hallucinations, or voices that make demands, are not uncommon and are often very upsetting. Not all auditory hallucinations are negative, and some individuals have voices telling them that they are wonderful, gifted, or that they have special powers or abilities.

Visual hallucinations have similar characteristics. They can be either nondescript (for example, flashing lights or moving shapes) or apparent real images of faces, animals, or monsters. Visual hallucinations are more common in children and become less common in later adolescence and adulthood. Feeling insects crawling on the skin is a common tactile hallucination, and olfactory hallucinations are typically foul smelling. Gustatory hallucinations, or hallucinations of taste, are rare in individuals with psychotic disorders.

Delusions are false beliefs that remain fixed despite being far-fetched or having considerable evidence to the contrary. Delusions can only be understood within their cultural and ethnic context. Thus certain religious or ethnic beliefs, although they may appear odd to those outside that culture, would not be considered delusions.

Interestingly, individuals within the cultural or ethnic group are often able to readily identify delusional beliefs when someone within that same group deviates from the cultural norms. Psychosis is a worldwide phenomonen that crosses all ethnic and religious

KEY FACTS

Description

Psychotic disorders are those disorders that are associated with psychosis, or an alteration of a person's thoughts and perceptions.

Causes

Although the underlying cause of psychotic disorders are as yet unknown, there are both genetic and environmental factors associated with these illnesses.

Symptoms

An alteration in someone's thoughts and perceptions, causing hallucinations, delusions, and disorders of thought and speech.

Diagnosis

The diagnosis of the psychotic disorder will require a thorough history, physical and neurological examination, laboratory studies, and often imaging studies of the brain.

Treatments

The treatment of psychotic disorders often includes antipsychotic medications. Supportive or cognitive behavioral therapy is also important.

Pathogenesis

Psychotic symptoms are related to the brain chemical known as dopamine.

Prevention

Little is known about the prevention of psychotic disorders, although there is emerging evidence that avoiding marijuana will reduce the chance of developing schizophrenia.

Epidemiology

Rare during childhood, and the primary age of onset is late adolescence and early adulthood. Males tend to present with symptoms earlier than females.

lines and can be found equally on all continents. Delusions can be divided into those that are false but yet fall within the realm of possibility (for example, "the government is plotting to kill me"), and those that are unrealistic ("the government has implanted chips in the brains of everyone at birth so that they can know and manipulate our thoughts").

The most common types of delusions that people have are paranoid delusions, such as the feeling that others want to cause harm. Other types of delusions include grandiose delusions (having special powers or abilities), somatic delusions (feeling that the body has some disease or illness), or religious delusions (having a special relationship with God that others do not have). Most individuals who suffer with delusions do not have insight into the possibility that their belief system is distorted. Thus, their actions will reflect their beliefs. For instance, an individual who fears that his food is poisoned may avoid eating certain types of food. Although delusions can alter one's beliefs, most individuals with psychosis are not aggressive.

An additional symptom that may or may not be present in individuals with a psychotic disorder is called a formal thought disorder. This refers to the disruption in the flow or processing of a person's thoughts and becomes apparent during normal conversation. The severity of the thought disorder can be quite variable, ranging from rather mild disruptions in thought, such as a long latency between asking a question and obtaining a response, to a complete lack of communication or speaking gibberish ("word salad").

Additional symptoms of a thought disorder include moving rapidly between one topic and another (flight of ideas), rapid or pressured speech, creating new words (neologisms), or suddenly switching to a completely unrelated topic during conversation (tangentiality).

Diagnosis

When individuals develop obvious symptoms of psychosis, it is first very important for physicians to correctly determine if there is an underlying medical or substance use disorder.

Psychosis can have many causes, and the treatments differ, depending on the diagnosis. In order to obtain an accurate diagnosis, the physician will perform a thorough history and physical examination, laboratory tests, and often brain imaging studies. Although nonpsychiatric medical illnesses that cause psychosis are quite rare, they will only worsen if not identified and treated.

In addition, psychiatric disorders such as bipolar disorder, major depressive disorder, substance abuse, post-traumatic stress disorder, or borderline personality disorder may have psychosis as a secondary symptom. Substance abuse is one of the most common causes of psychosis and can be identified either through the history or by laboratory studies.

Once it is determined that the psychosis is a part of a psychotic disorder, there are differences between the psychotic disorders (see box below) that help solidify the diagnosis.

PSYCHOTIC DISORDERS

Brief psychotic disorder is a condition in which the psychotic symptoms develop suddenly, usually within a day or two. The psychosis may follow some tragic event or a period of considerable stress and disappear as quickly as it came. The psychosis must come and go within a month for it to be considered a brief psychotic disorder.

Schizophrenia is a devastating illness that affects approximately 0.5 to 1 percent of the world's population. Along with psychotic symptoms, schizophrenia is also associated with a lack of motivation, withdrawal from social interactions, a flattening of facial expressions, and greater difficulties performing cognitive tasks.

Schizoaffective disorder is similar to schizophrenia and is a hybrid of schizophrenia and a mood disorder. It is defined by the presence of both psychosis and a mood disorder in the same individual, but at different times.

Schizophreniform disorder is similar to schizophrenia, except that the symptoms are present for less than six months.

Delusional disorder is a condition in which an individual experiences only nonbizarre delusions, without hallucinations or a thought disorder.

Shared psychotic disorder is an illness in which delusional beliefs are transferred to another. It usually involves two family members or a married couple. The person who first develops the delusion is typically more dominant; the person who adopts the delusions tends to be more suggestible.

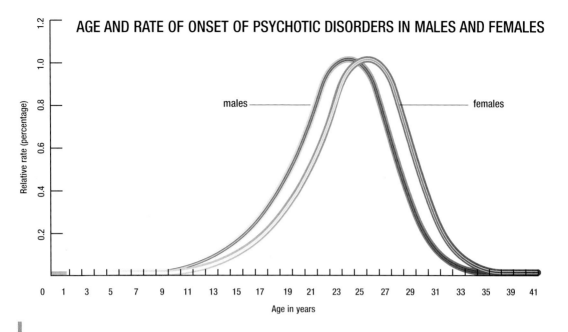

AGE AND RATE OF ONSET OF PSYCHOTIC DISORDERS IN MALES AND FEMALES

males ——————— females

Relative rate (percentage)

Age in years

The graph shows that the incidence of psychotic disorders peaks between age twenty and thirty.

Treatments

The treatment will be dependent on the diagnosis. Psychotic symptoms that are a result of nonpsychiatric medical disorders should resolve when the medical illness is treated. For psychotic disorders, the mainstay of treatment is an antipsychotic medication. Antipsychotic medications were first used during the 1950s and dramatically altered the lives of many individuals with psychotic disorders.

Since the 1980s, newer medications have been developed with fewer side effects. These antipsychotic medications are also used for psychosis in the presence of mood disorders. Treatment of shared psychotic disorder requires the separation of the two or more individuals who adhere to the delusion. This may result in rapid improvement in the individual who adopted the delusion.

Cognitive behavioral therapy

There is emerging evidence that people with a psychotic disorder may benefit from a specific type of therapy called cognitive behavioral therapy (CBT). The goal of CBT is to assist patients to recognize when they are experiencing hallucinations and delusions and to help them learn that it is a part of their illness. The support and encouragement of parents and friends is also very important to help a person suffering from a psychotic disorder.

Pathogenesis

Long-term treatment is usually needed, and recurrence is likely. Individual outcomes vary but seem worse if the person is young when the disorder begins.

Prevention

There is emerging evidence that individuals who are genetically predisposed to develop a psychotic disorder increase their risk with the use of marijuana during early and middle adolescence. Being familiar with the symptoms of psychosis may promote early identification and treatment.

Epidemiology

The most common age to develop psychotic disorders is during late adolescence and early adulthood. Psychotic disorders are rare during childhood. Males tend to have an earlier age of onset than females, although the rates are equal in delusional disorders.

Finally, it is important to note that upward of 15 percent of children and adolescents may experience mild hallucinations, such as hearing their name called. These events are considered to be normal developmental events and are not psychosis.

Tonya White

See also
- Bipolar disorder • Depressive disorders
- Mental disorders • Personality disorders
- Schizophrenia • Substance abuse and addiction

Rabies

Rabies is a life-threatening viral disease that mainly involves the central nervous system. The illness is usually transmitted to humans from the bite of a rabid animal. Rabies is a rare but feared disease that has been documented in every country except Australia and Antarctica and in all U.S. states except Hawaii.

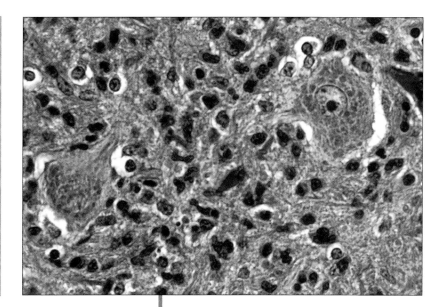

This magnified and colored microscopic image of cerebellar tissue from someone who died of rabies shows characteristic negri bodies, which are found in the brain in cases of rabies. The negri bodies are the dark round structures with basophilic granules at the center.

Rabies can be contracted through contact with animals infected with rabies virus or by contact with the virus in a research laboratory. Rabid animals usually spread the illness to humans through a bite wound. In some cases, the bite goes unnoticed, particularly instances involving bat bites. It is thought that such bite injuries can go undetected because of the small teeth of a bat. There is a possibility of aerosol transmission of the virus from bats to humans.

Nonbite transmission can occur through scratches made by a rabid animal, by the animal licking over an open wound or mucous membrane, or by exposure to brain fluid or tissue that is infected with the rabies virus. Rabies is not transmitted by simply petting a rabid animal or by contact with blood, urine, or feces of a rabid animal; nor is it transmitted from person to person. In a few cases, rabies has been transmitted by corneal transplantation.

The type of rabies virus (varies by species), the body site where the virus enters, and the dose of virus introduced at the entry site are all factors in risk of infection and progression of illness. The immune status of the host also plays a role.

Animal control and vaccination programs account for the low rates of rabies in the United States compared to developing countries. Most animal rabies cases in the United States are identified in raccoons, skunks, foxes, and bats. Except for the woodchuck, rodents and lagomorphs (hares) usually do not transmit rabies.

Symptoms and signs

Rabies starts out as a nonspecific, flulike illness. Symptoms usually begin within 20 to 90 days after exposure to the virus, but can occur within only a few days or up to one year or more after this exposure. Fever, headache, and malaise are common symptoms. Pain, numbness, and tingling may occur at the injury site. As the illness progresses, the person develops changes in behavior, hallucinations, and agitation. Difficulty in swallowing develops from neurological dysfunction, leading to fear of water. Excessive salivation, convulsions, cardiac arrhythmias, respiratory failure, and death usually follow. In almost all cases, once classic symptoms appear, death results.

Diagnosis

Early symptoms of rabies are nonspecific and difficult to distinguish from common, benign illnesses, making diagnosis difficult and often untimely. In animals, diagnosis of rabies is made by examining postmortem brain tissue. In humans, multiple specimen sources are examined, including serum and spinal fluid for antibody to the virus. The virus may be grown in culture in a laboratory. Saliva specimens may be analyzed for the presence of rabies viral genetic material.

Treatments

There is no effective treatment once symptoms appear. Wounds inflicted by a potentially rabid animal should be washed with soap and water. Immediate medical attention should be sought. The geographical location of the incident, the animal involved and its vaccination status, and whether or not provocation was involved is important. Capture of the animal and testing of post-mortem tissue, or, in the case of a domesticated animal that has documented up-to-date rabies vaccine status, confinement and observation for a specified period of time are needed. In the latter case, the animal is watched for any signs of rabies.

For potential exposures to rabies, immune globulin and five doses of rabies vaccine are administered. This is referred to as post-exposure prophylaxis. Immune globulin provides antibody to the virus and is administered around the site of the wound. The vaccine induces the body to produce antibody to rabies virus, a situation that takes some time. The vaccine is administered in the upper arm and is given over a period of 4 weeks.

Pre-exposure prophylaxis, used by those at high risk of exposures, such as veterinarians, field biologists, and laboratory personnel working with rabies virus, involves the administration of three doses of rabies vaccine given over three to four weeks. The recipient's antibody levels are monitored periodically, with boosters administered as needed to maintain adequate antirabies antibody levels in the blood.

Pathogenesis

Once rabies virus enters the body through a bite or mucous membrane contact, the virus multiplies in the muscle cells. No symptoms appear during this time. The virus spreads along nerves, traveling to the spinal cord. At this time, the person may have numbness, tingling, and discomfort along the path of the nerve. The virus eventually infects the central nervous system. Since salivary glands are supplied with a dense amount of nerve tissue, excessive salivation may be seen. Inflammation of the brain, or encephalitis, and cardiopulmonary failure follow. Death usually occurs within one week after the onset of signs and symptoms.

Prevention and epidemiology

No vaccine is available. Every year, about 40,000 people in the United States receive rabies pre-exposure prophylaxis and about 18,000 people receive post-

---

KEY FACTS

Description
Viral infectious disease of mammals.

Cause
Rabies virus.

Risk factors
Contact with animals infected with the virus, or with rabies virus in a laboratory setting.

Symptoms
Nonspecific, flulike initially, then hallucinations, excessive salivation, convulsions, and death.

Diagnosis
In animals, postmortem brain tissue is examined for presence of the virus. In humans, blood and cerebrospinal fluid are examined.

Treatments
Rabies vaccine for those at risk of exposure to rabies; vaccine plus immunoglobulin (preformed antibodies) for someone exposed to rabies.

Pathogenesis
The virus enters at the site of injury, or perhaps via mucous membrane inoculation, and travels to the central nervous system. Inflammation of the brain and death usually follow.

Prevention
Avoid contact with unknown or wild animals, keep pets' vaccines up to date. Seek immediate medical attention for exposures to potentially rabid animals.

Epidemiology
In the United States, rabies causes only 1–2 deaths yearly; worldwide, the virus causes more than 35,000 human deaths every year.

---

exposure prophylaxis. The best way to avoid rabies is to avoid contact with wild animals and with unknown animals. Those who are planning travel to a country where rabies is a problem should visit their physician in the event that rabies pre-exposure prophylaxis is required. Pet owners should keep their pets' vaccines up to date. Any openings in the home through which animals could enter should be sealed. If someone is bitten or exposed to an animal that could potentially be infected with rabies, immediate medical attention should be sought.

Rita Washko

See also
- Arrhythmia • Brain disorders • Infections
- Infections, animal-to-human • Infections, viral • Respiratory system disorders

Radiation sickness

Radiation sickness, also known as acute radiation syndrome (ARS), is caused by exposure to an excessive amount of radiation. The exposure may be in a series of doses over time (chronic) or in a single large dose (acute). The larger the dose, the greater the risk of developing radiation sickness. The effects are felt first in each cell. With very high doses of radiation, many cells are affected, and the tissues cease to function. Eventually the body is unable to repair itself, and if the damage is great enough, the person will die.

Radiation is the process of emitting energy in the form of waves or particles. There are various types of radiation, which are distinguished according to their properties of emitted energy and matter. Radiation occurs naturally in the environment, so everyone is exposed to some daily radiation without harmful consequences. For example, routine cases of exposure to artificial radiation are living near a nuclear power plant or undergoing a medical test, such as an X-ray. This kind of radiation occurs in amounts too small to cause any damage.

Radiation is normally classified into ionizing and nonionizing types. Nonionizing radiation comes in the form of light, radio waves, microwaves and radar, which are relatively harmless. These types of radiation generally do not cause tissue damage. On the other hand, ionizing radiation is radiation that produces immediate chemical effects (ionization) on human tissue. X-rays, gamma rays, and particle bombardment (neutron beam, electron beam, protons, and mesons) emit ionizing radiation. This type of radiation is used for medical testing and treatment, industrial testing, manufacturing, sterilization, weapons and weapons development, and many other uses.

Too much exposure to excessive ionizing radiation can cause serious health problems. Any living tissue in the human body can be damaged by radiation, but some body parts are more sensitive to radiation than others. These are the breasts, thyroid gland, reproductive organs, and bone marrow. The body's cells attempt to repair the damage, but if the damage is too severe, radiation sickness will result.

The major factors that determine the severity of radiation injury are the amount and length of time of radiation received and the length of exposure time. For example, a person exposed to ionizing radiation in a focused medical procedure such as a knee X-ray will usually not suffer any symptoms of radiation sickness since the procedure is short, localized, and radiation exposure is minimal. However, a person can be exposed to radiation anywhere radioactive materials are used. Someone exposed to a large nuclear plant leak such as the Chernobyl nuclear reactor accident is likely to suffer from severe radiation sickness if the radiation was in the atmosphere for long periods of time and exposure occurred to the whole body. Thus, the larger and longer the dose, the greater the risk for radiation sickness.

Causes and risk factors

Ionizing radiation causes cells to die by damaging DNA, which becomes so impaired that it can no longer function and support the biochemical processes that keep the cells alive. Children and fetuses are more sensitive to radiation because they are growing more rapidly, and there are more cells dividing and a greater opportunity for radiation to disrupt the process. Anyone can be exposed to radiation if radiation sources or radioactive materials are used, such as in nuclear power plants, medical centers, research laboratories, or if radioactive material is removed from mines.

The degree of radiation sickness depends on the dose and the rate of exposure. Exposure from X-rays or gamma rays is measured in units of roentgens. For example, a total body exposure of 100 roentgens causes radiation sickness. A person with a total body exposure of 400 roentgens will get radiation sickness; death occurs in half of these individuals. A dose of 100,000 rads (radiation absorbed dose) causes almost immediate unconsciousness and death within an hour. The severity of symptoms and sickness depends on the type and amount of radiation, the duration of the exposure, and the body areas exposed. Symptoms of radiation sickness usually do not occur immediately following exposure.

A person who is contaminated with radioactive materials will expose others. Contaminated materials must be handled by specially trained people. Once the radioactive material has been removed, the person cannot spread radiation.

Signs and symptoms

Cell death is manifested in the body through the symptoms of radiation sickness. Symptoms of radiation sickness usually do not occur immediately following exposure but over the course of a few days or months. These symptoms appear gradually and include nausea and vomiting; diarrhea; skin burns (radiodermatitis); weakness; fatigue; loss of appetite; fainting; dehydration; inflammation (swelling, redness or tenderness) of tissues; bleeding from the nose, mouth, gums, or rectum; low red blood cell count (anemia); and hair loss.

Because it is difficult to determine the amount of radiation exposure from accidents, the best indications of the severity of the exposure are the length of time between the exposure and the onset of symptoms, the severity of symptoms, and severity of changes in white blood cells. Generally, the higher the amount of radiation, the greater the severity of early effects and greater possibility of later effects, such as cancer. The effects of radiation exposure on the body vary according to the circumstances in which they occur. Radiation sickness can be acute or chronic. The acute form of the disease can develop quickly, within a few hours or days of exposure. A set of symptoms appear in an orderly fashion. A person with acute radiation sickness has usually been exposed to large amounts of radiation over a very brief period of time. This happens in the case of a nuclear plant accident or a nuclear bomb explosion. It may take several days or weeks to develop the chronic form of the disease. A person with chronic radiation sickness has usually been exposed to lower doses over a longer period of time, as in the case of radioactive outcome from a nuclear explosion or accident. It may also be caused by long-term exposure to radiation in the workplace. Chronic sickness is usually associated with delayed medical problems such as cancer and premature aging, which may happen over a long period of time.

The main phase of the intestinal form of the sickness typically begins two to three days after radiation exposure with abdominal pain, fever, and diarrhea, which progress rapidly in severity for several days to dehydration, total exhaustion or weakness, and a fatal, shocklike state. The main phase of the hematopoietic (production of blood cells) form of the illness usually begins in the second or third week after radiation exposure with fever, weakness, infection, and hemorrhage. If damage to the bone marrow is severe, death from infection or hemorrhage may follow four to six weeks after exposure unless corrected by transplantation of unexposed bone marrow cells.

The diagnosis is based on the symptoms and a person's report of radiation exposure. There is no effective treatment cure for radiation sickness after exposure. Only supportive treatments to alleviate symptoms can be offered; there is no medication that can prevent or reverse the damage caused by radiation.

Recovery from radiation injuries may take months or years. Chronic problems, such as damage to the chromosomes, may be permanent and can last a lifetime. A person who has been exposed to radiation will be monitored closely. Laboratory studies of blood samples, including a complete blood count, will reveal how well the body is working to recover. Physical exams will also be done to check for the development of late effects from the radiation poisoning.

Rashmi Nemade

KEY FACTS

Description

Damage to living tissue as a result of excessive exposure to ionizing radiation.

Causes

Accidental or intentional exposure to radiation.

Risk factors

Working with or around radioactive materials and equipment, as well as receiving medical treatments that require radiation. Children and fetuses and people who work with radiation and radiation equipment are at risk.

Symptoms

Nausea, vomiting, diarrhea, hair loss, weakness, bleeding, swelling of mouth or throat, or both, fatigue, skin ulcers, and low blood count.

Diagnosis

History of exposure to radiation, physical signs and symptoms, and a complete blood count.

Treatments

No effective treatment for reversing the effects. Treatment is aimed at relieving symptoms.

Prevention

Avoiding unnecessary exposure to radiation.

Epidemiology

A person is exposed to about 0.002 grays of radiation from natural, medical, and work-related sources per year. One gray is the absorption of 1 joule of radiation energy by 1 kilogram of matter.

See also
• Environmental disorders • Occupational disorders

Raynaud's disease

Raynaud's disease or phenomenon (RP) is described as an episodic vasoconstriction of the arteries and arterioles of the hands or digits.

Raynaud's phenomenon is considered primary if there are no other symptoms, or secondary if systemic symptoms are part of another, often more serious disease. Attacks are usually caused by an exaggerated response to cold temperature or emotional stress. Provoking factors may be caused by shifts from warmer to colder temperatures, such as air conditioning or the frozen food section of a supermarket. An attack may occur after stimulation of the sympathetic nervous system, such as by sudden startling. There are no known risk factors for Raynaud's disease. Intermittent, sudden pallor or blue digits are usually present. Most often the hands are involved, but attacks can occur in the toes, ears, nose, face, and nipples. An episode may be described as a sharp demarcation of white or blue, lasting about 15 to 20 minutes, after which the skin reddens.

Criteria for the diagnosis of primary Raynaud's phenomenon include attacks brought on by cold or emotional stress, attacks involving both hands, and lack of tissue death or gangrene. The patient should have normal nail-fold capillaries, normal erythrocyte sedimentation rate, and negative serologic findings, such as antinuclear antibodies. Potential causative or aggravating factors should be excluded, including chemotherapeutic agents, interferon, estrogen, nicotine, cocaine, and clonidine. Environmental causes should be investigated, such as frostbite or repetitive occupational stress.

Clues to the presence of secondary RP include age of onset at more than 40, male gender, painful severe events with insufficient blood supply to tissues, ulceration, and asymmetric attacks. Signs and symptoms of systemic disease (myalgias, fever, weakness, weight loss, rash, and cardiac or pulmonary symptoms) suggest secondary Raynaud's phenomenon. Further investigation can include complete blood count, general chemical analyses, urinalysis, antinuclear antibodies, rheumatoid factors, and complement levels. Positive findings may suggest a rheumatological disease, such as scleroderma or lupus. Referral to a rheumatologist is usually appropriate. In patients who demonstrate single-digit involvement, absent pulses, or asymmetric attacks, vascular disease should be considered and evaluated.

Avoidance of triggers is the best prevention, and the entire body should be kept warm. Therapies aimed at reduction of emotional stress and elimination of medications known to exacerbate RP can be preventive. Smoking should be avoided in patients who suffer from RP. Temperature-related biofeedback may be beneficial for some patients. Calcium-channel blockers have been widely used to treat Raynaud's phenomenon. Patients with secondary RP should seek treatment for an underlying cause. Sometimes, but rarely, blood flow to the digits is permanently reduced, leading to gangrene.

Surveys suggest that the prevalence of Raynaud's phenomenon in the United States is about 3 to 5 percent in most ethnic groups. It may be more common in young women, younger age groups, and family members. There are geographic variations related to climate. The severity and frequency of attacks are influenced by temperature, with more attacks during the winter.

Kathleen Stergiopoulos

KEY FACTS

Description

Episodic vasoconstriction of the arteries and arterioles of the digits.

Causes

An exaggerated response to cold or emotional stress.

Risk factors

More likely to occur in colder climates.

Symptoms and signs

Excessive sensitivity to cold and intermittent pallor or cyanosis of the distal portions of hands and toes.

Diagnosis

By history and physical exam.

Treatments

Calcium-channel blockers. Vasodilator drugs.

Pathogenesis

Rarely, ulceration of the digits occurs, which can lead to gangrene.

Prevention

Avoidance of triggers.

Epidemiology

Prevalence of 3 to 5 percent in most U.S. ethnic groups. More common in young women.

See also

- Arteries, disorders of

Repetitive strain injury

Repetitive strain injury (RSI) describes a spectrum of musculoskeletal pain disorders as a result of occupational overuse or repetitive motion. Such overuse injuries can occur in people who do repetitive movements over a long time, for example, when using a computer, handheld instrument, or tool. RSI may also occur in occupations that require a person to maintain a fixed position for long periods of time. RSI can eventually become a chronic condition, in which the person suffers pain even when he or she is not carrying out the repetitive action that originally caused the pain.

RSI is also known as repetitive stress injury, repetitive strain injury, work-related upper limb disorder (WRULD), and occupational overuse syndrome. Specific disorders that may fall under the classification of RSI include adhesive capsulitis, bursitis, carpal tunnel syndrome, cervical spondylosis, writer's cramp, cubital tunnel syndrome (ulnar nerve entrapment), De Quervain's syndrome, Dupuytren's contracture, epicondylitis, ganglion cyst, peritendonitis, rotator cuff syndrome, tendonitis, tenosynovitis, trigger finger or thumb, and thoracic outlet syndrome.

Nonspecific disorders may affect muscles, tendons, bursae, or joints of the neck, shoulders, upper back, elbows, wrists, or hands, or all of them. "Diffuse RSI" refers to a nonspecific pain syndrome in which pain is present in several areas, attributed to underlying nerve damage as a result of repetitive motions. Occupations commonly associated with RSI disorders include working for long periods of time without rest breaks at a computer, desk, or assembly line.

Causes

Repetitive motion and prolonged tension in muscles that are held in a continuous position are believed to cause microtrauma to underlying tissues, which injures muscles, tendon sheaths, ligaments, nerve sheaths, or other structures, resulting in swelling and pain.

Swelling of muscles or tendon sheaths is believed to reduce blood flow to the affected tissues and the surrounding area, exacerbating the symptoms. Repetitive motions aggravate the underlying microtrauma to tissues and prevent healing.

KEY FACTS

Description
Spectrum of soft tissue injury disorders of the neck, shoulders, upper back, arms, wrists, or hands.

Causes
Occupations or activities that require prolonged repetitive motion or a prolonged fixed position, such as work with a computer, a handheld instrument, or a tool.

Risk factors
An ergonomically unsound work station, poor posture, excessive workload, prolonged periods of work without rest, repetitive movements with work (such as typing), repetitive forceful hand motions (such as twisting or gripping), prolonged body vibrations (such as from power tools), fatigue, cold work environments, and psychosocial stressors.

Symptoms
Sharp or dull pain, soreness, stiffness, tingling and numbness, loss of sensation, limited range of motion, weakness, fatigue, or persistent tension in the neck, shoulders, upper back, elbows, wrists, or hands. Pain may develop in the back or lower extremities or be referred from one area to another.

Diagnosis
Thorough history and physical exam.

Treatment
Depends on the specific underlying syndrome and its cause. Options include rest, anti-inflammatory medications, anti-convulsant medications for neuropathic pain, deep tissue massage for acute pain and trigger points, stretching or strengthening exercises, specialized orthopedic braces for immobilization, or surgery.

Pathogenesis
Repetitive microtrauma to muscles, tendon sheaths, and nerve sheaths of the neck, upper back or upper extremities, causing swelling and pain. Reduced blood circulation after soft tissue swelling exacerbates symptoms.

Prevention
Good posture, frequent breaks from prolonged fixed positions, adaptive technology in the workplace, and maintenance of general good health through physical activity.

Epidemiology
Exact prevalence and incidence is unknown because of underreporting and misdiagnosis. Reporting varies by industry.

Risk factors

Risk factors include an ergonomically unsound work station, poor posture, and excessive workload. Working for long periods without rest and using repetitive movements or repetitive forceful hand motions (twisting or gripping) are also contributing factors, as are prolonged body vibrations (such as from power tools), fatigue, cold work environments, and psychosocial stressors.

Symptoms

Symptoms may accumulate over long periods of time and include recurring sharp or dull pain, soreness, stiffness, tingling and numbness, loss of sensation, limited range of motion, weakness, fatigue, or persistent tension in the neck, shoulders, upper back, elbows, wrists, or hands. Pain may be referred from one area to another, such as when nerve impingement in the neck or shoulder causes pain in the forearm or hand. Less commonly, pain may also be referred to the back or lower extremities.

Symptoms in the arms or hands may worsen when lying in bed. Routine daily activities such as driving, carrying groceries, housework, or gardening may worsen symptoms. Without treatment, symptoms may become continuous and progress to long-term injury and disability.

Diagnosis

Diagnosis is often difficult and is based upon a thorough history and physical examination by a physician familiar with RSI syndromes. Injuries are not identifiable with X-rays or other radiological studies since the injuries involve soft tissues. Several different specialists may be involved with the diagnosis and treatment plan, such as occupational therapists, physical therapists, physiatrists, surgeons, massage therapists, and alternative medicine practitioners.

Treatments and prevention

Treatment of RSI will vary and will depend on the specific underlying syndrome and its cause. Possible treatment options include rest, anti-inflammatory medications, anti-convulsant medications for neuropathic pain, deep tissue massage for acute pain and trigger points, stretching or strengthening exercises (or both), biofeedback techniques, or specialized orthopedic braces for immobilization. Surgery is considered a last resort. Cessation of hand activity both at work and in routine daily activities may be required for a period of time to prevent worsening of symptoms and to promote healing of affected tissues.

Adaptive technology such as specialized keyboards, computer mouse replacements, and speech recognition software may be considered for certain work environments. Computer users are encouraged to decrease the risk of RSI by adjusting their work stations so that the top of their computer screen is at eye level, to keep their arms at a 90-degree angle to the computer keyboard, to use a chair back that supports the spine and tilts the pelvis forward, and to keep feet flat on the floor. People who type for prolonged periods are encouraged to avoid bending their wrists or resting their hands on the keyboard. People in occupations at risk for RSI are encouraged to take frequent breaks to stretch and increase blood circulation to muscles. General physical activity to maintain flexibility is encouraged, as is a healthy diet, as well as smoking cessation to promote general health.

Epidemiology

RSI has a significant economic impact; research in the United States reveals that in Washington State alone, compensation for workers affected by RSI was in the region of $20 billion, and one-third of worker's compensation costs in the United States are directly related to RSI. Added to that is the burden of the cost of lost revenue and the cost to employers when workers take sick leave.

Although statistics regarding RSI are controversial, it seems clear that RSI is almost always occupational in nature, and the huge increase in the use of computers in the workplace and computers at home puts people at risk for the condition. In the United States, around 50 percent of injury claims for upper limb disorders involve a computer. A European survey showed that 30 percent of workers suffered from backache and 17 percent, about 25 million people, complained of muscular pain in the arms and legs. The British Health and Safety Executive reported that around half a million workers complained of some type of neck or limb disorder. In 2002 in the United Kingdom, 5.4 million working days were lost in sick leave as a result of RSI.

Ergonomically designed workstations, combined with appropriate strategies in the workplace, are essential in order to combat RSI.

Joanne L. Oakes

See also
- Backache • Bone and joint disorders
- Environmental disorders • Muscle system disorders • Nervous system disorders
- Occupational disorders • Spinal disorders

Respiratory system disorders

Every time someone takes a breath, the respiratory system is exposed to an environment that teems with pollutants, irritants, pathogens, pollens, molds, and other foreign material. Each of these is a risk not only to the respiratory system, but to the body's general health. There are a wide variety of respiratory disorders: obstructive diseases, such as asthma; infections, such as pneumonia; as well as cancer, inflammatory diseases, and interstitial disease. Some respiratory disorders are relatively benign, while others can be life threatening.

When air is breathed in through the nose or mouth, it passes downward through the throat (pharynx) to the larynx. The larynx (voice box) is situated at the level of the Adam's apple and contains the vocal cords, which control sound production by their movement. At the top of the larynx is a small leaflike flap of tissue, the epiglottis, which folds over the opening of the larynx during swallowing to prevent food, liquid, or foreign material from entering the lungs. Instead, what is swallowed slides down the esophagus, which lies behind the respiratory air passages, and into the stomach. If the epiglottis fails to close off the larynx, at least some of what is swallowed will enter the major airway (trachea) that extends down from the larynx.

The air passages are so well supplied with sensitive nerve endings that the person immediately begins coughing, which is the body's mechanism for clearing the airway of anything but air. This is often referred to as "something going down the wrong way." A cough is produced when the vocal cords close, trapping air in the lungs. As the pressure in the lungs builds up, the vocal cords suddenly open, allowing the air, and possibly the irritating material, to be ejected forcibly.

The part of the respiratory system that ends at the bottom of the larynx is considered the upper airway. An infection of these passages is often referred to simply as a URI (upper respiratory infection). By the time inhaled air reaches the lower part of the respiratory system, it has been humidified and warmed to approximately body temperature by the mucous membrane lining the nose and throat, and it is free of airborne particles of greater than microscopic size.

After passing through the larynx, inhaled air continues into the trachea (windpipe), which extends downward from the larynx. The tubelike trachea is the largest and longest airway, or air passage, and is surrounded by C-shaped rings made of cartilage, a flexible, fibrous connective tissue that protects and supports the trachea. In an average-size adult, the trachea is approximately 4 to 5 inches (10 to 12 cm) long, so at approximately the midlevel of the sternum, the flat bone that can be felt in the upper chest, the

RELATED ARTICLES

BRONCHIECTASIS

Scarring and deformity of the air passages, known as bronchiectasis, occurs in association with several diseases and is characterized by recurrent infections and excessive mucus production.

In adults, several diseases, including immune defects (which cause infections), cystic fibrosis, allergic bronchopulmonary aspergillosis, and early childhood infections, are the most common causes of bronchiectasis. In children and adolescents, cystic fibrosis is the most common cause, with immunodeficiencies, gastroesophageal reflux, and ciliary dyskinesia syndromes comprising most of the other cases.

Bronchiectasis most often begins in childhood, although symptoms may not be noticeable early in the disease; later, it is often misdiagnosed as asthma or pneumonia.

Three types of bronchiectasis have been described. Cylindrical bronchiectasis is the most common type and may be found after an attack of acute bronchitis. This type involves slight widening of the air passages and may be reversed with timely treatment. In the varicose type, the air passages are both distended and collapsed, while the most severe type, the cystic type, involves irreversible stretching and ballooning of the passages.

Symptoms include coughing, which becomes worse when lying down because the trapped mucus shifts and irritates the lining of the air passages; shortness of breath; weakness; weight loss; and fatigue. With repeated infection, the mucus may become discolored, foul smelling, and possibly blood tinged. The thickness of the mucus makes it difficult to cough up. There may also be audible abnormal sounds of breathing.

Chest X-rays and CT scans, sputum cultures, and breathing tests may all be used to evaluate bronchiectasis, as well as testing for related conditions such as tuberculosis or cystic fibrosis. Treatment involves antibiotics for the infection, bronchodilating medication to open the air passages, and, in some cases, medication to thin the

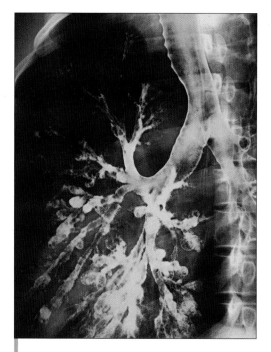

This colored bronchogram of a human lung shows bronchiectasis. The airways of the lungs, the bronchi and bronchioles (shown in red), are dilated and distorted, and some of the bronchi have bulbous enlargements. A bronchogram is obtained by performing a chest X-ray after injecting a colored contrast medium.

mucus. Physical therapy techniques to dislodge the mucus so that it can be coughed out of the air passages are often beneficial. Adults should avoid smoking, other irritants, and sedatives. Treating respiratory infections as soon as they occur may prevent bronchiectasis. Vaccinations against influenza, measles, and other infections may be a good preventive. Bronchiectasis is rarely fatal, but severe cases may be considered for lung transplantation.

trachea divides into two main stem bronchi, the right and left bronchi, which supply the right and left lungs. Beyond this point, each bronchus divides many times into smaller and smaller tubes (bronchioles) within each lung until they are as small as half a millimeter across. These bronchioles have circular muscles in their walls that allow them to narrow (constrict) and widen (dilate) to change the internal size, thus controlling the amount of air that can flow through them. At the very tip of the smallest bronchioles are air ducts that end as balloonlike air sacs (alveoli) with extremely thin walls containing tiny blood vessels (capillaries). It is here in the alveoli, via the capillaries, that oxygen passes into the blood, and carbon dioxide moves out of the blood into the alveoli to make its way upward through the respiratory passages to be exhaled. The millions of alveoli in the lungs form a surface for this exchange of more than 430 square feet (40 sq. m), or enough to cover half of a tennis court.

Each lung is composed of major divisions called lobes. The right lung has three lobes, but the left lung is slightly smaller and has only two lobes because of space taken up by the pericardial sac containing the heart. Each lung is covered by a thin membrane called the pleura. Another section of pleura lines the inside of the chest wall. Normally there is a small amount of fluid between the two layers of pleura that acts as a lubricant and allows the lungs to move freely within the chest.

The larger respiratory passages are lined internally by a thin mucous membrane containing tiny hairlike projections called cilia. The cilia move in a wavelike manner that can move unwanted or irritating material upward and outward so that it can be coughed out, blown out, or moved to the esophagus to be disposed of by swallowing. Without this seemingly simple mechanism, the lower respiratory system would be attacked by many more pathogenic organisms that are capable of producing infection and disease.

Infectious respiratory diseases

From the common cold to pneumonia, transitory infections or life-threatening disorders are usually caused by bacteria or viruses. In fact, some common infections may be due to either a bacterium or a virus. For example, common transient sore throats, often treated and relieved with lozenges or sprays, are usually caused by a variety of different viruses. However, the very serious "strep throat" is caused by the *Streptococcus* bacterium and requires active treatment with an appropriate antibiotic.

Although both may be pathogenic (disease producing), bacteria and viruses are very different organisms. Bacteria can live in or outside the human body and contain all the genetic material needed to reproduce and thrive independently under favorable conditions. Viruses are much smaller and must invade living cells in order to reproduce. However, viral infections cannot be cured with antibiotics, while appropriate antibiotics may effectively treat bacterial infections. It is imperative for the public to understand this difference and not insist that their health care provider prescribe an antibiotic to relieve symptoms of a viral infection. The antibiotic will not help viral symptoms, and inappropriate use may actually result in adverse effects, such as oral and vaginal yeast infections and severe diarrhea. Overuse of antibiotics inappropriately is known to be responsible for difficulty in treating diseases caused by bacteria that have become resistant to formerly effective medications.

Acute bronchiolitis. Bronchiolitis is a viral infection of the smallest air passages within lung tissue. The infection causes the bronchioles to swell, which makes breathing difficult. Children under age two are most affected, especially during winter and spring. Symptoms include a runny nose, slight fever of 101°F (38.3°C), loss of appetite, cough, rapid or shallow breathing, and possibly wheezing. The most common causes are the influenza virus and respiratory syncytial virus (RSV). Antibiotics are ineffective, and the infection must run its course of one to two weeks. Hospitalization may be necessary for more severe cases or if there are complications.

Usually, as with many respiratory infections, treatment consists of encouraging the child to drink clear fluids, bed rest initially, and acetaminophen for fever. Aspirin should be avoided. A cool mist vaporizer may ease the discomfort from the dry air passages and facilitate breathing if recommended by the health care provider. Because bronchiolitis is contagious through close contact, and saliva or mucus from sneezing or coughing is infectious, the child should not go to day care or school until fully recovered.

Emerging viral diseases

Among emerging viruses is a group of recently identified respiratory disease-causing viruses.

Respiratory syncytial virus (RSV) is one of the viruses that has been identified as causing respiratory diseases. It is the major cause of bronchiolitis and pneumonia in children less than three years old and so contagious that most children will have had RSV by the time they are four years old. Symptoms are similar to those listed under bronchiolitis, but they may last longer, up to three weeks. Antibiotics are not effective against this viral disease, but for severe cases that develop into pneumonia, an antiviral medication may be indicated.

If symptoms appear to worsen or fever rises above 101°F (38°C), the health care provider should be notified. Symptoms that compromise breathing warrant medical attention. RSV is most contagious for two to four days after the child becomes ill. As with all respiratory viruses, it is easily transmitted, and to protect other siblings, hand washing is important after caring for the ill child.

Human metapneumovirus (HMPV). This virus causes a variety of conditions, including mild upper respiratory infections as well as the more severe lower respiratory infections bronchiolitis and pneumonia. Upper respiratory infections may involve the nose, throat, and larynx, whereas lower respiratory tract infections involve the trachea, main stem bronchi, bronchioles, and alveoli. Although HMPV is believed to have been causing respiratory diseases for at least 50 years, it was first isolated and identified in the Netherlands in 2001.

Symptoms of HMPV include high fever, severe cough, difficulty breathing, rapid breathing, wheezing, vomiting, and diarrhea. It may also cause disease in elderly people, especially those with COPD. Researchers suggest that HMPV may stimulate asthma attacks in children known to have asthma. A recent study found that asthma was the most frequent diagnosis on discharge from the hospital among children who were HMPV-positive, while another study showed that 14 percent of cases involving HMPV infection had an exacerbation of asthma.

Severe acute respiratory syndrome (SARS). The 2002 outbreak of severe acute respiratory syndrome (SARS) was first reported in Asia; within a few months it had spread to two dozen countries in North America, South America, Europe, and Asia before being contained. Over 8,000 people became ill, of which 774 died.

The disease was caused primarily by a previously unidentified coronavirus (SARS-CoV), but there is a possibility that other infectious agents may have also been involved in some cases. Close person-to-person contact appears to be how most SARS spreads. The majority of new infections occurred in close contacts of patients, such as household members, health care workers, or other patients who were not protected by contact or respiratory precautions. The virus is transmitted by respiratory droplets produced when an infected person coughs or sneezes.

Droplets may be propelled up to 3 feet (0.9 m) through the air and land on the mucous membranes in the mouth, nose, or eyes of persons nearby. Another way of transmission is if someone touches a contaminated surface that the infected droplets have landed on, and then touches his or her mouth, nose, or eyes. However, the virus has also been found in the stool, so oral-fecal transmission may be possible, as with other known coronaviruses. In the outbreak in a Hong Kong hotel, the virus may have spread through the sewage systems of the buildings. Also, actual airborne spread (directly and widely through the air) has not been completely ruled out.

SARS usually begins with a general feeling of unwellness, headache, and body aches, accompanied by a fever of more than 100.4°F (38°C). Sometimes there are mild respiratory symptoms at the onset, but more often a dry cough develops two to seven days later. Most victims develop pneumonia, and some develop respiratory failure and require mechanical ventilation. The disease is most contagious during the second week.

A major problem in treatment and control of SARS is that there are as yet no diagnostic laboratory tests available that clearly and quickly identify the disease. The reason for this is that, unlike most viral infections, SARS patients do not show signs of the virus early in the infection; highly sensitive tests, able to detect the small amounts of virus present in the first few days of infection, are needed. These types of tests are under development in Canada, France, Germany, the Netherlands, Singapore, the United Kingdom, and the United States. Until viral presence in respiratory specimens and stool peak at approximately 10 days, detection largely depends on ruling out atypical pneumonia caused by other pathogens.

Although viral infections do not respond to antibiotics, and SARS is caused by a virus, initial treatment of the symptoms consists of broad-spectrum antibiotics along with supportive care, antiviral agents, and immunomodulatory therapy. Antibiotics appropriate for bacterial diseases with symptoms similar to early SARS are used until all other infections

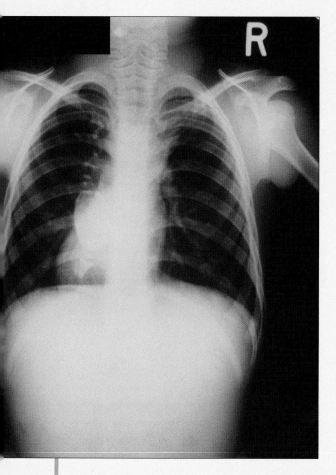

An X-ray of a child's chest area shows atelectasis (collapse of the lung) possibly because of enlargement of the bronchial tubes (bronchiectasis). As a result, the lungs are unable to clear the clogging mucus, which builds up.

are ruled out or there are definitive laboratory results indicating SARS. Additionally, some antibiotics are known to have immunomodulatory effects under other circumstances. Antiviral drugs with broad-spectrum effect may be used, but their effectiveness at nontoxic doses has not yet been proven for SARS. High doses may produce complications such as hemolytic anemia, especially in older people. When used for the treatment of SARS, antiviral agents are usually used in combination with corticosteroids.

Currently, a reverse transcription polymerase chain reaction (RT-PCR) is used to detect SARS-CoV in blood, stool, and nasal secretions when present. PCR is a type of laboratory test that is considered an important method for detecting infectious disease agents from specimens taken from symptomatic patients.

Serological tests can also be used for SARS and other infectious diseases to identify antibodies in the blood that are produced by the body's immune system after the person is infected. Viral cultures are another testing option.

The best prevention for SARS, like so many other contagious diseases, is frequent hand washing. For diseases like SARS that are spread by respiratory droplet, avoiding close contact with other people is important. This includes close conversation, for example, within 3 feet (0.9 m), sharing drinking or eating utensils, and avoiding direct physical contact. It does not mean briefly sitting across from someone or walking past other people.

Legionnaires' disease

Legionellosis, or Legionnaires' disease, is an example of a respiratory infection caused by a bacterium occurring naturally in the environment but that was not recognized as a pathogen until it was identified as the cause of a serious outbreak of respiratory disease, resulting in many affected individuals and several fatalities. Since then, it has been identified as the cause of multiple outbreaks throughout the world, the largest to date occurring in Spain in 2001. Many outbreaks have occurred as a result of cooling towers becoming infected with the bacterium.

The disease got its name when the bacterium was isolated and identified as the cause of multiple cases of respiratory infection that occurred among people attending a convention of the American Legion in Philadelphia in 1976. At least 220 people fell ill, resulting in 64 fatalities, all of whom were staying at the same hotel. In January 1977, scientists identified the bacterium and found it was breeding in the cooling tower of the hotel's air conditioning system, which spread it throughout the building. The bacterium was named *Legionella pneumophila*; since then, 46 species of *Legionella* have been isolated, but 90 percent of severe cases are caused by *L. pneumophila*.

How the bacterium spreads is not completely understood. There has been no evidence of person-to-person transmission, and although normally found in the environment in water and occasionally in soil, it appears that the bacterium must get deeply into the lungs to start an infection. Inhalation of small particles

ALPHA-1-ANTITRYPSIN DEFICIENCY

Alpha-1-antitrypsin deficiency is a hereditary disorder. Alpha-1-antitrypsin (AAT) is an enzyme produced by the liver to inhibit the action of other enzymes called proteases that break down proteins in the body when appropriate. Without enough alpha-1-antitrypsin, proteases may damage tissue, especially in the lungs and liver. AAT deficiency is usually identified in children who often do not reach adulthood as a result of the damage that occurs to these vital organs. It is estimated that 25 percent of children with AAT deficiency will die before the age of 12 because of liver damage. About 25 percent die by age 20, while another 25 percent have only minor liver destruction and live to adulthood. In the 25 percent who do not develop liver abnormalities, the disease does not progress.

The associated lung involvement is often severe, particularly considering the patients' young age, and is often misdiagnosed as asthma or conventional COPD. AAT deficiency may be detected with a simple blood test, and the World Health Organization recommends that all individuals with asthma or COPD be tested for the deficiency. Tests to evaluate the extent of lung involvement include pulmonary function tests, chest X-rays, and CT (computed tomography) scans.

Symptoms include frequent respiratory infections, shortness of breath, decreased exercise tolerance, rapid deterioration of breathing ability in nonsmokers, nonresponsive asthma, or year-round allergies. A family history of lung disease or liver disease is very significant.

Stopping or avoiding smoking is critical for patients who have AAT deficiency. Treatment with synthetic alpha-1-antitrypsin appears to improve survival and slow deterioration of lung function. Lung transplant is the preferred treatment in patients who have developed severe obstruction. Liver transplant is indicated for patients with severe liver involvement and has the added advantage of curing the disease, because the transplanted liver cells produce alpha-1-antitrypsin. AAT deficiency is also being investigated as a target for gene therapy.

---

of contaminated water, as in mists and aerosols, seems to be essential.

Legionella bacteria thrive in warm water, and it is believed that hot tubs, whirlpool spas, hot water tanks, large plumbing systems, and the cooling towers of air conditioning systems in buildings and ships provide ideal conditions. The bacterium can survive for months in warm moist conditions.

Legionnaires' disease usually begins 2 to 14 days after exposure with headache, muscle pain, and a general feeling of malaise, followed by high fever up to 104°F to 105°F (40°C–40.5°C) and shaking chills. Nausea, vomiting, and diarrhea may also develop. On the second or third day, dry coughing begins, followed by difficulty breathing and chest pain. The most severe cases develop an atypical pneumonia and may require hospitalization.

Unlike most respiratory infections, people with Legionnaires' disease often exhibit neurological symptoms. Mental changes, such as confusion, disorientation, hallucination, and loss of memory may occur to an extent that seems out of proportion to the seriousness of the fever. Because the pneumonia resulting from Legionnaires' disease resembles pneumonia from other causes, it is difficult to distinguish it from other pneumonias by symptoms or by X-ray findings alone. The diagnosis must be confirmed by laboratory tests that isolate the *Legionella* bacterium from the person's sputum. Now there is a fast and reliable test available to identify *Legionella* antigens in the urine. Blood tests are used to evaluate the amount of specific substances (antibodies) the body produces when attacked by pathogenic organisms or foreign proteins; however, these are done three to six weeks apart.

Treatment with appropriate antibiotics, those capable of penetrating into the human cell, is the basis of treatment, along with supportive therapy. Complete recovery can take several weeks.

About 5 to 15 percent of known cases of Legionnaires' disease have been fatal. Those most at risk of contracting the disease are the elderly; those with chronic lung disease; smokers; and those with depressed or weak immune systems from cancer and chemotherapy, kidney failure, diabetes, HIV, and post–organ transplant medication.

Pontiac fever. This disease is a much milder form of respiratory infection, which is caused by the same type of *Legionella* bacteria. Mild symptoms may last two to five days and usually disappear without treatment. The fever does not develop into pneumonia. It is not understood why the same species of Legionella is able to produce two different diseases.

Fungal infections of the lung

Fungi are extremely tiny spore-bearing organisms similar to yeast or mildew. They release heavily encased, long-lived seeds into the environment that are easily inhaled. Fungi are opportunistic and, although generally not considered pathogenic (disease producing), under favorable conditions they may grow within the lungs, causing infections difficult to cure.

Coccidioidomycosis. Referred to as simply *cocci*, coccidiodomycosis was first clearly identified during World War II when an alarming number of Army Air Corps personnel at airbases in the southwestern United States became ill with a condition the local inhabitants called desert fever, valley fever, or San Joaquin Valley fever. The cause turned out to be a fungus living in the soil that produced spores, which were blown around in dust and inhaled. The Air Corps reduced the incidence by laying more concrete, planting grass, and using irrigation to reduce dust.

The infection is not contagious, so it cannot be spread to humans by infected small desert animals or other humans. Visitors may easily develop the condition, but inhabitants engaged in dusty occupations, such as farm workers and construction workers involved in moving soil, are most likely to develop cocci. Archaeologists excavating in the area are also at risk. One bout of the infection confers immunity to further infection. A more serious condition develops if cocci spreads throughout the body (disseminates). Nonwhite people and those with impaired immune function are much more likely to develop the severe disseminated form. Blacks, Mexicans, and Filipinos new to the area are especially susceptible. The primary or simple form presents with flulike symptoms, and although any age group may develop cocci, those between ages 25 and 55 are most likely to develop symptoms, found equally among men and women. However, men and pregnant women are most susceptible to the serious type.

In the primary type, the condition is confined to the lungs. But as the inhaled spores that reach tiny alveoli start to grow, more and more spores are produced that may spread to other areas such as internal organs, brain, bones, and possibly skin. Wherever the spores become established, the body responds to these foreign substances with inflammation. Scars or cavities may develop into which calcium is eventually deposited.

As many as 70 percent of those infected may not have symptoms, but the remainder develop symptoms within one to three weeks. These include a cough and aches and pains, with fever as high as 104°F (40°C). Some individuals develop a measlelike rash a week or two after the fever. Usually these symptoms disappear within a month on two, but the person often lacks energy for several months. The disseminated type causes extreme fatigue along with a very high fever, cough, and flulike aches and may be fatal. In dark-skinned people, 10 to 20 percent develop disseminated cocci.

Diagnosis may be made on positive results of at least one of the following types of tests: presence of the cocci organism in the sputum or other body fluids; blood tests that show the presence of substances generated by the body in reaction to the fungus; and skin test. Chest X-rays may show abnormalities, but the shadows seen may be mistaken for those found with tuberculosis or other lung disease.

Diagnosis may be especially confusing in visitors who contract cocci but do not develop symptoms until they return home.

Treatment is supportive based on symptoms and may incorporate a number of medications. Surgical removal of a particularly diseased portion of lung, bone, or skin in disseminated cases may be necessary. A vaccine is under development.

Pneumocystis. Pneumocystis pneumonia (PCP), also called pneumocystosis, is an atypical pneumonia that is caused by a fungal organism widespread in the environment. Considered nonpathogenic to healthy individuals, in those with weakened immune systems caused by cancer, HIV/AIDS, solid organ or bone marrow transplantation, corticosteroids, or other medications that affect the immune system, the responsible organism (*Pneumocystis jiroveci*) may cause a serious lung infection.

PCP was relatively rare prior to the AIDS epidemic, but as many as 70 percent of patients with advanced AIDS developed PCP, and the infection became the most common cause of death in AIDS. Since treatment for HIV infection and preventive antibiotics for PCP have become available, the disease is less common.

The infection typically develops slowly, over weeks, in patients with HIV, but more explosively in others. In either population, fatal respiratory failure may occur. Symptoms include fever, cough, shortness of breath, and rapid breathing. The shortness of breath is most obvious with exertion.

Because many lung infections present with these symptoms, a detailed medical evaluation is often required to identify PCP. Chest X-ray may show abnormal findings, yet nearly 10 percent of patients with AIDS and PCP may have a normal chest X-ray. Sputum tests, using special stains to detect the *Pneumocystis jiroveci* organism, can be done. If these are negative, bronchial visualization and lavage (washing out) using a special instrument (bronchoscope) may be necessary for a diagnosis. Should all tests prove negative, biopsy of lung tissue may be required.

Antimicrobial medications, by mouth or intravenously (IV) in severely ill patients, are the first-line treatment for PCP. If the patient has decreased blood oxygen indicating severe PCP, corticosteroids are used in addition. The sickest patients may require mechanical ventilation.

Noninfectious respiratory disorders

There are several noninfectious respiratory disorders, including acute respiratory distress syndrome, asthma, and lung cancer

Acute respiratory distress syndrome (ARDS).

Acute respiratory distress syndrome, first recognized in the battlefield hospitals of the Vietnam War, is a life-threatening syndrome of low blood oxygen and chest X-ray abnormalities caused by a wide variety of insults and injuries to the lungs.

In approximately one-third of ARDS occurrences, the cause is extensive inflammation of the lung due to generalized infections throughout the body (sepsis) or severe pulmonary infections, such as pneumonia. Other causes may be as diverse as inhalation of saltwater or smoke; multiple blood transfusions;

overdoses of drugs such as heroin or methadone; or shock from any cause. ARDS may also occur after significant damage to another body organ, for example, damage to the pancreas may release proteins, including enzymes and cytokines, that are capable of then injuring the lungs and other organs (multiple organ system failure).

ARDS usually starts with shortness of breath and rapid shallow respirations. As the blood oxygen level decreases, the skin and nails may take on a bluish discoloration (cyanosis) as confusion and rapid heart rate develop. ARDS occurs in 15 to 20 percent of patients with any one of the major risk factors above; typically, it develops within 24–48 hours of the occurrence of the precipitating cause.

Oxygen administration is essential. Oxygen is delivered by nasal cannulae, face mask, or in severe cases, by mechanical ventilation. Care must be taken not to cause further lung injury from too much mechanical pressure. A supportive breathing technique using positive end expiratory pressure (PEEP) is effective. Simultaneously, the underlying cause of the ARDS must be treated, along with supportive therapy for other affected organs and careful fluid balance. This treatment may consist of antibiotics for infections, and rarely, anti-inflammatory corticosteroids. Experimental therapies continue to be investigated.

Without prompt emergency treatment, ARDS may be fatal in 90 percent of cases. With treatment, the fatality rate is 30 to 40 percent, mainly due to other organ failure. Over 150,000 cases of ARDS occur in the United States each year.

Asthma. This is a chronic lung disease in which the airways (bronchial tubes) to the lungs become inflamed, causing the tubes to narrow, which results in intermittent attacks of coughing, shortness of breath, and sometimes wheezing. An allergic response can trigger the inflammation and swelling that causes an attack. Trigger substances include mites, pollen, feathers, mold, and dander. Occupational asthma can be caused by substances that people regularly work with, such as chemicals, paint, latex, and glue. Each year nearly 500,000 individuals in the United States are hospitalized due to asthma, and more than 4,000 of these cases prove fatal. In 2005 the number of adults in the United States suffering from asthma was 15.7 million, that is, 7.2 percent.

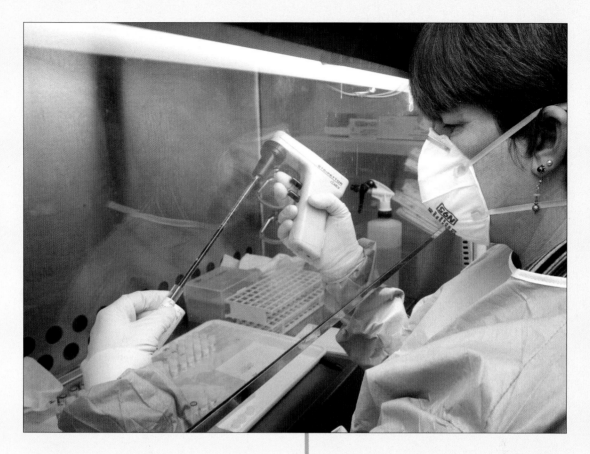

A worker in the Special Pathogens branch of the Centers for Disease Control and Prevention (CDC) processes specimens from SARS victims. The CDC has worked with the World Health Organization and other partners to address the SARS outbreak.

Asthma is also a common chronic disease of childhood. The National Council for Health Statistics estimated that in 2005 the number of children in the United States who had asthma was 6.5 million, or 8.9 percent. In that year, 3,780 children died from asthma, or 1.3 in 100,000.

COPD. Chronic obstructive pulmonary disease (COPD) is often a combination of two progressive respiratory diseases: chronic bronchitis and emphysema.The airways become obstructed by inflammation, which makes the air passages smaller, and the lungs become damaged, making breathing difficult. COPD is usually related to smoking. When irreversible changes in the lungs occur, the person will be short of breath and will experience fatigue, making everyday activities more difficult. Diagnosis is by X-ray or computed tomography scan. Drugs are available to help the symptoms, but there is no cure. Of the 24 million people in the United States who have COPD, in 85 percent it is a result of smoking.

Lung cancer. Lung cancer is the uncontrolled growth of abnormal cells lining air passages in one or both of the lungs. These abnormal cells form lumps or tumors that disturb normal lung function. The principal function of the lungs is to exchange gases such as carbon dioxide and oxygen. Normally, carbon dioxide exits from the bloodstream with each exhalation, and oxygen enters the bloodstream with each inhalation. With each breath, air is carried into and out of the lungs through the airways, comprising the trachea, bronchi, bronchioles, and alveoli. The trachea divides into the bronchi, which in turn branch into progressively smaller airways called bronchioles that end in alveoli, where gas exchange occurs. When there are tumors in any part of the airways, gas exchange is impaired and lung function is restricted. There are two major types of lung cancers: small cell lung cancer (SCLC) and non–small cell lung cancer (NSCLC). Sometimes a cancer in the lung may have characteristics of both types, which is known as mixed small cell–large cell carcinoma. Non–small cell lung cancer is the most common type of lung cancer; it accounts for 80 percent of all lung cancer cases. This type of cancer usually spreads or metastasizes to different parts of the body more slowly than SCLC.

The first symptoms of lung cancer are fatigue and shortness of breath; other symptoms include weight loss for no reason, a change in a persistent cough, and unaccountable aches and pains.

More than 80 percent of lung cancers are smoking-related; however, not all smokers will develop lung cancer. A person's risk of lung cancer diminishes if he or she stops smoking. Each year, more men and women die from lung cancer than from breast cancer and prostate cancer; lung cancer is the leading cancer killer in both men and women in the United States. In 2006 it was estimated that 31 percent of men and 26 percent of women suffering from cancer would have lung cancer. About 6 out of 10 people with lung cancer die within a year of being diagnosed with the disease. Lung cancer is predominantly a disease of the elderly. From 1998 to 2002 the median age at diagnosis was 70 years of age. African American men have an incidence rate of lung cancer that is 50 percent higher than that for Caucasian American men, and African American men are more likely to die from lung cancer than people in other racial or ethnic groups. Worldwide, the highest rates of lung cancer occur in North America and Europe, particularly eastern Europe.

Idiopathic pulmonary fibrosis

Idiopathic pulmonary fibrosis (IPF) is an idiopathic (cause unknown) disease that causes severe, progressive scarring (fibrosis) of the lungs; it is also known as cryptogenic fibrosing alveolitis. IPF affects more men than women, and it occurs most commonly in those aged 50 to 70, particularly if they have smoked. There are over 50,000 cases of IPF in the United States, with an estimated 15,000 new cases each year. Similar patterns of lung scarring are seen in patients with occupational exposures (asbestos), rheumatic diseases (scleroderma), and certain drugs (cancer chemotherapy), but the term *IPF* is reserved for cases in which no cause can be found. The scarring in IPF begins in the tissue between the air sacs (interstitium) but eventually damages and destroys the air-exchanging units themselves. The resultant scarring produces lungs that are stiff, difficult to inflate, and which lose the ability to efficiently transfer oxygen to the blood.

The principal treatment for IPF is oxygen, because many patients suffer from low blood oxygen and its complications, including fatigue, shortness of breath, and pulmonary hypertension (high blood pressure in the lungs and pulmonary arteries). Corticosteroids and cytotoxic agents (drugs used in cancer treatment, for example, azathioprine or cyclophosphamide) are often tried in IPF, but their effects are variable, and they can have severe side effects. Antifibrotic and immunomodulatory agents (colchicine, interferon gamma-1b, pirfenidone, and TNF receptor antagonist) have also been investigated for use in IPF, but no consensus has been reached about their effectiveness.

Lung transplantation has been a considered as a last resort for patients with severe IPF, but studies have shown that patients who receive lung transplants in this situation fare poorly. Some experts now think that early referral for transplantation is a better strategy.

Epidemiology

Around the world, different countries have many of the same respiratory diseases; statistics relating to them differ only in distribution and numbers. Some diseases are more prevalent in some countries than others. Nevertheless, there is a similarity between the diseases suffered in the developed world to those experienced in developing countries.

The causes of death were shared to some extent also. Eight of the ten leading causes of death in the United States were the same as those in other developed countries, and five leading causes of death matched those for developing regions.

For example, in the developed world, chronic lower-respiratory diseases are the fourth leading cause of death; in lower-income countries, lower-respiratory diseases are the third leading cause of death. In the developed world, COPD was the fifth leading cause of death; in the United States it is the fourth leading cause of death; and in lower-income countries, it is the sixth leading cause of death.

Nance Seiple

Retinal disorders

Retinal disorders are caused by injury, genetic mutations, hypertension, vessel occlusion, premature birth, glaucoma, diabetes, cancer, or unknown causes. Several disorders involve retinal cell degeneration due to retinal detachment or damaged blood supply and induced growth of abnormal, leaky vessels. Treatment of underlying disease and surgery to keep the retina attached to its source of oxygen and nutrients may slow vision loss.

The retina has connections to the brain. Adjacent to the whitish sclera of the eye is a vascular tissue layer known as the choroid, which feeds and supports the innermost lining of the eye, the retina. The retina is made up of the retinal pigment epithelium (RPE) layer, located next to the choroid, and the sub-adjacent multilayered neural retina. Photoreceptors (rods and cones) transform light energy into electrical impulses (see EYE DISORDERS). Rods are motion-sensitive and work best in dim light, whereas cones respond optimally in bright light and are highly concentrated in the macula, the small portion of central retina necessary for seeing fine details and color.

Electrical signals from photoreceptors travel through other retinal layers to the innermost sheet of retinal ganglion cells. Axons of these cells (see NERVOUS SYSTEM DISORDERS) collect together at the back of the eyeball and exit as the optic nerve, which transmits impulses from the retina to the brain, where they are interpreted. Thus, "seeing" an image involves collaboration between the outer layers of the eye (serving to focus the light): the retina, optic nerve, and brain. Vision may be affected if one or more of these components is compromised, or if information transfer from eye to brain is disrupted.

Retinal detachment occurs when the retina pulls away from its position against the choroid, causing the cells to degenerate due to lack of oxygen and nutrients. This can result from age-related shrinking of the vitreous, causing the layers to pull apart, or an injury that tears the retina, allowing fluid to pass through the tear under the retina, detaching it from the rest of the eye. A macular (central retina) pucker may also follow trauma, inflammation, or vitreous shrinking. Symptoms include blurry vision, seeing flashes, new floaters, or a shadow across the visual field. Retinal tears or detachments require immediate attention to prevent permanent vision loss, since the cells cannot survive away from the choroid.

Retinoschisis. Although sharing symptoms of retinal detachment, retinoschisis involves splitting of the retina into two layers. It is usually diagnosed after age 50 and frequently affects both eyes. If the affected area is stable, small, and peripheral, no treatment is recommended; larger, progressive, central conditions require treatment. A juvenile, congenital, X-linked form is less prevalent but affects the central retina.

Retinal cancers

Retinoblastoma is a rare retinal cancer detected in young children. Common symptoms are redness of the eye, irritation, pain, and loss of vision in the affected eye. It may be associated with mental retardation and slow growth. Mutations in *RB1*, a tumor suppressor gene (normally prevents uncontrolled cell growth) is associated with retinoblastoma; mutated genes are inherited (autosomal dominant) or occur spontaneously during embryonic life or later.

Choroidal melanomas originate in pigment-producing choroids cells; metastases originate elsewhere and spread to the choroid via its rich blood supply. The condition may be asymptomatic initially, then cause floaters, flashes, and retinal detachment.

Degenerative changes

Many changes affect the retina, including different types of macular degeneration and various syndromes.

Macular degeneration (MD). Age-related MD (ARMD), the leading cause of impaired vision in the elderly, involves a progressive degeneration of the central retina. Dry MD (90 percent of ARMD patients) is caused by damage to macular photoreceptors and retinal thinning. Wet MD is more severe, though less common. It occurs when new, leaky blood vessels form around a damaged macula, fluid leaks under the macula, and the retina may scar and detach. Blurry vision and a central blind spot develop in both forms of ARMD; straight lines appear wavy in wet MD. The vascular endothelial growth factor (VEGF) is required for growth of the vessels; when anti-VEGF antibody is administered as an intravitreal injection, it is effective in reducing leakage from blood from the abnormal vessels and slowing further loss of vision. Age, race (white, blue eyes), gender (female), smoking, high cholesterol, and family history are predisposing factors.

Stargardt disease (fundus flavimaculatus). This disorder is an inherited (autosomal recessive; also dominant), gradually progressive MD affecting both eyes, usually before age 20. Mutations in the *ABCR* gene cause degeneration of cones, blurry vision, deterioration of central vision (acuity stabilizes at 20/200), and reduced color vision, but peripheral vision is spared.

Best's disease (vitelliform macular dystrophy). This rare inherited disorder involves damage to the macula; it may be asymptomatic until the age of about 50. Mutations in the *RDS* or *VMD2* genes cause Best's MD.

Retinitis pigmentosa (RP), or retrolental fibroplasia, is a group of inherited disorders, detected before

---

KEY FACTS

Description

Disorders of the light-sensitive, inner layer of the eye.

Causes

Most unknown; some disorders are inherited; few contributing genes identified.

Risk factors

Diabetes, hypertension, family history, injury, premature birth, and age.

Symptoms

Blurry vision, flashes, new floaters, shadow across visual field, night blindness, tunnel vision.

Diagnosis

Eye exams with pupil dilation, imaging with fluorescent dye, tonometry, electroretinogram, electro-oculogram, family history.

Treatments

Laser microsurgery, cryotherapy, laser photo-coagulation to reattach the retina or arrest vessel leaking; vitreous removal; medically or surgically treating intraocular pressure (IOP), hypertension. Gene or stem cell therapies are in development.

Pathogenesis

Retinal cells or axons, or both, degenerate as a result of vitreous shrinkage, injury to eye, vessel damage or blockage, IOP, cancers originating in or metastasizing to retina. Visual impairments are sudden or progressive, permanent or resolvable.

Prevention

Regular eye exams, control of blood pressure, immediate attention to alterations in vision.

Epidemiology

1.8 million (0.66 percent) Americans have severe visual impairment stemming from retinal disorder.

---

age 30, that is linked with progressive photoreceptor degeneration. Symptoms of rod-cone dystrophy (more common) are an inability to adapt to dim light due to degeneration of rods with progressive peripheral vision loss. Less frequently, cones are affected first in cone-rod dystrophy; central vision and color perception are impaired, with later rod loss, sometimes accompanied by cataracts. More than 100 gene mutations cause RP, with differing inheritance patterns.

Usher syndrome. RP and severe hearing loss are both present, often at birth, in this inherited condition (autosomal recessive) associated with mutations in at least 10 genes related to balance, hearing, and vision. Peripheral vision deteriorates first, then central vision becomes blurred; cataracts may develop. Incidence is higher in Ashkenazi Jews and the Louisiana Acadian population.

Bardet-Biedl syndrome. Symptoms of this inherited disorder (autosomal recessive) include rapidly progressing RP in childhood, obesity, polydacytly (extra digits), short stature, broad feet, small genitalia (males); approximately 50 percent of affected individuals are mildly retarded and may exhibit kidney disease.

Choroideremia (tapetochoroidal dystrophy). This is a rare, inherited (X-linked) disorder associated with loss of *REP-1* gene, degeneration of choroid and retinal pigmented epithelial (RPE) cells, and photoreceptor loss. Choroideremia is diagnosed almost exclusively in male children, with initial peripheral vision loss, sometimes followed by central vision; degeneration continues throughout life.

Leber congenital amaurosis (LCA). This is an inherited (autosomal recessive) disorder, which is characterized by abnormal, prematurely degenerating photoreceptors and severe visual impairment in infancy. Keratoconus, cataracts, and retardation may also be present.

Retinal vessel occlusion

Blockage of the retinal artery, retinal vein, or their branches compromises the supply of blood, oxygen, and nutrients to and from the retina. Artery occlusion leads to sudden loss of vision in part of the visual field, then an irreversible death of retinal cells; blocked retinal veins cause backed-up blood flow, swelling, hemorrhaging of tiny vessels, and a gradual effect on vision. Occlusion results from a thrombus (blood clot) buildup, or an embolus (blood-borne floating clot or debris) lodging in vessel walls that may already be damaged from hypertension, diabetes, atherosclerosis, glaucoma, inflammation, malignancies, sickle-cell disease, medications, trauma, or radiation treatment.

Diabetic retinopathy

Retinopathy refers to a disease of the retina; many retinopathies are caused by retinal vessel abnormalities. Problems with glucose metabolism as a result of diabetes may damage blood vessels. Three stages of diabetic retinopathy are: nonproliferative, with damaged vessels and retinal swelling; macular edema, with leaky vessels and fluid collecting in the retina; proliferative, characterized by growth of abnormal vessels that bleed into the retina, damage cells, and lead to scar formation and retinal detachment. Symptoms, initially detectable in the second stage, include blurry vision, progressing to vision loss. Maintaining blood sugar levels may slow deterioration.

Hypertensive retinopathy. Hypertensive retinal atherosclerosis may result from chronic hypertension. At first, arterioles look constricted, then they hemorrhage. "Cotton wool" spots (retina deprived of blood) and yellowish lipid deposits (exudates) are visible on eye exam. Symptoms are managed by controlling blood pressure.

Familial exudative vitreoretinopathy (FEVR). Peripheral retinal vessels are not fully formed; the resulting oxygen loss (ischemia) induces formation of new vessels that are leaky, may cause retinal tears, fluid collection (exudates), and detachment. The condition may be congenital (present from birth). Mutations in the *FZD4* and *LRP5* genes are associated with 20 percent of the autosomal dominant inheritance of FEVR and in the *NDP* gene with the X-linked form.

Retinopathy of prematurity (ROP). A sporadic disorder, ROP resembles FEVR in that peripheral vessels have not fully developed by the time of the premature birth.

Other retinal disorders

Several other various conditions affect the retina. Some of them are inherited disorders.

Coat's disease (exudative retinitis). Typically diagnosed before age 10, Coat's disease primarily affects males. Retinal capillaries dilate and leak fluid that may collect under the retina, leading to detachment, usually in the central retina. Spontaneous arrest of disease progress is not uncommon.

Cystoid macular edema (CME). This disorder presents with swelling of the central retina, with fluid collecting in layers of the macula, which leads to distorted vision. CME is difficult to diagnose, but fluorescein angiography may allow detection. Anti-inflammatory medications applied directly to the eye are effective in reducing swelling.

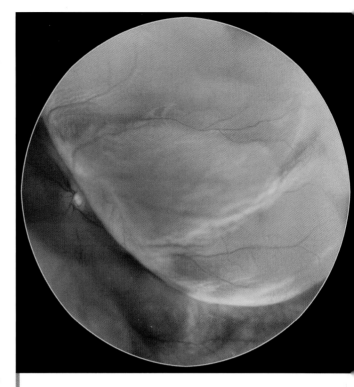

This retinal photomontage shows a retinal detachment, which is the separation of the sensory retina from the underlying pigment epithelium. The condition disturbs vision and usually requires immediate surgery to correct.

Central serous chorioretinopathy (CSC). CSC is characterized by a breakdown of RPE cells or choroidal vessels that supply the RPE, and fluid collection under the retina; vessel leaks may seal spontaneously. In the chronic condition, the retina thins, and may detach. CSC occurs mostly in males of 20 to 50 years and can be associated with stress.

Bieti's crystalline dystrophy (BCD). This is a rare autosomal recessive inherited disorder in which crystal deposits form on the cornea and retina, and the retinal layers and choroid progressively atrophy.

Color blindness is an inherited impairment in perceiving certain colors. It is much more common in males than females. Mostly, there is a loss of one or two types of cones (red-green color blindness is most common); fully color-blind individuals are rare. Occasionally, color blindness results from brain damage.

Coloboma. This is a rare birth defect in which the individual has a congenital gap (malformation) in the retina, optic nerve, iris, or lens.

Night blindness. Although people with this condition cannot see well in poor light, there may be no ob-

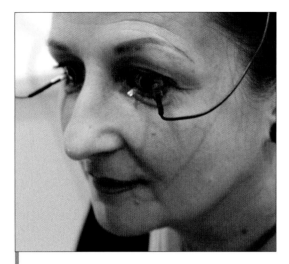

A patient with anomalies of the visual field undergoes electroretinography, an eye electrophysiology examination. Electrodes are placed on the cornea to allow measurement of the electrical response of the retina to light stimulation.

vious eye defect. Night blindness can be a result of vitamin A deficiency and may be a precursor to retinitis pigmentosa.

Glaucoma. This incurable disease is caused by degeneration of optic nerve axons, severing connections between eye and brain; retinal ganglion cells are secondarily damaged. Glaucoma may be caused by high intraocular pressure (IOP) but also occurs without it. Medication and surgery can relieve IOP.

Optic nerve atrophy (hypoplasia, optic nerve neuritis). The nerve is abnormal, due to a congenital degenerative condition (atrophy), underdevelopment (hypoplasia), or inflammation (neuritis). Retinal signals cannot be interpreted, leading to loss of vision.

Uveitis. In this condition there is an inflammation inside the eye, which affects the blood supply to the retina, often in otherwise healthy people. Symptoms include pain, itching, redness, floaters, and light sensitivity. Eye drops and anti-inflammatory medications are prescribed at once to prevent vision loss and scarring.

Diagnostic tests

These include tests of visual acuity and perimetry (to establish the extent of the visual field). Cat's eye reflex or whiteness in pupil, gonioscopy, ophthalmic examination with pupil dilation, and fluorescein angiography (injecting a fluorescent dye) are tests done to assess blood flow in the eye, as well as tonometry for IOP and blood tests for inflammation and cholesterol levels.

The Ambler grid is used for testing blurriness. Electroretinogram (ERG) measures the electrical response of retinal cells to a light stimulus; this is useful in differentiating between disorders such as RP and cone dystrophy. Electro-oculogram (EOG) is useful for evaluating disorders such as RP.

Treatments

A paramount concern is to treat conditions prior to the death of retinal cells. Regular eye exams, eye protection, and early detection are essential. For retinal detachment or vessel proliferation, treatments are laser microsurgery, laser photocoagulation, cryotherapy, or vitrectomy. If there is vessel occlusion, treatments include eye massage, breathing carbogen and rebreathing carbon dioxide to widen arteries, anterior chamber paracentesis (removing fluid), injecting clot-dissolving medications into the eye, and laser coagulation. Low vision aids are useful when peripheral vision is minimally affected. To slow RP progression, high doses of vitamin A are given (these are anecdotal reports). Many inherited disorders are not treatable; genetic counseling is recommended for these cases.

Preliminary experimental treatments are microretinal implants to replace photoreceptors; gene therapy for replacing or blocking defective gene action; neuroprotective proteins, survival factors, or stem cells to protect blood vessels and rescue photoreceptors.

Epidemiology

In the United States, 1.75 million people over age 40 have ARMD-related reduced vision; this may reach 3 million by 2020. The prevalence of retinitis pigmentosa is 100,000. Each year, 30,000 people (1 in 10,000) are diagnosed with retinal detachment; it is most common in severely myopic individuals. Around 10,000 to 15,000 people have Usher syndrome. An estimated 4 to 5.6 million (40 percent of diabetics) have at least some form of diabetic retinopathy; 65,000 per year develop stage 3 retinopathy. About 14,000 to 16,000 infants per year are affected with ROP; 400 to 600 infants become legally blind each year. Retinoblastoma (eye cancer) affects 1 in 15,000 to 20,000 live births (about 250 diagnoses yearly); around 1,300 retinal melanomas are diagnosed each year. One in 10 males is color-blind; it is rare in females.

Sonal Jhaveri

See also
- Cataracts • Diabetes • Eye disorders
- Genetic disorders • Macular degeneration

Rheumatic fever

Rheumatic fever is a disease of the joints and heart. It occurs as a result of an immune reaction following infection with specific types of streptococcal bacteria. It is acute but may become chronic and progressive.

After an episode of pharyngitis (painful inflammation of the throat) caused by streptococcal bacteria and commonly called "strep throat," acute rheumatic fever occurs in 0.4 to 3 percent of untreated people. The disease usually begins one to five weeks after the sore throat. Affected people develop fever, along with painful swelling of the large joints (such as knee, elbow, and hip). Some people may have a heart murmur, along with chest pain and shortness of breath. In some cases there may even be small, firm swellings under the skin, and a typical rash called erythema marginatum. The disease usually lasts 3 months and can be serious and life threatening. It may also be recurrent.

Diagnosis and treatment

Diagnosis of rheumatic fever is based on signs and symptoms and laboratory evidence of prior streptococcal infection, such as culture or detection of antibodies to the streptococcal bacteria. The disease is treated with high dose aspirin and sometimes steroid drugs. Aspirin should not be given to young children because of the risk of Reye's syndrome.

The long-term consequence of acute rheumatic fever is rheumatic heart disease, which is a disorder of the heart valves, or sometimes the outer lining of the heart. It occurs in 30 to 40 percent of patients if they had carditis and in 6 percent if they did not have carditis (inflammation of the heart or its linings). It is chronic and progressive. The most common abnormality in rheumatic heart disease is mitral stenosis, a tightening of the mitral valve of the heart. A rare complication of acute rheumatic fever is chorea, which is abnormal movements of the face, hands, and feet.

Individuals who develop chronic rheumatic heart disease need lifelong treatment with heart medications and may need surgical repair or replacement of the heart valves. Acute rheumatic fever may be prevented by prompt treatment of strep throat. Once acute rheumatic fever has occurred, chronic heart disease may be prevented by prolonged therapy with penicillin for 5 to 10 years or until adulthood. Efforts are ongoing to develop a safe and effective vaccine to prevent streptococcal infection and acute rheumatic fever.

Epidemiology

Acute rheumatic fever is most common in children between 5 and 15 years of age. Some complications of rheumatic fever such as mitral stenosis and chorea are more common in women. The disease is more common in African Americans compared to Caucasians. Although rare in the United States, rheumatic fever is widespread in the Middle East, India, selected areas of Africa, and South America, and in the aboriginal populations in Australia and New Zealand.

Pranavi Sreeramoju

KEY FACTS

Description
An acute disease affecting joints and sometimes the heart. It may become chronic and progressive.

Causes
An immune reaction following infection with streptococcal bacteria.

Risk factors
Crowded living conditions in a low-income country.

Symptoms and signs
Fever, rash, nodules under the skin, pain and swelling of the large joints, shortness of breath, chest pain, and heart murmur.

Diagnosis
From symptoms and signs, along with laboratory evidence for streptococcal infection.

Treatments
No specific treatments; rest, aspirin, and steroids depending on the severity of the illness.

Pathogenesis
Unknown.

Prevention
Treatment of streptococcal pharyngitis; once rheumatic fever occurs, prolonged treatment with penicillin for years to prevent heart disease.

Epidemiology
Rare in the United States, with incidence less than 1 per 200,000 people per year. Widespread in some low-income countries.

See also
• Bone and joint disorders • Infections, bacterial • Influenza • Heart disorders

Rheumatoid arthritis

Rheumatoid arthritis is a chronic systemic inflammatory disease characterized by inflammation of the small joints of the hands and feet. The disease begins in the lining, or synovium, of joints and results in damage to tissues such as adjacent bone, tendons, and ligaments. The prevalence is about 0.5 to 1 percent of the adult population worldwide. The disease can present at any age but usually begins between the age of 30 and 50. Females are affected two to three times more than males. Untreated, it is a cause of significant disability and premature mortality.

Rheumatoid arthritis is an autoimmune condition in which the body's immune system attacks the body's own tissues. The exact cause is still not known. It is thought to be the result of a combination of environmental and genetic factors. Infection occasionally precedes the onset of the disease; however, no specific virus or bacteria has been identified as the causative agent. Smoking is a contributing factor for the development of rheumatoid arthritis.

Symptoms and signs

Symptoms include joint pain, stiffness, swelling, and loss of function in affected joints. Symptoms are generally worse in the morning and after exercise and improve toward the end of the day. Early morning stiffness, generally lasting an hour or more, is an important clue to the fact that the condition is inflammatory in nature. The typical pattern of joint involvement is that of a symmetrical polyarthritis; that is, rheumatoid arthritis usually affects many joints on both sides of the body. The hands and feet are often the first to be affected. Wrists, elbows, shoulders, knees, ankles, and neck are also commonly involved. Other associated features include fatigue, fever, weight loss, and depression. Untreated, joint damage may result in permanent deformities. With long-standing disease of the cervical spine, there is a risk of joint instability and spinal cord compression.

Currently rheumatoid arthritis is classified according to the 1987 American Rheumatism Association (ARA) criteria. Those with early disease, however, may not have some of the features listed, such as rheumatoid nodules and the radiographic changes that occur later on. In people with long-standing disease, the inflammation may have settled, such that there is little swelling and morning stiffness. The criteria, therefore, are important for epidemiological purposes and helpful for identifying people with active disease. They cannot be used alone for making the diagnosis.

KEY FACTS

Description
Chronic systemic inflammatory disease, mainly targeting the synovial lining of the small joints of the hands and feet.

Causes
Rheumatoid arthritis is an autoimmune condition. The exact cause is unknown. It is thought to be caused by a combination of environmental and genetic factors.

Risk factors
Smoking is a contributing factor for the development of rheumatoid arthritis.

Symptoms
Symptoms include joint pain, swelling, loss of function, early morning stiffness, and fatigue. The typical pattern of joint involvement is that of a symmetrical polyarthritis, which predominantly starts in the hands and feet. Other organs, including the eye, heart, lungs, skin, nervous system, and kidney, may also be affected.

Diagnosis
History, physical examination, and other tests, including blood tests, X-rays, ultrasound, and MRI scans.

Treatments
Medication for pain relief and suppression of the inflammatory process. Physiotherapy, occupational therapy, orthotics, and surgery may be required.

Pathogenesis
The disease begins in the lining, or synovium, of joints, resulting in damage to tissues such as adjacent bone, tendons, and ligaments.

Prevention
Early diagnosis and treatment is the key to prevent disease progression.

Epidemiology
Affects 0.5 to 1 percent of the population worldwide. Women are more commonly affected than men.

THE 1987 ARA CRITERIA FOR RHEUMATOID ARTHRITIS

For a diagnosis of rheumatoid arthritis, at least four criteria must be fulfilled.

Symptom or sign	Description
Morning stiffness	Morning stiffness in and around the joints, lasting at least one hour before maximal improvement.
Arthritis in three or more joint areas	Soft tissue swelling or fluid (not bony overgrowth) observed by a physician, present simultanously for at least six weeks. Possible areas include right or left proximal interphalangeal (PIP), metacarpophalangeal (MCP), wrist, elbow, knee, ankle, and metatarsophalangeal (MTP).
Arthritis of hand joints	Swelling of wrist, MCP, or PIP joints for at least six weeks.
Symmetric arthritis	Simultaneous involvement of the same joint areas on both sides of the body (bilateral involvement of PIP, MCP, or MTP joints is acceptable without absolute symmetry) for at least six weeks.
Rheumatoid nodules	Subcutaneous nodules over bony prominences, extensor surfaces, or in juxta-articular regions, observed by a physician.
Rheumatoid factor (RF)	RF antibody found in 75 percent of sufferers and in 5 percent of normal controls.
Radiographic changes	Typical of rheumatoid arthritis on postero-anterior hand and wrist radiographs; it must include erosions or unequivocal bony decalcification localized in, or most marked, adjacent to the involved joints.

Rheumatoid arthritis is a systemic condition; many organ systems may be affected. This usually occurs in people who have had the disease for several years, and symptoms need to be differentiated from potential side effects of the medication used as treatment. Some of the extra-articular manifestations of rheumatoid arthritis include rheumatoid nodules, skin ulcers, anemia, peripheral neuropathy, pleural effusions, and lung nodules, and the eye condition keratoconjunctivitis sicca.

Diagnosis

The diagnosis of rheumatoid arthritis is usually made by a doctor after taking a careful history and a detailed examination. Further investigations help confirm the diagnosis. These include blood tests (to look for evidence of inflammation and antibodies) and X-rays (to look for evidence of joint damage).

Blood tests, such as the erythrocyte sedimentation rate (ESR) and C-reactive protein (CRP), are useful markers of inflammation. Levels rise, however, in the presence of any inflammation in the body and are therefore nonspecific.

Rheumatoid factor (RF) is an antibody found in the blood of approximately 75 percent of patients with rheumatoid arthritis. About 1 in 20 normal volunteers (5 percent) will have RF in the blood, and other inflammatory conditions may also cause a positive result. For this reason, results of the test must be interpreted with the clinical findings. Anticyclic citrullinated peptide (anti-CCP) antibody is a newer test for rheumatoid arthritis. It is as sensitive as rheumatoid factor but much more specific and can distinguish rheumatoid arthritis from other conditions. The anti-CCP antibody may predict who will develop the condition and identify who will be affected more severely.

Imaging is a useful diagnostic tool. Traditionally, X-rays have been the mainstay of radiological diagnosis as they clearly show characteristic changes as a result of damage caused by rheumatoid arthritis. These include bone erosions (bone pits), narrowing of the joint spaces, thinning of the bones (osteoporosis), and deformities. Early in the disease, however, X-rays may be normal; ultrasound and magnetic resonance imaging (MRI) are more sensitive. Unlike X-rays, they may also detect soft tissue inflammation and are more sensitve than clinical examination. They will probably play a more important part in the future management of patients with rheumatoid arthritis.

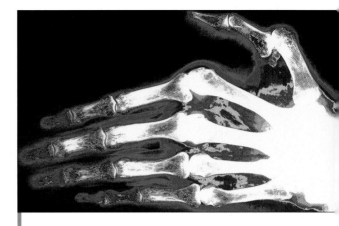

Rheumatoid arthritis, as revealed on the X-ray of this hand, causes the joints to become swollen and inflamed (red/pink and red/green) around the bone ends. The angles where bone ends meet have altered, causing deformity of the hand.

Treatments and pathogenesis

Joint damage occurs early in the course of the disease. Because effective treatment is available for people with rheumatoid arthritis, the aim is to make a diagnosis and start treatment as early as possible. The goals of therapy include alleviation of pain and management of the underlying condition to prevent further damage and disease progression and to maintain function and quality of life. Broadly, treatment can be divided into pharmacological and nonpharmacological therapies.

Pharmacotherapy, in the form of analgesics and non-steroidal anti-inflammatory drugs, may be needed for pain relief. Alone, however, they do not prevent joint damage. Glucocorticoids provide symptomatic relief and reduce the immune response, but with long-term use, risk of side effects increase. These include thinning of the skin, diabetes mellitus, cataracts, increased risk of infection, and osteoporosis. For this reason, short-term use of this drug is preferred.

Disease-modifying antirheumatic drugs (DMARDS) are effective to decrease the risk of disease progression and joint damage. Treatment should be commenced as soon as the diagnosis is made. DMARDS commonly used are methotrexate, sulphasalazine, hydroxychloroquine, and leflunomide. Newer biological agents target specific molecules in the inflammatory pathway of the disease. These include infliximab, etanercept, adalimumab, anakinra, and rituximab.

Nonpharmacological therapy encompasses multidisciplinary care. Nurse practitioners and support groups provide education, advice, and emotional support for patients and their families. Physiotherapists may assist with pain relief and exercise programs. Occupational therapists make splints and assistive devices and provide practical advice on lifestyle and the work environment. Orthotists and podiatrists help with foot care. People with long-standing rheumatoid arthritis may develop chronic deformities requiring surgery.

The activated immune system targets the synovium, a thin membrane that lines certain joints. The inflamed lining becomes swollen, thickened, and vascular, and starts to invade local tissues. Cartilage, bone, ligaments, and capsule may be damaged as a result of this process. Recently there has been much progress in the understanding of the complexities in the inflammatory process. As a result, newer therapies have been developed to target factors such as molecules or cells directly involved in the inflammatory process.

In some, the condition may remit spontaneously. Others may experience recurrent flare-ups. The majority, if untreated, will develop chronic disease. Predictive factors for progression include the duration of disease, the number of joints involved, and the presence of rheumatoid factor and anti-CCP antibodies.

At present the aim is to diagnose and treat rheumatoid arthritis as early as possible to prevent disease progression. There is ongoing research to predict the onset of rheumatoid arthritis with the aim of targeting the disease prior to, or at symptom onset.

Jackie Nam and Richard J. Wakefield

See also
- Arthritis • Bone and joint disorders
- Immune system disorders • Osteoarthritis

Rickettsial infections

The term *rickettsiae* embraces a broad group of potentially lethal microorganisms that have caused devastating epidemics among the world's population. Dr. Howard Ricketts, for whom the bacteria are named, died from epidemic typhus, a type of rickettsial infection that he was researching. Rickettsiae are small bacteria associated with arthropods. Rickettsial infections vary in severity but can be life threatening.

Most rickettsia are carried by arthropod vectors, with the exception of Q fever (caused by *Coxiella burnetti*), which is transmitted through exposure to body fluids of infected animals. *Ehrlichia chaffeensis* and *Anaplasma phagocytophilum* cause human monocytic ehrlichiosis and human granulocytic anaplasmosis, respectively, and are transmitted by ticks during ticks' blood meals. Epidemic typhus is a louse-borne disease caused by *Rickettsia prowazekii*, while scrub typhus is caused by *Orienta tsutsugamishi* and is transmitted by mites. Rickettsialpox is a mite-borne illness caused by *Rickettsia akari*.

Risk factors

Most rickettsial diseases are transmitted to humans by bacteria-harboring arthropod vectors (ticks, mites, fleas, and lice) during feeding, and the greatest risk of acquiring these infections occurs with exposure to these vectors. Animals and humans can be infested with these arthropods and transmit them to others. Areas of poor sanitation, such as impoverished or rural communities, have higher infestation levels and higher rates of infection among the inhabitants.

Symptoms and signs

Symptoms vary depending on the specific infection. The incubation period varies from one to three weeks. Patients often do not recall exposure to an insect vector. High fever, headache, muscle aches, and lymphadenopathy are often seen. Rash may be prominent (vesicular in rickettsialpox, macular in epidemic and scrub typhus and monocytic ehrlichiosis) or absent (granulocytic anaplasmosis). Patients may also develop a localized area of dead tissue, often black in color, at the site of an arthropod bite, also called an "eschar." An eschar is prominent in rickettsialpox and scrub typhus. Pneumonia can occur in Q fever. As the bacteria replicate, patients may develop inflammation in the blood vessels, heart muscle, lungs, liver, and central nervous system, leading to widespread organ dysfunction.

KEY FACTS

Description

A group of bacterial infections distributed worldwide that range in severity from a mild flulike illness to multi-organ failure and death.

Causes

Bacteria that are usually transmitted to humans through the bite of an infected arthropod. Common pathogens include *Ehrlichia chaffeensis*, *Anaplasma phagocytophilum*, *Coxiella burnetti*, *Rickettsia prowazekii*, and *Rickettsia akari*.

Risk factors

Exposure to bacteria in lice, fleas, and mites poses the greatest risk. Infestation levels are likely to be higher in areas of poor sanitation.

Symptoms

Vary widely depending on the specific infection. A lesion or ulcer may develop at the site of the bite. Fevers, muscle aches, and diffuse rash may also occur. In very severe cases, patients can develop pneumonia and organ failure.

Diagnosis

Blood tests measuring antibody; skin biopsies. Treatment should not be delayed while these tests are in progress.

Treatments

Antibiotics; doxycycline and tetracycline are most effective. Chloramphenicol is a second choice.

Pathogenesis

The infecting organisms target the inner lining of blood vessels or blood leukocytes (white blood cells). Inflammation develops, leading to leakage of fluid into surrounding tissues and possible damage to various organs.

Prevention

Avoidance of arthropod vectors and appropriate hygiene and sanitation practices. There is no vaccine available.

Epidemiology

Worldwide distribution, determined by their vectors. Often occur as outbreaks due to poverty, overcrowding, or animal exposure.

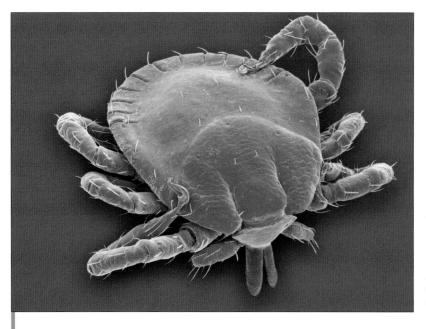

This brown dog tick larva (Rhipicephalus sanguineus) has mouthparts adapted to suck blood. Although it prefers dogs, it will feed on many mammals. It can transmit Rocky Mountain spotted fever and tularemia to humans.

neutrophils. All induce inflammation and clotting abnormalities, leading to fluid discharge into tissues. Severe infection can damage multiple organs. Without treatment, complications like pneumonia, central nervous system damage, and gangrene of the extremities can occur.

Prevention

Avoidance of insect vectors that carry the bacteria is the best method of prevention. In wooded areas, protective clothing and insect repellant should be applied to skin and clothing. The body should be carefully inspected for ticks. If found, these should be removed immediately using tweezers. Good hygiene and sanitation help eradicate carriers in areas of high infestation. Control programs for animals, both wild and domestic, may be necessary. Avoiding contact with fluids from potentially infected animals helps prevent Q fever.

Thrombocytopenia, leukopenia, and hepatitis can be seen in most rickettsial infections. Because of the potential lethality, *Rickettsia prowazekii* (epidemic typhus) is listed as a potential agent of bioterrorism.

Diagnosis and treatments

Rickettsiae are difficult to culture. Rickettsial infections can be diagnosed with various blood tests that detect components of the host immune response, specifically antibody levels that fight the infection. Testing for antibodies to rickettsial antigens provides a retrospective diagnosis. Polymerase chain reaction assays on blood are useful in diagnosing ehrlichiosis. Biopsies of skin lesions are helpful in rickettsialpox and scrub typhus, but these tests are time consuming, labor intensive, and not available at all medical institutions.

Treatment should be started immediately if rickettsial infection is suspected. Irreversible complications and death may result when therapy is delayed. The treatment of choice is doxycycline or tetracycline.

Pathogenesis

Most rickettsiae target the vascular endothelium in the wall of blood vessels and cause a vasculitis (inflammation of blood vessels). *Orienta, Ehrichlia* and *R. akari* multiply in blood monocytes, and *Anaplasma* targets

Epidemiology

Rickettsial infections can be found all over the world. Their geographic distribution is determined by their vectors, and specific infections are limited to certain areas. Ehrichiosis and anaplasmosis are predominantly found in the United States in the southeastern, south central, and mid-Atlantic regions, with an annual incidence of two to three cases in 1 million. Q fever occurs worldwide wherever there is animal exposure (for example, farmers and slaughterhouse workers are at risk). Epidemic typhus has killed millions of people since the Middle Ages but is now limited to a few locations in Africa, Asia, and Central and South America. Rickettsialpox has been reported in the United States, South Africa, and eastern Europe.

Joseph M. Fritz and Nigar Kirmani

See also
- Infections, bacterial • Rocky Mountain spotted fever • Typhus

Risk factors and analysis

Risk is the probability that exposure to a hazard will lead to an undesired consequence. We are constantly at risk—at home, during transportation, at work and schools, while in a hospital, or even on vacation. Health risks, which are a part of everyday life, include accidents, illnesses, and injuries as a result of infections, pollution, radiation, natural disasters, crime, animals, and recreational activities.

At its simplest, risk is the idea that something bad might happen—a probability of an adverse outcome, or a factor that raises this probability.

Risk is different for different people. For example, school-age children are at risk for contracting an illness from classmates. A bungee jumper is at risk for injuries related to the sheer physical stress of bungee jumping or crashing at the bottom of the jump. A person taking medication is at risk for developing side effects. People everywhere are exposed all their lives to an almost limitless array of risks to their health, whether in the shape of communicable or noncommunicable disease, injury, consumer products, microorganisms in food, hazardous chemicals,

violence, or natural catastrophe. Risk may be self-inflicted; for example, someone who smokes, drinks too much, or takes recreational drugs is jeopardizing his or her health by these activities.

Sometimes whole populations are in danger, as in the case of waterborne illnesses; at other times, only an individual is involved, such as in the case of a genetic disorder.

There is more to risk than calculating the statistical chances of a certain outcome. Risk involves not only issues of probability, but also consequence, hazard, and exposure. Thus, risk is the probability that exposure to a hazard will lead to a harmful consequence. The facts about risk are compiled from scientific analysis in the areas of toxicology, epidemiology, and statistics. Studies in these areas inform the public about what kinds of risks are encountered in daily life.

Common risks people face in everyday life

There are risks to health everywhere: at home, while traveling, in the workplace or classroom, while in a hospital, or even on vacation. Risks are associated with the location, as well as the activities taking place. Health risks include accidents, illnesses,

RELATED ARTICLES

and injuries due to infections, pollution, radiation, natural disasters, crime, animals, and recreational activities. These are simply a part of life. Accidents happen. Unintentional injuries, including motor vehicle crashes, were the fifth largest cause of death in the United States and the leading cause of death for people from ages 1 to 38 years in 2004. Some accidents that cause death are falls, poisoning, drowning, fire, choking, firearms, occupational, natural and environmental accidents such as extreme cold or heat, medical errors, and injuries caused by animals. Accidents are a particular health concern because, unlike the four largest causes of death (heart disease, cancer, stroke, and chronic obstructive pulmonary disease), accidents kill people at any age. The average ages of those who die from the four largest causes of death range in the 70s, whereas the average age of someone killed in an accident is 50 years.

Common activities in everyday life, such as eating and drinking, pose risks as well. Food- and water-borne illnesses and risks that may be associated with food irradiation, artificial food and drink additives, and genetically modified foods are risks that people take every time they eat or drink. Infectious agents can use food and water as a vehicle to infect an individual or whole populations. Pathogens commonly found in food and water are salmonella, E. coli, and cryptosporidium. They are particularly dangerous when circulated in large groups of people, such as through restaurant food or a common water source.

Each year, roughly one in four Americans suffers from some kind of food poisoning, resulting in 76 million illnesses each year and 5,000 deaths. The risks connected to food irradiation, artificial additives, and genetically modified foods are highly contentious and a matter of risk perception (see below). These areas of food consumption are still under study, so their exact risks are as yet unknown.

Respiratory problems

Like eating and drinking, breathing is essential to life. However, breathing can be adversely affected because there is a risk of air pollution both indoors and outdoors. People spend about 90 percent of their time indoors: at home, at work, at school, in stores, medical facilities, recreational facilities, or in some kind of vehicle. Air pollutants are more likely to be concentrated in indoor areas because of the limited volume of air.

Many public health experts deem indoor air pollution to be one of the biggest environmental risks that we face. Some common indoor pollutants are carbon monoxide, secondhand smoke, bacteria, mold, mildew, animal dander, droppings from dust mites, pesticides (insecticides, herbicides, disinfectants used in cleaning), and particles, which may be asbestos, lead, and combustible particles, such as those emitted from stoves, water heaters, and boilers. Radon is a less common hazard.

Symptoms of air pollution can be difficulty in breathing, coughing, headaches, nausea, and

PATTERNS OF RISK PERCEPTION

Most people are less afraid of risks that are natural than those that are human-made. For example, more people are afraid of radiation from nuclear waste than radiation from the sun.

People tend to be less afraid of risks that they choose to impose on themselves than risks over which they have no control, for example, risks associated with smoking as opposed to risks from air pollution. Another example is driving an automobile; although driving is much riskier than flying, most people are less afraid of driving than flying because of a perception of control. Risky behaviors are acceptable if they also confer some benefits; for example, the risk of a tidal wave is outweighed by the anticipated enjoyment of a beach vacation.

People are more afraid of risks that have been highly publicized, such as terrorism. Prior to the terrorist attacks of September 11, 2001, awareness and fear of terrorism in the U.S. population were low; it was perceived as something that occurred in foreign places. After that date, the risk became real. Thus, the American population is more aware of terrorism, which contributes to more fear, even though the statistical reality of the risk may still be very low. Although a risk may have existed previously, an increase in awareness results in a heightened and possibly exaggerated sense of risk.

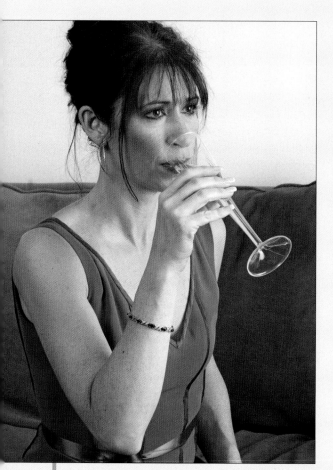

People who have an occasional drink at a social occasion can enjoy it without ill effects. However, when drinking alcohol becomes a regular habit, it is time to acknowledge that help is needed.

general sluggishness. Because the effects of air pollution are so generalized and gradual, many people do not realize that the air they breathe is causing their illnesses.

Smoking

Ironically, the leading risk factor for several diseases such as lung cancer, heart disease, and other chronic diseases is a self-inflicted lifestyle, that is, smoking. Cigarette smoking is the most important preventable cause of premature death in the United States. It accounts for more than 440,000 of the more than 2.4 million annual deaths. Cigarette smoking causes over 90 percent of all lung cancers and is related to the risk of cancers of the bladder, kidney, pancreas,

lip, mouth, tongue, larynx, throat, and esophagus. Furthermore, smokers have a higher risk of developing a number of chronic disorders such as atherosclerosis (buildup of fatty substances in the arteries),which is a chief contributor to coronary heart disease, heart attack, and stroke.

Occupational hazards

People are also exposed to risks through their work. Occupational diseases can be caused by exposure to toxic, irritating, or cancer-inducing substances, and damage to hearing can be caused by sustained high levels of noise or vibration. Common occupational hazards are back pain, neck pain, carpal tunnel syndrome, and respiratory disorders. Back pain is likely for those whose jobs involve heavy lifting. Neck pain and carpal tunnel syndrome are likely for those who sit at computers for long hours. Job-related respiratory illnesses are often related to some kind of indoor or micro-environmental pollution. For example, black lung disease is the result of working in the closed confines of a coal mine.

Controlling risk

Eating, drinking, and breathing healthfully can control many of the risks above. Healthy lifestyle choices could prevent numerous diseases in the United States; these include eating a properly balanced diet, maintaining a healthy weight, taking multivitamins, staying physically active, eliminating tobacco and alcohol use, limiting sun exposure, and being aware of one's family history in order to have regular screenings. Medical risks that can be minimized but not completely eliminated include cancer, heart disease, and sexually transmitted diseases. Typically, minimizing these risks involves simply avoiding the factors that cause these risks. For example, preventing heart disease involves eating a low-fat diet and exercising; preventing STDs involves using condoms and avoiding casual sex.

However, some medical risks cannot be controlled, such as genetically inherited diseases and medical errors. Medical errors occurring in a hospital, such as the administration of a conflicting drug, are usually unavoidable by the person concerned because the authority to perform this task lies with someone else. Many risks are intensified when people travel away from their homes. Whether travel is for business or pleasure, the simple act of changing locations can increase risks and anxiety for people. In a new location, the food, water, and air can be different, and pathogens may be encountered to which a person has no antibodies. If an illness occurs while traveling, there is a risk of having to deal with unfamiliar health care surroundings, particularly if travel is outside one's home country.

Thus, everyday activities are accompanied by some kind of risk. Although risks are probabilities that particular behaviors will lead to unfortunate consequences, risk is most profoundly subject to one's perception, assessment, and management. Statistics, experts, and the media help to characterize and communicate these risks. Together these allow people to interpret the risks in their lives and live with them.

Risk perception

Risk is everywhere, life is hazardous, and to live is to risk dying; however, risk is also a perception. Risk perception is the subjective judgment that people make about the characteristics and severity of a risk. For example, some people fear flying because of the potential risk of crashing, but the reality is that more people crash while driving. The perception of risk and the anxiety associated with it is what compels a person toward a particular behavior.

Scientists studying human behavior have discovered psychological patterns in the subconscious ways people "decide" what to be afraid of and how afraid they should be; this has to do with their perception. However, there is typically a balance between the perception of risk and the management of it. People manage their behavior to reflect the risk that they perceive.

In the modern world, risk perception is influenced by the quality of the information and analysis one receives. The media is in a unique position to inform and influence whole populations regarding particular risks. Television, newspapers, magazines, and the Internet all contribute in disseminating information and risk analysis to the population.

For example, after September 11, 2001, the overall risk of terrorism has probably not changed from before September 11th, but the heightened perception of risk has influenced people's compliance with new security regulations.

Where do the facts, interpretation, and perceptions about risk come from?

As one tries to judge what is risky and what is not, one may look to science for the answers. There are three sciences that are involved in studying risk: toxicology, epidemiology, and statistics. Although these three disciplines offer data on the risks in life, it must be remembered that the three fields are inherently imprecise.

For example, toxicology is the study of poisons. For this very reason, toxicologists cannot test the risk of various poisons on humans. Thus, they must extrapolate this information from laboratory animal studies. In epidemiology, scientists study populations of people in which a threat has already occurred or where people have already been exposed. Thus, epidemiologists study what has happened, or is currently happening, to real populations in the world, and try to make sense of which hazards and exposures might be associated with which consequences. Like toxicology, epidemiology is not an exact science because it can only provide assumptions, not absolute proof, that some particular exposure may be what is causing some particular consequence.

In addition to the findings of toxicology and epidemiology, risk analysts also look for clues among large sets of statistics. Data collections are compilations of real-world information, on either morbidity or mortality. The limitation of statistics lies in data collection. Not all details about particular incidents may have been reported or collected. For example, not every person who suffers from food poisoning goes to the doctor, and not every company honestly collects emissions data. Numbers are also subject to interpretation and can be presented in such a way as to present a particular kind of argument. For example, public health officials may use statistics associated with the risks of obesity to recommend healthier lifestyle guidelines.

Thus, toxicology, epidemiology, and statistics supply facts about risks and can provide valuable insights, but their results are uncertain and open to interpretation. Perceptions of risk come from data

SCREENING

The best protection and prevention against many diseases and disorders is early detection. Routine health screening can reduce the incidence of stroke, aneurysm, vascular disease, osteoporosis, and many other diseases. Almost every ailment has an advocacy organization that publishes screening guidelines. For instance, the American Cancer Society provides various screening recommendations for different types of cancer in different populations. In the case of colon cancer, it is recommended that beginning at age 50 years, both men and women should be screened for colon cancer. If a positive result is found in a screen, additional tests are performed to diagnose the disorder. Thus, health care screening is one way in which the medical system communicates risks to the general public. If people are aware of the need to receive screening, they are likely to handle medical problems early and avoid advanced stages of disease.

found by these sciences; interpretations are made by scientists and public health officials and by people's experiences of living in the world.

Risk assessment

In the context of public health, risk assessment is the process of quantifying the probability of a harmful effect to individuals or populations from certain human activities.

In most countries, the use of specific chemicals or the operation of specific facilities (for example, power plants and manufacturing plants) is not allowed unless it can be shown that these chemicals or facilities do not increase the risk of death or illness above a specific threshold. For example, the American Food and Drug Administration (FDA) required in 1973 that cancer-causing compounds must not be present in meat at concentrations that would cause a cancer risk greater than one in a million lifetimes.

In the estimation of the risks, two mathematical steps are involved. The first step, called hazard identification, determines the probability that a specific dose of the pollutant (such as a chemical, radiation, or noise) will have a harmful impact on an exposed individual. In addition, the genetic or other differences between individuals mean that hazards may be higher for particular groups. These groups are called susceptible populations, such as infants or the elderly. To account for the largely unknown effects, a cautious approach is adopted by including safety factors in the estimate of the hazard.

The second step, called exposure quantification, determines the amount of a contaminant (dose) that individuals and populations will receive. Exposure is assessed by locations, lifestyles, and other factors likely to influence the amount of toxin that is received.

Susceptible populations are treated with greater caution. The results of the two steps above are then combined to produce an estimate of risk. Because of the different susceptibilities and exposures, risk varies within a population. However, the decisions based on the outcome of risk assessment must be based on one number only.

In general, if the risk is higher for a particular subpopulation because of increased exposure rather than susceptibility, this group must not be considered by rules applicable to the general population. The group should be protected instead by ad hoc regulations. This is often the case for workers subject to occupational risk. For example, the risk of lung cancer for coal mine workers is higher than for the general population because of exposure to breathable carcinogens in coal mines.

Acceptable risk increase

The idea of not increasing lifetime risk by more than one in one million has become commonplace in public health discourse and policy. How consensus settled on this particular figure is unclear. In some respects, this figure has the characteristics of a mythical number. In another sense, the figure provides a numerical basis for what to consider a negligible increase in risk. Compare, for example, the one in a million increase in cancer risk of many regulations with the typical one in four lifetime risk of death by cancer in developed countries.

In the interest of public health, the risks versus benefits of the possible alternatives must be carefully considered. In fact, risk-benefit analyses are often performed for new medical technologies and therapies. For example, it might well be that treating drinking water results in a high number of minerals and chemicals that contribute to poor general health in some individuals. However, this risk must be balanced against the available alternatives of no water treatment, which has implications for the potential risk for spread of infectious diseases.

Unless or until creativity and technological development offer superior methods for water treatment, the choice based on risk assessment must be taken as being that of the lesser evil.

Risk management

Generally, risk management is the process of measuring or assessing risk and developing strategies to manage it. In the case of health, strategies include avoiding the risk, reducing the negative effect of the risk, and accepting some or all of the consequences of a particular risk. Traditional risk management focuses on risks stemming from physical causes (such as natural disasters, fires, and accidents). In ideal risk management, a prioritization process is followed whereby the risks with the greatest loss and the greatest probability of occurring are handled first, and risks with lower probability of occurrence and lower loss are handled later. In practice, the process can be very difficult, and balancing between risks with a high probability of occurrence but lower loss versus a risk with high loss but lower probability of occurrence can often be mishandled. In the case of an individual, a person assesses the risk versus benefits and manages the risk involved.

For example, riding a motorcycle poses a risk of accidents and head injuries. The risk can be managed by wearing a helmet while riding, or riding only on country roads. The individual handles the greatest risk of head injury by wearing a helmet.

Protection from heath risks

Protection from health risks is mainly handled by communication, screening, and insurance. Health

agencies communicate risks to the general population, so that the public can be aware of risks that may affect their lives. For example, the warning labels that exist on alcohol and cigarettes inform people about the risks of drinking alcohol and smoking cigarettes while pregnant. By educating the public and creating awareness, public health agencies can help people avoid potential risks, thereby protecting them. Routine health screening allows for the early detection of health problems, thus reducing the risk that they will occur in advanced forms.

While health insurance does not necessarily protect people from health risks, it is instrumental in the first two modes of protection and alleviates the risk of health care costs.

Obesity puts people at risk of many diseases that are preventable. They are pulmonary disease, heart disorders, diabetes, and high blood pressure. Also, obese people feel uncomfortable in hot weather and find it hard to exercise.

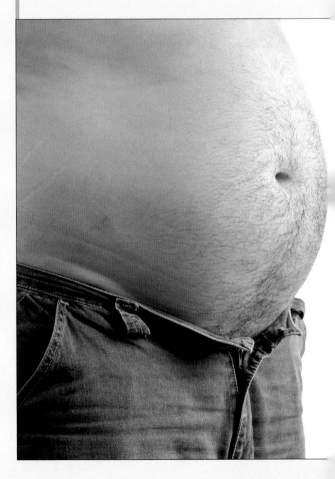

Health risk communication

There are many challenges involved in communicating health risks. Advances in medicine and biotechnology continue to fuel debates about risks and benefits.

Stem cell research, vaccine development, and genomic manipulation are just a few of the areas that are under recent attack. Even public health successes that have significantly decreased morbidity and mortality, such as vaccination, air bags, and fluoridation, are surrounded by controversy.

Risk communication emphasizes the process of exchanging information and opinion with the public. The imprecise nature of science and experimentation leads to mistrust among the public and therefore doubts, criticism, and debate follow. It is in this debate that risk communication about a particular area is formed. The purported link between autism and the measles, mumps, and rubella vaccine was an example of such a debate.

Genetic testing

Since medicine has entered the genomic area, it has become easier to find out the risk of inheriting diseases based on genetic testing. This ability has facilitated the field of genetic counseling. Genetic counselors are health professionals with specialized graduate degrees and experience in the areas of medical genetics and counseling. Genetic counselors work as members of a health care team, providing information and support to families who have members with birth defects or genetic disorders and to families who may be at risk for a variety of inherited conditions. These risks can exist for an unborn child, as well as an adult who is at risk for developing a genetic disease.

Genetic counselors identify families at risk, investigate the problem present in the family, interpret information about the disorder, analyze inheritance patterns and risks of recurrence, and review available options with the family.

Genetic counselors also provide supportive counseling to families, serve as patient advocates, and refer individuals and families to community or state support services. They serve as educators and resource people for other health care professionals and for the general public. In this way, genetic counselors serve to protect people from passing on potential genetic risks to their offspring.

Gene tests (also called DNA-based tests), the newest and most sophisticated of the techniques used to test for genetic disorders, involve direct examination of the DNA molecule itself. A DNA sample can be obtained from any tissue, including blood. Other genetic tests include biochemical tests for gene products, such as enzymes and other proteins, and microscopic examination of stained or fluorescent chromosomes.

Genetic tests are commonly used for prepregnancy, prenatal, or newborn diagnostic testing, as well as presymptomatic testing for adult-onset disorders such as Huntington's disease, certain cancers, and Alzheimer's disease. In the case of risk to an unborn child, carrier screening can be done prior to conception to identify unaffected parents who may carry one copy of a defective gene. If a disease requires two copies of a gene to be expressed, both parents are screened and informed of their potential risk of having a child that may become affected by the particular disease. For example, cystic fibrosis is the kind of disease in which parents unknowingly can be carriers of the gene that causes this disorder. In this case, if family history indicates that these parents might be carriers, they could undergo carrier screening. If both parents are found to be carriers, there is a 1 in 4 chance that they will have a baby with cystic fibrosis. Genetic counselors can provide this information, as well as counseling, for a couple going through this process. If the couple decides to proceed with conception knowing the risks, then prenatal tests can be conducted to determine whether the baby is healthy or will have cystic fibrosis.

Prenatal testing can include testing the embryo or the fetus. One form of genetic test for the embryo is preimplantation genetic diagnosis (PGD), which screens for genetic defects among embryos used in in vitro fertilization. With PGD, DNA samples from embryos created in vitro by the combination of a mother's egg and a father's sperm are analyzed for gene abnormalities that can cause disorders. Fertility specialists can use the results of this analysis to select only mutation-free embryos for implantation into the mother's uterus. If conception occurs in vivo, that is, in the body, the fluids surrounding the fetus are tested to give information regarding the genetic makeup of the fetus. These tests are called chorionic villus sampling

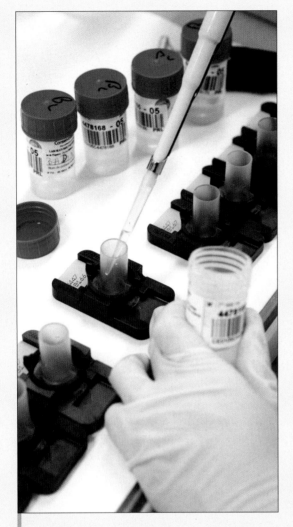

A laboratory worker is working on cervical smears, which are in a liquid phase. They are prepared for centrifugation and analysis. If all the cells appear normal, no further action is taken; if there are abnormal cells, a series of investigations will follow to assess the problem.

and amniocentesis. If the fetus tests positive for a particular disorder, parents are faced with the dilemma of whether or not to terminate the pregnancy. With PGD, couples are much more likely to have healthy babies.

In adult genetic testing, a patient's DNA sample is scanned for mutated sequences. Based on this information and family history, the risk of someone developing a particular disorder is determined. Knowing one's risk for developing disorders can lead individuals to adopt behaviors to reduce risks. For example, if an individual has been tested for the risk of developing breast cancer, she may wish to make a change in her diet to include more cancer-fighting foods. In general, knowledge gained from genetic testing can help people to minimize risks.

Health insurance

Health insurance is a type of insurance whereby the insurer pays the medical costs of the insured if the insured becomes sick due to covered causes or due to accidents. The insurer may be a private organization or a government agency. Market-based health care systems, such as that in the United States, rely primarily on private health insurance. A health insurance policy is a legal, binding contract between the insurance company and the customer. It is generally purchased year by year, with generally no assurance of renewability, and if renewable no guarantee that premium rates will not increase.

Before buying health insurance, a person typically fills out a comprehensive medical history form that asks whether the person smokes, how much the person weighs, and if the person has ever been treated for any of a long list of diseases. Applicants can get discounts if they do not smoke and live a healthy lifestyle, which might encourage some people to quit smoking or make other improvements in their lifestyle. The medical history is also used to identify persons with preexisting medical conditions. For example, a preexisting medical condition can be diabetes. In this case, an insurance company may charge a higher premium because of the risks related to paying the medical expenses of a diabetic patient.

Because health insurance companies take risks when they insure people, they have a vested interest in educating the public about health risks. For this reason, many health insurance companies provide education programs, will help pay for health club memberships to promote healthier lifestyles, and provide free screening procedures. All of these activities reduce the risk of health problems, as well as the companies' risk of paying for health care.

Thus, risk is a common part of life—how much risk depends on people's lifestyles, where they live, and where they travel. On a daily basis, everyone faces risk, subconsciously assesses it, and manages it by making behavioral changes.

Rashmi Nemade

River blindness

River blindness, or onchocerciasis, is a chronic parasitic illness found mainly in tropical Africa that causes intense suffering and can lead to visual impairment and blindness. The disease is found only in humans and has been the focus of control and eradication efforts by international health and aid agencies.

River blindness gets its name from the fact that the disease is transmitted along fertile river areas, mainly in Africa but also in several Latin American countries and Yemen, and can lead to blindness. About 123 million people live in areas where the disease is endemic. It is the second leading infectious cause of blindness and thus is a preventable cause of blindness. The illness has been blamed for adversely affecting the socioeconomic status of people living in endemic regions, because populations may abandon areas where the blackfly lives and breeds. In the United States the disease is rare; it has been diagnosed only in immigrants or travelers who spent time in endemic areas.

Causes and risk factors

The parasitic worm *Onchocerca volvulus* causes the debilitating illness river blindness. It is transmitted by the bite of an infected *Simulium* blackfly, found mainly in tropical Africa near fast-flowing waters. Humans are the only known host. Risk of contracting the illness is only in areas where the blackfly lives.

When an infected blackfly bites a human, usually only one to two of the larval forms of the parasite are injected into the skin. Multiple bites can occur and are common in regions endemic for this illness. In humans who contract this disease, the intensity of their illness (number of the parasitic worms) is related to the number of such bites.

Symptoms and signs

The earliest symptom is severe itching, or pruritis. The itching can become so severe that it interferes with sleep and results in social isolation. Scratching can produce skin trauma such as excoriations and can result in thickened, dry skin. Skin nodules are common, especially overlying bony prominences, as are skin rashes and depigmentation. Skin color changes resulting from depigmentation in some areas and normal-looking skin in others has been referred to as "leopard skin." Lymphadenoapthy (enlargement of lymph nodes) in the groin and femoral areas may become quite pronounced, resulting in elephantiasis of the genitalia. General debilitation can occur. The most feared outcome is blindness. Because the probability of blindness is related to the length of illness, the peak age when affected is 40 to 50. Even though the illness

KEY FACTS

Description
Chronic parasitic illness involving mainly the skin, lymph nodes, and eyes.

Cause
Onchocerca volvulus, a parasite transmitted by the bite of infected blackflies.

Risk factors
Risk increases with time spent in areas where the disease is endemic.

Symptoms
Severe itching, skin nodules, swelling of the groin lymph nodes, possible blindness.

Diagnosis
Identification of larvae in skin snips or of adult parasitic forms from the deeper skin nodules. In some cases, examination of the eye with a special lamp allows identification of the parasite.

Treatments
Ivermectin, an oral medicine, for 10 years or more.

Pathogenesis
Infected blackflies deposit larval forms of the parasite into human skin. There, the parasites mature and produce offspring (microfilariae) that then migrate to other tissues. Microfilariae live up to 30 months; an inflammatory response to dying microfilariae is responsible for the human tissue damage, including blindness. The life cycle is completed when an infected human is bitten by a blackfly, which takes up the parasite and thus can continue the cycle.

Prevention
Avoidance of areas where the vector blackflies live; insecticides to control blackfly populations.

Epidemiology
More than 18 million people are currently infected; up to 1 to 2 million have been blinded by the disease.

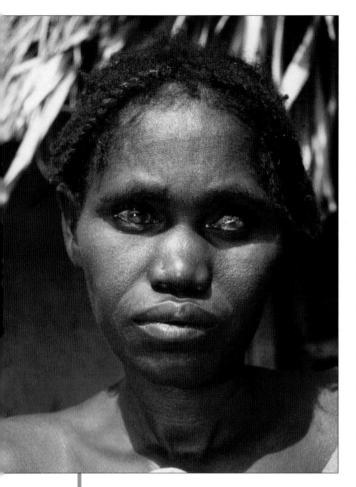

This young woman in Sudan has been blinded by onchocerciasis (river blindness). The blindness in this condition is caused by the death of the worms in or near to tissues of the eye. It can be effectively treated if caught in time.

is not life threatening, the overall life expectancy among those who are affected by river blindness is only about one-third of that found in uninfected people.

Diagnosis and treatments

Diagnosis is made by identification of larvae in skin snips or adult worms in deeper tissue specimens. In some cases, examination of the eye using a special lamp called a slit lamp may reveal the parasite. Once to twice a year, ivermectin, an oral medication developed initially for use in veterinary medicine, is effective against the larval forms but ineffective against adult worms. This antiparasitic medication reduces further transmission of the disease, improves symptoms such as pruritis, and reduces the possibility of blindness. When there is intense involvement of the eye by the infecting parasite, pretreatment with prednisone (an anti-inflammatory medication similar to cortisone) may be required to protect the eye from the inflammatory effects of the dying parasites.

Since the adult forms may live in the human for up to 14 years, treatment must be continued for as long as 15 years. Treatment is well tolerated. Excision of accessible subcutaneous nodules may help some patients.

Pathogenesis

Once an infected blackfly bites a human and deposits the infective larval forms of the worm in the skin, the parasites mature over a 6 to 12 month period. Female adults grow to a size of 8 to 31½ inches (20 to 80 cm) and are surrounded by a fibrous capsule. They are fertilized by the smaller, adult males, which are 1 to 2 inches (3 to 5 cm) long. The males travel from capsule to capsule. About one year after the initial infection, females produce new larvae, called microfilariae. Each female can produce 1,000 to 3,000 microfilariae per day. These microfilariae migrate through the human body, remain alive for 6 to 30 months, and subsequently incite an inflammatory response by the host's tissues as they are dying. It is this inflammatory response that causes tissue damage, particularly when the eye is involved, leading to visual impairment and possible blindness.

The life cycle is completed when a human infected with this illness is bitten by a blackfly that ingests the microfilariae; these larvae go on to mature within the blackfly into larvae that can infect humans.

Prevention and epidemiology

No vaccine is available. Arrest of the disease rests on controlling blackfly with insecticide programs. Mass treatment programs have been implemented that consist of once or twice yearly ivermectin treatment of people in endemic regions. Travelers to areas where the disease is endemic are advised to use insecticide repellants and to wear long sleeves and pants to reduce the risk of bites. It is felt, though, that short-term travelers to these endemic regions are at low risk of contracting the illness since a minimum of several months in these areas is required before infection occurs.

Rita Washko

See also
- Blindness • Filariasis • Giardiasis
- Infections, animal-to-human • Infections, parasitic • Liver fluke • Malaria
- Schistosomiasis • Trichomoniasis

Rocky Mountain spotted fever

First described in the late 1800s, Rocky Mountain spotted fever is caused by the bacterium *Rickettsia rickettsii*. It is transmitted to humans by tick bites and is the most lethal tick-borne illness in the United States.

Ticks acquire the bacterium *Rickettsia rickettsii* after feeding on infected animals, then transmit the organism to humans during feeding. There are no specific risk factors for this disease, but heavy tick exposure increases the risk of acquiring the infection.

Symptoms and signs

Patients typically develop symptoms 2 to 14 days after the tick bite. Initial symptoms may include fever, headache, nausea, muscle aches, joint pain, and diarrhea. A rash is common and typically develops between the third and fifth day of the illness. It usually first appears over the ankles and wrists as flat areas of red discoloration but later spreads to the trunk, palms, and soles. Patients may develop inflammation in the blood vessels, heart wall, lungs, and central nervous system, leading to widespread organ dysfunction. Gangrene of the extremities and seizures are possible late complications of this disease.

Diagnosis and treatments

There is no reliable diagnostic test in the early stages of illness. Blood tests can be obtained to confirm the diagnosis, but they are highly specialized and time-consuming. Treatment should not be delayed while blood tests are in progress. Typically, the diagnosis is made based on detailed history (especially with history of tick exposure) and clinical presentation.

Antibiotics should be started as soon as this condition is suspected; doxycycline is the drug of choice. Other antibiotics may be effective, although there is less experience in the clinical setting.

Pathogenesis

Once in the bloodstream, the bacteria replicate in the cells lining the blood vessels. Focal areas of bacterial and cellular infiltration within the blood vessels lead to damage of the vessel wall and surrounding tissue.

Prevention and epidemiology

Avoidance of ticks is the most effective prevention. In a tick-infested area, protective clothing and tick repellents should be used. If a tick is found, it should be removed as soon as possible under the guidance of a physician. Currently there is no available vaccine.

Despite its name, most cases of the disease are reported from the southern Atlantic region. Two-thirds of cases occur in children younger than 15. From 1994 to 2003, the average number of cases reported to the Centers for Disease Control and Prevention was 585 per year. The mortality rate is 2 to 4 percent.

Joseph M. Fritz and Bernard C. Camins

KEY FACTS

Description
Acute bacterial infection transmitted to humans through tick bites.

Causes
Rickettsia rickettsii carried by tick vectors.

Risk factors
Heavy tick exposure.

Symptoms
Fever, headaches, muscle and joint pain, vomiting, diarrhea. Rash on extremities, then spreads.

Diagnosis
Based on clinic presentation.

Treatments
Antibiotics.

Pathogenesis
Organism gains access to the bloodstream via tick bite. It creates inflammation within blood vessel wall and damages surrounding tissues.

Prevention
Avoidance of tick exposure, tick repellent, protective clothing, and careful inspection for potential tick bites. No available vaccine.

Epidemiology
Several hundred cases per year in the U.S.

See also
- Filariasis • Infections, animal-to-human
- Lice infestation • Rickettsial infections
- Toxoplasmosis

Roundworm infections

Roundworm infections and schistosomiasis are among the most prevalent infections of humans. There are an estimated 2 billion cases worldwide. Most occur in areas of poverty in the developing nations of the tropics and subtropics, where they account for approximately 40 percent of the global burden of disease from all tropical infections, excluding malaria.

As a result of acute complications, roundworm infections account for approximately 150,000 to 200,000 deaths annually. There are approximately 1.221 billion (26 percent), 795 million (17 percent), and 740 million (15 percent) cases of ascariasis, trichuriasis, and hookworm infection, respectively. Significantly more people are considered at risk for acquiring these infections. Among the 4.8 billion people living in the regions of Latin America and the Caribbean, sub-Saharan Africa, the Middle East and North Africa, South Asia, India, East Asia and the Pacific Islands, and China, it is estimated that 88 percent, 67 percent, and 67 percent are at risk for ascaris, trichuris, and hookworm infection, respectively.

Causes and risk factors

Of all the roundworms that infect humans, the most important are the intestinal roundworm (*Ascaris lumbricoides*); the human whipworm (*Trichuris trichiura*); and the human hookworms, *Necator americanus* and *Ancylostoma duodenale*. All three, collectively known as the soil transmitted helminths (STHs), are directly transmitted, either through ingestion of the eggs (*A. lumbricoides* and *T. trichiura*) or invasion of the infective larvae through skin (the hookworms). Risk of infection is in areas of poverty and poor sanitation, where eggs or larvae, or both, are found in the environment. The eggs are extremely tough and may remain in the environment for several years. There have been occurrences in the United States of humans becoming infected with a similar species of ascaris, *A. suum*, caught from close contact with pigs, and frequent cases in immigrant populations, but these are parasites that are usually only found in humans.

Risk factors

Both genetic and environmental factors are included in risk factors for roundworm infections.

Genetics. An increasing number of studies suggest that helminth infection and disease are under genetic control. Recent studies estimate that 28 to 50 percent of variation in egg counts can be quantitatively attributed to genetic factors, while shared environment accounts for between 3 and 13 percent, depending upon population and parasite.

Behavior and occupation. Specific occupations and behaviors influence the prevalence and intensity of helminth infections, particularly for hookworm, in which the highest intensities occur among adults. Engagement in plantation-style agricultural pursuits, for example, remains a common denominator for hookworm infection. In some cases, hookworm infections are attributed to widespread use of feces as fertilizer.

Poverty, sanitation, and urbanization. STH transmission depends on environments contaminated with eggs in feces or larvae. Consequently, helminths are intimately associated with poverty, poor sanitation, and lack of clean water. In most cases, it is difficult to separate these different risk factors. Self-evidently, the provision of safe water and improved sanitation are essential for the control of helminth infection. The social and environmental conditions in many unplanned slums and squatter settlements of developing countries are ideal for the persistence of *A. lumbricoides* and *T. trichiura*. In contrast, high rates of hookworm infection are typically restricted to areas where rural poverty predominates.

Climate, water, and season. Adequate warmth and moisture are key features for each of the STHs, with wetter areas exhibiting increased transmission. In some endemic areas, STH infections exhibit marked seasonality.

Symptoms and signs

Clinical appearance of these infections often lacks specific symptoms and is rarely recognized by the infected person, even when causing significant health damage. Intensity of infection, and thus morbidity, is directly related to the number of worms harbored. Therefore, individuals with moderate and large numbers of worms suffer from the most severe morbidity.

T. trichiura may cause trichuris dysentery syndrome, which is associated with chronic dysentery, rectal prolapse, anemia, and growth stunting. Hookworm infection can contribute to anemia-related deaths, such as malaria.

The nutritional consequences of STH infections are of great significance, particularly for children and pregnant women. Hookworms, for example, have long been recognized as an important cause of intestinal blood loss, which leads to iron deficiency.

Pathogenesis

It is estimated that infection with an individual *Ancylostoma* can lead to blood loss of 0.15 milliliters each day, as well as the associated pain and chronic diarrhea caused by the adults attached to the intestinal surface by abrasive mouth parts. Ascaris infection is associated with pneumonitis that is caused by migrating larvae in the lungs; gut symptomology is related to the numbers of adults present, for example diarrhea, intestinal colic, and gut perforation. Adult migration to other areas of the intestinal system, such as the pancreas, stomach, and liver, can cause peritonitis and secondary bacterial infections. In addition to their health effects, these infections adversely affect physical and mental growth in childhood and cause iron-deficiency anemia, particularly among women still in their reproductive years. The infections therefore can hinder economic development.

The iron-deficiency anemia (IDA) that accompanies moderate and heavy hookworm burdens is sometimes referred to as *hookworm disease* or *hookworm anemia*. The pathophysiology of hookworm anemia occurs through the attachment of hookworms' cutting organs to the intestinal mucosa and submucosa and the subsequent rupture of intestinal capillaries and arterioles. IDA during pregnancy has been linked to adverse maternal or fetal consequences, or both, including prematurity, low birth weight, and impaired lactation. There is increasing evidence that hookworm infection also contributes to anemia in schoolchildren and preschool children. Some of this anemia can be reversed through repeated and regular chemotherapy.

STH infections are associated with reversible deficits in growth and physical fitness in school-age children; they are most pronounced in children with the heaviest infections and can lead to poor performance in tests of cognitive function.

The most striking epidemiological features of human helminth infections are aggregated distributions in human communities; predisposition of individuals to heavy (or light) infection; rapid reinfection following chemotherapy; and age-intensity profiles, which show that most worms are found in very young age groups (with the exception of hookworm).

For all of the major human STH infections studied to date, worm burdens exhibit a highly aggregated (overdispersed) distribution so that most individuals harbor just a few worms in their intestines, although a few hosts harbor disproportionately large worm burdens. As a general rule, approximately 80 percent of the worm population is harbored by 20 percent of the host population. This overdispersion has many consequences, both in terms of the population biology of helminth and the public health consequence for the host, since heavily infected individuals are simultaneously at highest risk of disease and the major source of environmental contamination. One feature that may help explain overdispersion is that individuals tend to be predisposed to heavy (or light) infections.

KEY FACTS

Description
Infection by parasitic worms.

Causes
Ingestion of eggs of worms or invasion of the skin by larvae.

Risk factors
Poverty, poor sanitation, and inappropriate hygienic measures.

Symptoms
Dysentery syndrome, rectal prolapse, anemia, and growth stunting.

Diagnosis
Direct examination of the feces for worm eggs.

Treatments
Anthelmintic drugs.

Pathogenesis
Hookworm infection can contribute to anemia-related deaths, such as malaria. Ascaris infection is associated with pneumonitis, and invasion of the intestines can cause peritonitis and secondary bacterial infections. Physical and mental growth in childhood is affected, and iron-deficiency anemia is likely.

Prevention
Improved sanitation and health education.

Epidemiology
Around 20 percent of the worm population in infected tropical areas is borne by 80 percent of the population. There appears to be a genetic predisposition for heavy or light infections.

Predisposition to infection has been demonstrated for all four major STHs.

Following treatment, rapid reinfection commonly occurs. The rate of reinfection is species specific and depends on the life expectancy of the helminth species, intensity of transmission within a given community, and treatment efficacy and coverage. Reinfection rates are inversely correlated with the magnitudes of each of these factors, which, in turn, can help to determine the frequency at which chemotherapy must be applied.

The age-dependent patterns of infection prevalence are generally rather similar among the major helminth species, exhibiting a rise in childhood to a relatively stable plateau in adulthood. Maximum prevalence is usually attained before five years of age for *A. lumbricoides* and *T. trichiura*, and in young adults with hookworm and schistosome infection. For *A. lumbricoides* and *T. trichiura* infections, the age-intensity profiles are typically convex in form, with intensity peaking in children between five and fifteen years of age. In contrast, the age-intensity profile for hookworm exhibits considerable variation, although intensity typically increases with age until well into adulthood, and then plateaus. In both South China and in Southeast Asia, it is also common to find the highest intensities among people over 60 years old.

Improved sanitation is the only definitive intervention to eliminate STH infections. STH infections are not usually a public health problem when sanitation standards are appropriate. Improvement of the sanitation standards has a repercussion on environmental contamination and reinfection levels. However, to be effective, sanitation should cover a high percentage of the population. Therefore, because of the high costs involved, implementation of this strategy is difficult when resources are limited. Moreover, when used as the primary means of control, it can take years or even decades for sanitation to be effective. Small-scale sanitation interventions (for example, the construction of latrines in schools) that are normally the only feasible sanitation interventions in low-income endemic countries are important as a model, but may have very limited impact on transmission of STH infections.

Health education aims to reduce transmission and reinfection by encouraging healthy behaviors such as by recommending the use of latrines and promoting self-protection from reinfection (through hygienic measures such as washing hands and proper food preparation). By periodical treatment, without a change in defecation habits, it is impossible to attain a

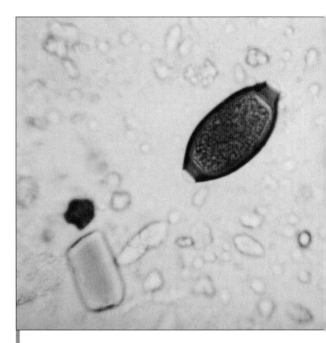

A colored micrograph depicts an egg from the whipworm Trichuris trichiura, *the causal agent of trichuriasis, which is contracted by the ingestion of embryonated eggs. The trichuriasis human intestinal infection is more frequent among children who live in a tropical area where there are poor sanitation practices.*

stable reduction in transmission. Health education can be provided simply and economically and presents no contraindications or risks. Furthermore, it has benefits that go beyond the control of helminth infections. In this perspective, it is reasonable to include this component in all helminth control programs.

Diagnosis and treatments

Diagnosis for all the STHs is by direct examination of feces to look for the presence of eggs.

Ascaris eggs are the largest; they are golden brown in color with a single cell inside. Trichuris eggs have a brown smooth shell with bipolar plugs. Hookworm eggs are barrel shaped; they are usually in the four- to eight-cell stage in fresh feces.

Anthelmintic drug treatment. The most commonly used drug for the treatment of STH infections is either albendazole (400 mg) or mebendazole (500 mg). Both agents are benzimidazole anthelmintics, administered as a single tablet regardless of size and age. Repeated chemotherapy at regular intervals in high-risk groups can ensure that the levels of infection are kept below those associated with morbidity. High-risk groups for STH infections are children and women of reproductive age. Repeated chemotherapy with anthelmintic drugs will frequently result in immediate improvement in child health and development (including iron and hemoglobin status, physical growth, cognition, educational achievement, and school absenteeism). For ascaris and trichuris infections, for which intensity peaks among school-age children, frequent and periodic anthelmintic treatments may reduce transmission over time.

Other roundworm infections

Dracunculis medinensis, the tissue-dwelling Guinea worm, is found in areas of sub-Saharan Africa; however, due to a Global Eradication Program, the numbers of infections are dropping, and in 2005 there were just an estimated 11,000. Infection is indirect; the intermediate host is a water flea or cyclops, which contain infective L3 larvae, and the water fleas are ingested in unfiltered drinking water. The larvae penetrate the gut wall and migrate to the subcutaneous tissue, then develop into adults. After copulation the females migrate to the lower extremities and produce infected L1 larvae that are released into the water when the female induces a blister in the skin that ruptures. Diagnosis is by seeing the females emerging through the skin, usually in the ankles and legs. For Guinea worm infections, there is no effective chemotherapy, but the life cycle can be broken by filtering drinking water and changing bathing habits. The adults, once they have emerged from the skin, can be gently removed (usually by twisting around a matchstick, over several days). The blisters are painful and often become secondarily infected. Adults develop more than eight to ten months after the initial infection and produce infective larvae for three to four weeks.

The pinworm or threadworm, *Enterobius vermicularis*, is the most common intestinal roundworm found in temperate areas. Epidemiologically, it most often affects children, with 500 million infections yearly; prevalence in some populations in the United States is as high as 12 percent. Infection is by ingestion of eggs, released at night, when the female worm migrates to the anal region and releases eggs. This causes irritation, and the patient scratches the area, transferring eggs, which can be ingested or inhaled later. Autoinfection can also occur as eggs hatch on the anus and the larvae migrate back into the intestine. The infection thus can be spread rapidly between family members and school or nursery peers, due to poor hand washing behavior. Most infections are generally asymptomatic. Treatment

is with a single dose of a benzimidazole anthelmintic, as for the STHs, but all bedding and towels should also be washed to eliminate infective stages from the environment. Diagnosis is by using a piece of sticky tape around the anal region at night and then microscopic examination to check for eggs.

The dog roundworm, *Toxocara canis*, and the cat roundworm, *T. cati*, only infect humans as an accidental, or zoonotic infection. *T. canis* is found worldwide, including in the United States (reports estimate 2 to 5 percent prevalence in healthy adults in urban Western countries); most at-risk areas are in children's parks where dogs have been allowed to defecate. If children pick up the eggs in dog feces and inadvertently ingest them, the eggs hatch and larvae emerge to migrate around the body, where they cause granulomas and die. The disease is a form of visceral larval migrans and is most serious in the liver, lungs, and eyes, where the granulomas can lead to endophthalmitis with retinal degeneration. Diagnosis is difficult and is by demonstration of larvae by biopsy or seeing the larvae migrate across the eye, either reported by the patient or during a regular eye check or by serologic testing (ELISA). Treatment is with benzimidazole anthelmintics and outcome is usually good, unless there is severe eye involvement.

Trichinosis is caused by *Trichinella spiralis* and is a worldwide infection. Short-lived adults in the guts of a wide range of animal hosts produce invasive L1 larvae that migrate around the voluntary muscles of their host and encyst. Humans become infected by eating the muscle containing the cysts (frequently undercooked pork or wild game), although the number of cases in the United States per year is in the tens. Pathogenesis is due to the migrating and encysting larvae, which in heavy infections lead to diverse symptoms, such as muscle ache, nausea, fever, and even cardiac and central nervous system damage. Definitive diagnosis is by demonstration of encysted parasites in muscle, or detection of parasite DNA in polymerase chain reaction (PCR), which copies DNA, allowing it to be analyzed. There is no specific treatment; mebendazole can be administered to kill larvae, but should be given in conjunction with a steroid, such as prednisone, to prevent a reaction to the dying larvae.

Helen Roberts

See also
- Anemia • Filariasis • Infections
- Infections, parasitic • River blindness
- Schistosomiasis • Tapeworm infestation

Rubella

Rubella is also known as German measles. However, it is not caused by the same virus that causes measles. Rubella is highly contagious; it is transmitted through the air or by close contact with an infected person. Children and adults who contract this viral infection will usually experience mild symptoms and a rash. A rubella virus vaccine helps prevent the spread of this infection.

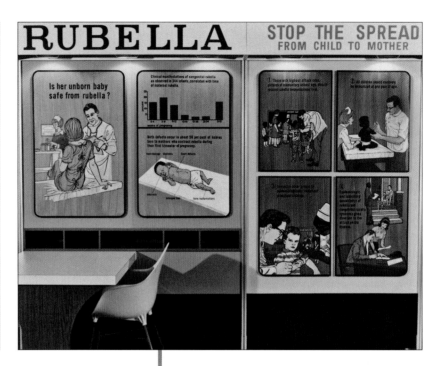

Rubella, commonly known as German measles or three-day measles, is a viral infection that mainly causes a skin rash and fever. It is caused by an RNA rubella virus, not the same virus that causes measles. *Rubella* is a name derived from the Latin and means "little red." It became known as "German measles" ever since it was first described in the German medical literature.

Causes and risk factors

Rubella is a viral illness mainly spread through the air by droplets of fluid from the infected person. The fluid contains the virus; coughing, talking, sneezing, hugging, and sharing food and drinks with an infected person can spread the virus. Also, if someone touches a surface contaminated with viral droplets and then touches the nose, face, eyes, or mouth afterward, they can become infected. From the time of exposure to an outbreak with the infection is usually 13 to 20 days. Rubella usually causes a mild infection in children and adults. If contracted in the first months of pregnancy, it can lead to severe abnormalities in the unborn child. Rubella vaccine is used in over one-half of all countries worldwide. It remains a common viral infection, and the risk of exposure to rubella outside the United Kingdom and United States can be high.

Posters in a clinic highlight the dangers of rubella. If a woman who has not previously had rubella contracts the disease during the first few months of pregnancy, the rubella virus can cause severe birth defects in the unborn child.

Symptoms and signs

A person infected with the rubella virus may have one or more symptoms. They may have rash with skin redness or inflammation, fever, headache, general discomfort (malaise), bruising, runny nose, loss of appetite, and swollen lymph nodes. Many infected people have few or no symptoms at all. The rash usually appears on the second day of infection; it begins on the face and spreads downward on the body. The rash can itch and may last up to three days. Complications can occur, usually more often in adults than children. Over one-half of adult females who contract rubella develop a type of arthritis that mainly affects the fingers, wrists, and knees. These joint symptoms may last up to one month after the infection. Hemorrhaging is a rare complication that occurs more often in children with the rubella infection. Most patients do recover.

If a pregnant woman becomes infected with the rubella virus, it may cause congenital rubella syndrome, with potentially severe birth defects for the unborn child. The infection may lead to premature delivery or death, or both, to the child. Children who are infected with the rubella virus before birth may be born with abnormalities of the heart and eyes; deafness; mental retardation; and growth retardation. Deafness is the most common abnormality of congenital rubella infection. Cataracts and glaucoma can result from congenital rubella syndrome. Diabetes mellitus often occurs in affected children.

Diagnosis

A blood test for rubella antibodies is usually performed on a woman who is or wants to become pregnant to determine whether she is at risk for a rubella infection. Several laboratory methods are available to detect the rubella antibodies. The most common test is the enzyme-linked immunosorbent assay (ELISA).

KEY FACTS

Description

A contagious viral infection with mild symptoms and a skin rash.

Causes

A virus spread through the air or by close contact.

Risk factors

Contact with infected people. It can be transmitted to an unborn child by a mother with a rubella infection, causing severe disease in the unborn child (fetus).

Symptoms

There may be fever, headache, runny nose, general discomfort, and a skin rash. When rubella occurs in a pregnant woman, it can cause congenital rubella syndrome with mental and growth retardation in the newborn, as well as other abnormalities.

Diagnosis

Laboratory blood test for rubella antibodies; a nasal or throat swab for viral culture.

Treatments

There is no treatment. Medication may be given to reduce fever. Congenital rubella syndrome requires treatments for any abnormalities.

Pathogenesis

This viral infection usually has mild symptoms that occur over a three-day period. When rubella occurs in a pregnant woman, it may cause severe abnormalities in the infant, such as deafness and mental retardation.

Prevention

Vaccination; isolation of infected people.

Epidemiology

Rubella occurs worldwide.

Prevention and treatments

When a person has a rubella infection, antibodies are made by the body's immune system to fight and kill the rubella virus. These antibodies remain in the blood for years. In the clinical laboratory, testing is available to detect the presence of rubella antibodies in a person's blood, verifying that the person either had been infected with the rubella virus or had received the vaccination available for rubella. If the rubella blood test is negative for antibodies in a woman who wants to become pregnant, she can receive the rubella vaccination to help protect her against contracting the rubella infection. However, she needs to wait one month after she receives the rubella vaccination before becoming pregnant to provide full protection for her baby against the rubella virus. A pregnant woman cannot receive a rubella vaccination during her pregnancy, since it may be harmful to the unborn child. If a pregnant woman has not had a rubella infection or received the rubella vaccination, she must avoid anyone who has or may have rubella.

The rubella vaccination is given as a single preparation, combined with the measles and mumps vaccine. It is referred to as the measles, mumps, and rubella (MMR) vaccine. In some countries, it is a measles, mumps, rubella, and varicella combination vaccine called the MMRV. At least one dose of rubella vaccine, as the combination MMR or MMRV, is usually recommended for all children. The first dose of MMR or MMRV is usually given on or after the first birthday, followed with an additional dose given at age 4 to 6 years, before a child enters school.

A woman of childbearing age who is not pregnant should be immunized with MMR if she has not been immunized previously or had a rubella infection. Rubella is a very safe vaccine. A mild fever or joint pains, or both, are the most common complaints that follow rubella vaccination.

Rubella infection does not require any special treatment. The infected person usually needs a few days of rest at home. Since it is highly contagious, the infected person needs to avoid public places until one week after the rash has disappeared.

Kathleen Becan-McBride

See also
- Chicken pox and shingles • Childhood disorders • Diphtheria • Infections
- Infections, bacterial • Infections, viral
- Measles • Mumps • Scarlet fever
- Whooping cough

SARS

Severe acute respiratory syndrome, or SARS, is an acute viral infection of the respiratory tract marked by a high fever of more than 100.4°F (38°C). Other symptoms include chills, headache, body aches, dry cough, an overall feeling of discomfort, and diarrhea. Most people infected with the virus develop pneumonia. Some people with SARS will have difficulty breathing and will not be able to get enough oxygen into the blood. About 10 percent of people infected with SARS may die.

A coronavirus called SARS-associated coronavirus (SARS-CoV) is the cause of SARS. This disease was unknown before the first outbreak began in southern China in 2002. It was, however, not reported in the world press until 2003. It developed into the first new serious contagious illness of the twenty-first century. SARS was notable because it spread so rapidly and unexpectedly. Public health efforts contained the disease, and the first epidemic ended in 2003. SARS seems to spread in several different ways. It can spread in the respiratory droplets produced when an infected person sneezes. Like the common cold, it can spread when a person touches an object like a telephone or a doorknob that a person with SARS contaminated from a touch or a sneeze. There is also some suggestion that the virus may travel in the air. This may explain how some buildings seem to be at risk if they have poorly designed sewer systems—air coming from the sewer pipes may carry the virus through the building. People are not at risk to get SARS unless there is an outbreak. If this occurs, then people who have close contact with infected people are at risk. Close contact is defined as being near someone or having direct physical contact.

A diagnosis of SARS is made if the patient has a temperature of more than 100.4°F (38°C), cough, difficulty breathing, pneumonialike symptoms, body aches, and a feeling of general discomfort.

Treatment and prevention

Treatment for SARS is similar to that for viral pneumonia, but people with SARS are treated in isolation. Health care workers have to wear protective equipment, including filter masks. Although antiviral medications and antibiotics have been tried, there is currently no known effective treatment for the infection. SARS is only a concern when an outbreak occurs, when people can take simple steps to reduce the chance of infection. The most important thing is to wash the hands frequently and avoid touching the eyes, nose, or mouth with hands. A disposable tissue should be used to cover the mouth and nose when sneezing.

Pathogenesis and epidemiology

Because people have no immunity to the SARS virus, unless they are treated promptly there is a risk of death, particularly in groups such as the elderly or those who have a compromised immune system.

The cumulative number of cases worldwide from the start of the outbreak in China in November 2002 until December 2003 was just more than 8,000.

Richard Bradley

KEY FACTS

Description
Viral infection of the human respiratory tract.

Causes
Infection by SARS-associated coronavirus.

Risk factors
Direct, close contact with an infected person.

Symptoms
Fever over 100.4°F (38°C), headache, body aches, dry cough, a feeling of discomfort, and pneumonia.

Diagnosis
Lab tests of blood, nasal secretions, or feces.

Treatments
Experimental use of antiviral treatments. No approved treatments are available yet.

Pathogenesis
Humans lack immunity to SARS-CoV, and severe symptoms develop quickly.

Prevention
Hygienic practices such as frequent hand washing and covering one's mouth when sneezing.

Epidemiology
Around 8,000 cases occurred worldwide between November 2002 and December 2003.

See also
- Infections, viral • Pneumonia
- Respiratory system disorders

Scarlet fever

Scarlet fever is an infectious disease caused by streptococcal bacteria. Usually, this infection involves the throat, in which case it is called pharyngitis. In some cases it involves the skin; then it is called impetigo. Symptoms are fever and rash.

Scarlet fever is an illness affecting young persons, mainly children. Cases of this illness have declined over time, even though cases of strep pharyngitis have not undergone similar decreases. Reasons for this are unknown.

Causes and risk factors

Infection of the throat with toxin-producing group A *Streptococcus* (strep) precedes scarlet fever. In some cases, strep infection of the skin leads to scarlet fever. Not everyone who becomes infected with group A *Streptococcus* develops scarlet fever, however. The disease is transmitted through contact with the secretions of someone infected, including respiratory droplets produced by coughing or sneezing. Touching something that has been contaminated with such infectious secretions, followed by touching one's mouth, eyes, or nose, can also cause this illness.

Symptoms and signs

Sore throat, fever, and a bright red, finely textured, and raised rash (sandpaper rash) are most common. With impetigo, the skin sores are red and weeping and then crust over (honey-crusted lesions). On examination, a strep throat infection appears as red, swollen tissue in the back of the throat. White or yellow patches called exudates may be present. The normal bumps on the tongue may become exaggerated (strawberry tongue), and the area surrounding the mouth may appear pale. The creases of the skin may look darker than usual, referred to as Pastia's lines. Other common symptoms include chills, body aches, and headache. Nausea and vomiting may occur. The rash usually starts in the central areas of the body, then spreads over the rest of the body, and persists for several days. Afterward, the skin of the fingertips and toes may peel.

Diagnosis is made by physical exam and a throat culture that tests positive for group A *Streptococcus* or, in the case of impetigo, a culture of skin lesions that tests positive for this organism. Antibiotics such as penicillin are used as treatment. Fever can be treated with acetaminophen. Bed rest and increased fluid intake are recommended. With appropriate treatment, persons are usually cured within about one week.

Pathogenesis, prevention, and epidemiology

For scarlet fever to develop, the strep bacteria must be a strain that produces toxin and the person must be sensitive to this toxin. In a few cases, infection with the bacteria staphylococci can cause scarlet fever. If treated appropriately, complications are rare. Otherwise, complications may include pneumonia, sinusitis, ear infections, inflammation of the kidneys, or rheumatic fever.

Hand washing, avoiding contact with people who have the illness, and avoiding the sharing of drinking cups and eating utensils can prevent this illness. Group A *Streptococcus* infections are very common in the United States; there are about 10 million cases yearly.

Rita Washko

KEY FACTS

Description
Illness consisting of rash and fever.

Cause
Group A *Streptococcus* bacteria.

Risk factors
Contact with infected persons or their airborne droplets created by coughs, sneezes, exhalations.

Symptoms
Fever, sore throat, or skin infection and rash.

Diagnosis
Physical exam and a throat or skin culture that is positive for Group A *Streptococcus*.

Treatments
Antibiotics.

Pathogenesis
If treated appropriately, complications are rare.

Prevention
Frequent hand washing; avoid sharing utensils.

Epidemiology
Once considered a serious threat, the frequency has dropped over time.

See also

• Infections, bacterial • Pneumonia • Skin disorders • Throat infections

Schistosomiasis

Schistosomiasis is a common parasitic disease that affects an estimated 200 million people worldwide, with a majority of infected individuals residing in Africa. Fresh water and availability of intermediate hosts help to maintain the continuous transmission of this infection to humans. Schistosomiasis is a disease of the developing world, where limited access to health care, sanitation, and clean water continue to be a challenge.

People with certain occupations involving constant freshwater exposure, for example fishing or farming, are at higher risk for this parasitic tropical disease. School-aged children and women using freshwater for domestic purposes are more likely to be affected with a significantly higher burden of the infection. Children with schistosomiasis may have disrupted growth and development.

As with any parasitic disease, the life cycle of this organism includes several stages; egg, larval, and adult stages. For effective passage of the parasite, there are intermediate and definitive hosts for this infection. The eggs are released in the stool or urine by an infected person; the eggs hatch in freshwater into miracidium, a larval stage, and infect the intermediate host, the snail. In the snail, miracidium produces many cercariae (also a larval stage of the parasite), which are released back into the water. Cercaria can survive in freshwater for up to 48 hours. In order to continue the parasite cycle, cercariae must reach the definitive host, which is human or, in some cases, another mammal. Cercariae can penetrate the intact skin in seconds. Inside the human body, cercariae undergo further transformation and become mature adult worms that start sexual reproduction. One of the unique features of schistosoma is the presence of both sexes; usually most of the trematodes are hermaphrodites. The male worm wraps itself around the female worm, and egg production begins about four to six weeks after the original skin penetration by cercariae has occurred.

Causes

Schistosomiasis is caused by several species that are endemic to many countries. *Schistosoma hematobium* is prevalent in Africa and the Middle East; *Schistosoma mansoni* has wide distribution in South America, the Caribbean, Africa and the Middle East; and *S. japonicum* is prevalent in Southeast Asia. Less common schistosomal species known to cause human disease are *S. mekongi* in Southeast Asia and *S. intercalatum* in Central and West Africa. *S. hematobium* is a cause of urinary schistosomiasis; the rest of the species affect the gastrointestinal system. On rare occasions avian schistosoma species can cause severe dermatitis in humans, also known as swimmer's itch, without causing an invasive disease.

Pathogenesis

Pathogenesis of schistosomiasis is defined by the body's immune reaction, which is induced by both immature worm stages, but more so by the eggs. Acute infection occurs several weeks after the first encounter with the parasite and is characterized by an acute inflammatory response to cercaria. It is more common in people visiting endemic areas for the first time and who harbor a high burden of the parasite. The severity of illness depends on the heaviness of the infestation and the amount of eggs produced. After cercariae enter a human body, they loses the tail and become schistosomula that pass through a migratory phase in the lungs and liver, further develop into a worm, and establish themselves in the blood vessels supplying either the gastrointestinal tract or the urinary bladder (*S. hematobium*). The adult worms feed on blood and can persist for years and produce hundreds to thousands of eggs daily. Depending on the species, eggs are passed through either urine or stool. Only a small fraction of eggs are excreted; the rest are trapped in the tissues, inducing a granulomatous inflammatory response, which leads to formation of scarring tissue. Such serious scarring or fibrosis can develop in the bowel, urinary bladder, and in blood vessels supplying the liver and lungs. Fibrosis leads to disruption of normal blood flow and further damage of the tissues supplied by this blood flow. Similar processes can occur in any other human body tissues since eggs can travel along the circulation.

Symptoms and signs

Acute schistosomiasis (Katayama fever) develops two to eight weeks after the first exposure. It is characterized by fever chills, muscle aches, abdominal pain, and diarrhea. It is often accompanied by enlargement of the liver and spleen as well as lymph node enlargement. Infiltrates in the lungs can be seen on a chest X-ray as a result of the passage of the organism via the lungs. Increased white blood cell counts in peripheral blood are common. These symptoms typically resolve within several weeks. In patients with a chronic form of the disease, the severity of the infection depends on the parasite burden and the extent of egg production. Some individuals may have no symptoms or only mild symptoms. The eggs can be deposited in any human body tissues. With heavy infection, abdominal pain, anemia, and diarrhea are common. Granulomatous inflammation induced by eggs can block the blood flow in the liver, leading to the development of liver fibrosis, or in the lungs to cause pulmonary hypertension.

In cases of infection with *S. hematobium*, the adult worms establish themselves in the blood vessels supplying the bladder. Eggs deposited in the urogenital system result in granuloma formation that may cause obstruction of urinary flow, which could eventually lead to kidney failure. The most common symptom of urinary schistosomiasis is the presence of blood in the urine (hematuria). In women, the egg deposition can occur in the vulva and cervix, which leads to increased susceptibility to sexually transmitted diseases, including HIV infection. *S. hematobium* is associated with bladder cancer and a urinary tract infection caused by salmonella organisms. Salmonella bloodstream infections are also common in schistosomiasis caused by other species. *S. japonicum* is known to invade the central nervous system (CNS) and cause a seizure disorder; other schistosoma species rarely invade the CNS.

Diagnosis

Schistosomiasis is highly prevalent in endemic areas; therefore any history of freshwater exposure in the endemic area should raise a high level of suspicion for this infection, even if the symptoms are subtle or absent. Besides history of an exposure, diagnosis is based on identification of eggs in either stool or urine, or in tissues samples from bowel or bladder lining (mucosa). Serological tests detecting antibodies against schistosomes are also available. The test will be positive regardless of active or past status of the infection; therefore it is a useful aid in diagnosis but not a definitive diagnostic test. Serology could also be useful in assessing overall infection rates in an endemic area. Once the presence of the infection is established, further testing is necessary to evaluate the extent of the tissue damage caused by egg deposition and resulting organ dysfunction. Peripheral blood analysis can also show an elevated eosinophil count and anemia. In cases of urinary schistosomiasis, hematuria (blood in the urine) is one of the major signs of schistosomiasis.

Treatments

Schistosomiasis is treated by administration of an antiparasitic agent called praziquantel. Alternative agents are also available. Single treatment can be high-

---

KEY FACTS

Description

Schistosomiasis (bilharziasis) is a parasitic disease caused by a helminth (worm).

Causes

Schistosomiasis is caused by five species of a trematode flatworm or fluke. *S. mansoni, S. japonicum, S. mekongi,* and *S. intercalatum* cause intestinal disease. *S. hematobium* causes urogenital disease.

Risk factors

Freshwater exposure in endemic areas depends on the snails that serve as an intermediate host for the parasite. People traveling to endemic areas are at risk of developing acute schistosomiasis.

Symptoms

Schistosomiasis can present itself as an acute or chronic illness. Chronic presentation is more common among people residing in the endemic areas. Depending on the anatomic location of the adult worms, the disease can manifest itself in various ways. Schistosomiasis affects either the urinary bladder or the gastrointestinal system.

Diagnosis

Examination of stool or urine for presence of eggs produced by the adult worms is a major means of diagnosis, along with the history of freshwater exposure in an endemic area.

Treatments

Schistosomiasis is effectively treated with the antiparasitic drug praziquantel.

Pathogenesis

The worms have a layer of protein on their surface that makes them highly resistant to the body's immune system. The eggs deposited in various human body tissues illicit inflammatory response that results in tissue damage.

Prevention

The best way to prevent schistosomiasis is to avoid exposure to water contaminated by flatworms.

Epidemiology

Schistosomiasis is endemic in tropical and subtropical areas of Africa, South America, the Caribbean, and Asia. It is the second most common tropical disease in Africa after malaria.

LIFE CYCLE OF SCHISTOSOMIASIS

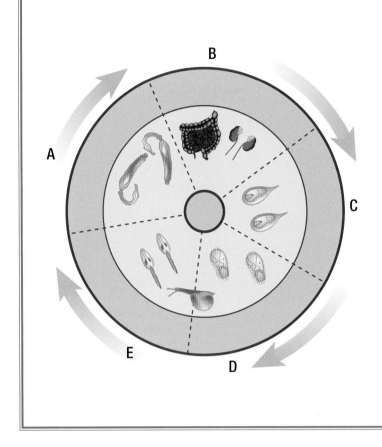

A Cercariae, a larval stage of the parasite, penetrate skin of humans or mammals who are swimming or in contact with infected water. Cercariae travel to the bloodstream, where they become adult worms.

B The male and female adult worms establish themselves in the veins of the gastrointestinal tract and bladder and produce thousands of eggs, which are passed in the feces or urine.

C The eggs pass into sewage systems or directly into water systems and end up in rivers and lakes.

D The eggs hatch into a larval stage called miracidium and enter freshwater snails.

E Miracidium produce cercariae in the snails, which are released back into the water. Cercariae can survive in freshwater for up to 48 hours.

ly effective in chronic schistosomiasis. Although the treatment is not curative, it does significantly decrease the burden of the egg production. In such cases repeated treatments may be necessary. In acute schistosomiasis, medications, such as corticosteroids that help to reduce the intense inflammatory response, are necessary in addition to antiparasitic agents. In acute infection a repeat round of medication may be necessary since praziquantel has no effect on the immature worm stages (like schistosomula) in the human body.

Prevention

For travelers to the endemic areas, avoidance of freshwater exposure is a major way to prevent schistosomiasis. In areas with suboptimal sanitation, where water supply is not treated, certain measures can be preventive, for example, heating or filtering the water. There is currently no vaccine available for schistosomiasis.

Schistosomiasis Control Initiative is an effort supported by the World Health Organization that is launched to control the infection rates in the areas en-

demic for schistosomiasis. The aim of this initiative is to treat for schistosomiasis and intestinal helminths 75 percent of school-age children and other persons at risk by the year 2010. Initially launched in Uganda, this initiative is currently expanding to several other African countries. The program involves assessment of schistosomiasis prevalence and morbidity, determining areas with high infection rates, and mass administration of a single dose praziquantel provided on a regular basis. Such strategy helps decrease the transmission rates and morbidity in the affected population.

Other more costly preventive measures are the improvement of sanitation and providing a safe water supply, as well as the elimination of snails that carry the larval stage of the parasite.

Diana Nurutdinova

See also
• Anemia • Bladder disorders • Diarrhea and dysentery • Infections, parasitic • Respiratory disorders

Schizophrenia

Schizophrenia is one of the most devastating of all the mental illnesses. It is the most common of the psychotic disorders, affecting about 0.5 to 1 percent of the population in the United States. It also presents during late adolescence and early adulthood, a time when individuals are making the transition from adolescence to adulthood. Schizophrenia affects all cultures around the globe equally. As such, it is an illness that can be found described in various writings in many countries throughout history.

The term *schizophrenia* was first coined by Eugen Bleuler in the early 1900s and was not meant to describe a splitting of personalities, which is a common misperception, but rather a splitting of psychic processes. Individuals who are psychotic have a distortion, or a split from reality. This typically takes the form of hallucinations or delusions, which are two of the primary symptoms in schizophrenia.

However, individuals may have no delusions or hallucinations and still receive a diagnosis of schizophrenia. In these cases, other symptoms of schizophrenia predominate, such as a reduction of the emotions seen in facial expressions (affective flattening), withdrawing socially from others, a loss of interest in activities (anhedonia), disorganized or catatonic behavior, and a disruption in the thought processes (thought disorder). This wide diversity of symptoms may be the result of several different causes.

Schizophrenia is an illness that is surrounded by many misconceptions. These misconceptions may have arisen through television shows and movies that have depicted individuals with schizophrenia as having either multiple personalities or psychopathic traits. Individuals with personality or trait disorders have very different symptoms from those with psychotic disorders. There is also a misconception that individuals with schizophrenia are overly aggressive. Although individuals with schizophrenia have engaged in horrible crimes, as is true of individuals without schizophrenia, people tend to perceive them as more aggressive than they really are. This is perhaps due to attempts by some people to avoid prosecution for their crimes by attempting to obtain a diagnosis of schizophrenia in order to plead not guilty by reason of insanity.

Causes and risk factors

Although the actual cause of schizophrenia is not known, it involves both genetic and environmental factors. People are born with certain genes that may put them at risk for developing schizophrenia, but they do not develop the illness without specific environmental influences. It is likely not just one gene or one environmental factor that places an individual at risk, but rather a number of different factors that all contribute in some way to the development of the illness. These differences in the genes and environmental factors account for the variability in the types of symptoms that people experience.

As an example, consider an individual who has a grandmother with schizophrenia and whose mother developed influenza infection while he was developing inside her womb. He had no other difficulties during early childhood and seemed to be no different from any other child. As a teenager he used marijuana and cocaine. Finally, when he was 18 years old, he began to exhibit psychotic symptoms that became worse over eight months until he was brought to the hospital for an evaluation. Both influenza during pregnancy and the use of marijuana in early to mid-adolescence have been shown to increase the risk of schizophrenia. Thus, it is possible that this individual would have never developed schizophrenia if the influenza infection and drug use had never taken place.

To simplify a complex situation, both genes and environmental factors could be considered as a dose. If someone gets a high dose of genes that lead to schizophrenia, then it takes fewer environmental factors to develop the illness. On the other hand, certain genes may be protective; that is, they are protective in spite of the dose of environmental factors. There is still a considerable amount of research to be done to understand the cause of the disorder, and many questions remain unanswered.

Symptoms

The symptoms of schizophrenia have been categorized as either positive and negative symptoms.

Positive symptoms are those symptoms that are expressed outwardly by the individual. These include delusions and hallucinations and disorganized thoughts. Hallucinations commonly include hearing voices, feeling odd sensations, and smelling foul odors. Delusions are exaggerated or distorted beliefs, such as the idea that one is being conspired against or a belief that one has special powers. These can range from the plausible ("The police are trying to kill me") to the completely implausible ("My parents are aliens who abandoned me on earth when I was a child"). Positive symptoms are more likely to improve with medication, and thus individuals with only positive symptoms do better than those with negative symptoms.

Unlike positive symptoms, which come and go throughout the course of the disease, negative symptoms are often always present. They are also less responsive to medications and are linked to how well one functions in one's environment (for example, greater negative symptoms are associated with greater difficulties in areas such as work and social relationships). Negative symptoms include apathy, a lack of motivation, poverty of speech, inability to experience pleasure, and flattened affect (lack of emotional expressions or response).

Cognitive deficits are also prevalent in people with schizophrenia and are closely tied to the negative symptoms. These deficits include impaired memory and attention and greater difficulty with what are termed *higher order brain functions*. These higher order brain functions include the ability to solve problems and to use abstract reasoning. Since memory, attention, and problem-solving skills are all important for both school and vocation, and since cognitive symptoms are linked to negative symptoms, it is not surprising that individuals with greater negative symptoms tend to have greater difficulties with vocational issues.

Finally, individuals with schizophrenia may have difficulties ordering their thoughts. This is known as a formal thought disorder.

Course of schizophrenia

There are four phases of schizophrenia. These include the pre-illness, the prodromal, the active, and the residual phase. Although individuals will experience all of these phases, the duration in each phase can vary significantly from individual to individual.

Pre-illness phase. During the pre-illness phase, some individuals, but not all, may exhibit minor difficulties with memory, attention, and their motor skills. These symptoms are common in the population, and so most people with deficits in these areas will not go on to develop schizophrenia.

Prodromal phase. *Prodrome* is a term to describe an early symptom of illness that heralds what is yet to come. Symptoms in the prodromal phase are variable and nonspecific. The phase includes symptoms such as worsening academic performance, social withdrawal, attention problems, conduct problems, and difficulties

---

KEY FACTS

Description

Schizophrenia is a disorder that includes a combination of hallucinations, delusions, disordered thought, lack of motivation, flattening of affect, and disruptions in social functioning. Not all of these symptoms are present in everyone with schizophrenia, and there is considerable variability in the severity of the symptoms.

Causes

The cause of schizophrenia is not yet known. Evidence shows that both genetic and environmental factors play a role in who will get the illness and who will not.

Symptoms

An alteration in a person's thoughts and perceptions, including hallucinations, delusions, and disorders of thought and speech. Cognitive deficits are also commonly associated with schizophrenia.

Diagnosis

The diagnosis of schizophrenia requires a thorough history, physical and neurological examination, laboratory studies, and often imaging studies of the brain.

Treatments

Antipsychotic medications are the mainstay for treating schizophrenia. Supportive therapy and sometimes cognitive behavioral therapy are also important.

Pathogenesis

Psychotic symptoms are related to the brain chemical known as dopamine.

Prevention

There is no direct evidence that schizophrenia can be prevented. Evidence is emerging that avoiding marijuana will reduce the chance of developing schizophrenia.

Epidemiology

Affects 0.5 to 1 percent of the population worldwide. It affects males and females equally, although females have a slightly later age of onset.

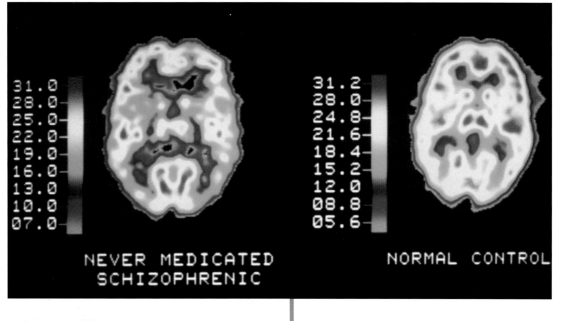

NEVER MEDICATED SCHIZOPHRENIC

NORMAL CONTROL

with hygiene. What is meant by nonspecific is that these symptoms could also be seen in someone who has other illnesses, such as major depression, bipolar affective disorder, or in someone who is actively using drugs. The duration of the prodrome varies from several days to several years.

Active phase. The active phase is the time period when the diagnosis of schizophrenia is made. During the active phase, individuals meet the criteria that are shown in the box on page 758. Normally, an individual with schizophrenia experiences several active stages over the course of his or her life, with periods of relative remission, or a residual period, in between.

Residual phase. The time between active stages is called the residual phase. Although a person may experience low-grade hallucinations and delusions during the residual stage, they often display negative symptoms and cognitive deficits.

Diagnosis

An accurate diagnosis is obtained through a similar approach to that used for psychotic disorders. It is first important to eliminate any nonpsychiatric medical conditions that would have symptoms similar to those seen in schizophrenia. There are several rare conditions that do this, and since the treatments are often quite different from those for schizophrenia, it is important to make sure that tests are done to ensure that these do not account for the symptoms.

Once a nonpsychiatric medical condition is ruled out, schizophrenia is diagnosed by a careful psychiatric

A positron emission tomography scan shows a horizontal slice of the brain from a normal person (right) and a schizophrenic (left) after a radioactively labeled substance was introduced into the body. In this scan, red shows a high level of activity; blue or purple indicates low levels of activity. The scan reflects the function of tissues rather than the structure.

history and examination of the patient's mental status. The criteria that are used during the examination are the same for any age and are shown on page 758. Diagnosis during the prodromal period is very difficult, since the symptoms overlap with other psychiatric disorders.

Once a patient is in the active stage of the illness and it has been determined that the symptoms are not a result of a nonpsychiatric illnesses, the diagnosis is often readily made.

Treatments

The mainstays of treatment for individuals with schizophrenia are the antipsychotic medications. These medications have been widely studied in adults and have been shown to work well in controlling the positive symptoms and thought disorder.

The negative symptoms are more difficult to treat, being less responsive to medications. As individuals are different, not everybody responds equally to the same medication and dose.

Sometimes an individual takes several medications before they find one that works. However, it will soon be possible to test a person's genes and be able to

DIAGNOSTIC CRITERIA FOR SCHIZOPHRENIA FROM THE DSM-IV

There are several characteristic symptoms of schizophrenia, and to make a definitive diagnosis, two or more of the symptoms must each be present for a significant portion of time during a one-month period, or less if the condition has been successfully treated.

Symptoms

Typical symptoms of schizophrenia are: delusions; hallucinations; disorganized speech; grossly disorganized or catatonic behavior; negative symptoms such as affective flattening (lack of emotional response), alogia (lack of speech), or avolition (lack of any motivation).

Making a diagnosis

Only one of the above symptoms is required if the person has delusions that are bizarre or hallucinations that consist of a voice keeping up a running commentary on the person's behavior or thoughts, or two or more voices conversing with each other.

In addition, there must be social or occupational dysfunction, or both; continuous signs of the disturbance persisting for at least 6 months; and evidence to show that the disturbance is not due to the direct physiological effects of a substance, such as a drug of abuse or a medication, or a general medical condition.

---

determine which medications will be most efficacious. Two different types of therapies have been shown to be helpful in individuals with schizophrenia.

The first therapy, which should be provided to all patients, is supportive psychotherapy. This therapy works to support the patient and often the family in all facets of dealing with the illness and its effects. It involves educating the patient and family early on about the illness and getting them connected to any support systems in the community. It is often helpful for those diagnosed with schizophrenia to meet regularly with their psychiatrist or therapist to discuss the issues and problem solve.

The second type of therapy is called cognitive behavioral therapy. This therapy, which also is useful for those with anxiety and mood disorders, helps the patient understand the distortions in how they perceive things. For example, it will work so that the patient understands that when he hears voices, they are a result of his illness and he should try to ignore them. Since not all patients have insight into their illness, this tends to work best with those who understand that they are ill.

Finally, it is very important that physicians ask whether or not their patients with schizophrenia are having thoughts of harming themselves. Approximately 5 percent of individuals with schizophrenia commit suicide, and those who do are more likely to do so during the first six months of the illness. Those who have insight into their illness seem to be at a greater risk. Also, some individuals with schizophrenia experience auditory hallucinations that tell them to kill themselves. It is important to understand the devastating effects of the perceived stigma of having schizophrenia. Such stigma can result from unfair reporting in the media of incidents involving schizophrenic patients. An isolated occurrence may be described as if it were common, which can foster attitudes of intolerance toward, and rejection of, people with mental problems. Because people with schizophrenia find it difficult to find employment or housing, they become socially isolated. Studies in 2005 show that stigma in developed countries is universal, that stigma is attached to mental illness in many different socio-cultural communities worldwide, and that the negative consequences of stigma are increasing.

Epidemiology

Schizophrenia affects approximately 0.5 to 1 percent of the population. If this statistic is extrapolated in a school of 1,000 people, 5 to 10 people in that school will one day develop schizophrenia. The prevalence of schizophrenia is the same in all countries across the globe. Thus, schizophrenia affects an extremely large number of people worldwide.

Males and females are affected equally, although females tend to develop the illness at older ages than males. The disease generally develops in the late teens or early twenties. Onset of schizophrenia prior to the age of 12 is rare, and the incidence increases afterward.

Tonya White

See also
• Bipolar disorder • Depressive disorders
• Personality disorders • Psychotic disorders
• Substance abuse and addiction

SCID

SCID (severe combined immunodeficiency) is a rare disorder in which the immune system's two major weapons against disease—antibodies and T cells—are genetically missing or disabled. Babies born with SCID usually experience multiple and persistent infections, such as pneumonia and oral thrush, and may fail to develop physically at a normal rate.

SCID is a group of inherited disorders distinguished by a lack of immune response. It is the most serious of the primary immunodeficiencies. It occurs when a child lacks lymphocytes (B and T lymphocytes), which are the specialized white blood cells that the body uses to fight infection. During fetal development, lymphocytes are made in the bone marrow. Some lymphocytes move to the thymus gland behind the breastbone, where they become T cells; others remain in the bone marrow to become B cells. Each specialized type of cell is responsible for a particular immune response: T cells attack antigens (microorganisms and foreign substances) and help the body reject unfamiliar tissue. T cells are also needed to trigger the B cells that produce antibodies to fight specific invaders.

There are many causes of SCID. The most common type is that in which the X chromosome harbors a genetic defect; the mechanism that allows T and B cells to receive signals from growth factors is flawed. Since a male child has only one X chromosome inherited from his mother, SCID is more common in males. In females, typically there is one normal X chromosome that compensates for the defective one.

Symptoms of the disorder can vary from mild to life threatening. Typical signs of SCID are an increased vulnerability to infection and failure to grow and gain weight. A baby with SCID may have persistent bacterial, viral, or fungal infections—such as ear infections, sinus infections, mouth thrush, and pneumonia—that may not respond well to treatment. Infants with SCID may also have persistent diarrhea.

Early diagnosis of SCID is uncommon because routine white blood cells counts are not performed on newborns. After multiple infections, if SCID is suspected, T- and B-cell counts are done. SCID can be successfully treated if it is identified early; otherwise, the disease is often fatal within the first year of life. Patients with SCID can be treated with antibiotics and immune serum to protect them from infections, but these treatments cannot cure the disorder. Until recently, SCID eventually ended in death; now, with advances in biomedical research, SCID patients have hopes of surviving much longer. Bone marrow transplantation, if performed early, is an effective treatment for SCID, and it will help rebuild a defective immune system.

Another treatment for SCID is a hematopoietic stem cell transplant. This is a procedure in which blood-forming stem cells (early cells found in the bone marrow where blood cells develop) are placed into the body in the hope that these new cells will help rebuild the immune system.

Rashmi Nemade

KEY FACTS

Description

A rare disorder in which the immune system components are genetically missing or disabled.

Causes

Genetic defects.

Risk factors

Children with a family history of SCID.

Symptoms

Many infections in first few months of life, and persistent diarrhea.

Diagnosis

Positive family history of SCID and blood tests.

Treatments

Bone marrow transplant, special diet, and stem-cell transplantation.

Pathogenesis

Until recently, SCID was always fatal.

Prevention

None, since it is an inherited disease.

Epidemiology

Occurs in approximately 1 in 5,100,000 births and is most common in boys; 50 percent of all cases are linked with the X chromosome.

See also
• Genetic disorders • Immune system disorders • Infections • Pneumonia

Scleroderma

Scleroderma, which means "hard skin," is a rare autoimmune, chronic, and progressive disease. The disease causes tightening and thickening of the skin, as well as blood vessel damage, inflammation, and immune system changes.

Scleroderma is not a single disease but a set of related disorders with similar symptoms. Scleroderma is typically described as a rheumatic autoimmune disorder of the connective tissues. Autoimmune diseases occur when the body's tissues are attacked by its own immune system. Scleroderma is characterized by the formation of scar tissue (fibrosis) in the skin and organs of the body, which results in thickness and firmness. It is a chronic, degenerative disorder with vascular weakening and tissue loss. Scleroderma can be damaging, debilitating, and deadly. In the most serious cases, the disease causes severe harm and severe complications for the body's digestive, respiratory, and circulatory systems.

Scleroderma is one of a group of arthritic conditions called connective tissue disorders. There are two main types of scleroderma, localized and systemic. The systemic forms can affect the skin, blood vessels, and internal organs. The systemic forms are also referred to as systemic sclerosis. The localized type of scleroderma is limited to the skin and deep tissues below the skin. The localized forms affect only the skin; they do not affect the internal organs or reduce life expectancy.

Causes and risk factors

The cause of scleroderma is unknown. Exposure to chemicals and other substances, including detergents, herbicides, plastics, silica, silicone prostheses, and various drugs, such as cocaine, increase the risk of developing scleroderma. Researchers have found that genetics, fetal cells, and viruses might also be factors.

Signs and symptoms

Scleroderma has been dubbed the "disease that turns people into stone." The systemic forms of scleroderma cause scar tissue (fibrosis) to be created, resulting in hardening of affected areas in the skin or internal organs, or both. The fibrosis eventually causes the skin or organs to harden. Symptoms vary widely between people, in course and severity. Pain, ranging in severity from uncomfortable to debilitating, is a common characteristic of the disease. In general, symptoms such as heartburn, high blood pressure, constipation, and muscle aches are common. Specific symptoms include hardening of skin; pain, stiffness, and swelling of joints; ulceration of fingertips or toes; difficulty swallowing; dryness of mucous membranes; weight loss; diarrhea; constipation; and shortness of breath.

Diagnosis of scleroderma is difficult because the symptoms mirror rheumatoid arthritis or lupus. Currently there are no treatments or cures for scleroderma, only therapies for symptoms. Aspirin and nonsteroidal anti-inflammatory drugs can help treat the inflammation and pain of scleroderma. Physical therapy and skin and joint protection techniques also help.

Rashmi Nemade

KEY FACTS

Description
An autoimmune disorder of connective tissue.

Causes
Unknown.

Risk factors
Exposure to chemicals or stress on the hands.

Symptoms
Hardening of skin, damage to blood vessels, stiffness and swelling of joints, ulceration of fingertips or toes, difficulty swallowing, weight loss, diarrhea, constipation, shortness of breath.

Diagnosis
History, examination, skin biopsy, and blood tests.

Treatments
To alleviate symptoms. Physical therapy.

Pathogenesis
Caused by the overproduction of a protein called collagen, which results in excess deposits of the protein throughout the body, especially the skin.

Prevention
Reducing exposure to chemical agents.

Epidemiology
Approximately 300,000 people in the U.S. are affected. Women aged 20 to 40 are three times more likely to be affected than men.

See also
- Immune system disorders • Lupus
- Muscle system disorders

Sexual and gender identity disorders

A sexual dysfunction or disorder can be defined as a problem in someone's desire to engage in sexual activity, or an inability to experience the natural unfolding of the sexual response cycle. Such disorders can cause personal distress or relationship problems. Gender identity disorder is a condition that is characterized by two components. First, the person has a persistent belief that he or she should be, or actually is, a member of the opposite sex. Second, there is a feeling of distress or inappropriateness that the person has about her or his birth sex and the accompanying role, body characteristics, and appearance. Both criteria must be present to establish the diagnosis.

Media bombardment of erotic images and frank discussion of previously taboo topics create the impression that sexual activity in modern society is a well-understood, uncomplicated endeavor. In reality, many people, including those who display no other physical or psychological problems, have distressing sexual dysfunctions. It is very difficult to know precisely how widespread these difficulties are, and estimates vary considerably.

One large survey revealed that 43 percent of women and 31 percent of men reported some form of sexual disturbance in a previous one-year period. Sexual dysfunctions include disorders of desire and disorders of arousal.

Disorders of desire

There are two disorders of desire. The first is hypoactive sexual disorder, a condition that is diagnosed in individuals with little or no interest in sexual activity. It affects approximately 20 percent of women and 10 percent of men.

If a hormone deficiency is thought to be a causative factor, testosterone may be used in treatment. However, the disorder is more often a result of depression, stress, or relationship problems. These disorders require psychotherapeutic treatment.

The other disorder of desire, sexual aversion disorder, is diagnosed in individuals who avoid sexual contact or become anxious when confronted with a

KEY FACTS: GENDER IDENTITY DISORDERS

Description
A disorder in which someone feels that they are, or should be, a member of the opposite sex.

Causes
Thought to be a neurodevelopmental condition in the prenatal brain.

Risk factors
Unknown.

Symptoms
A wish or a belief expressed by a child, at between two and four years of age, that he or she belongs to the other sex. Boys may prefer female role playing and dressing in girls' clothes. Girls may refuse to wear feminine clothes, such as dresses, and reject stereotypical norms, such as playing with dolls or playing house. Adults want to change their appearance to fit in with the other gender.

Diagnosis
Evaluation of symptoms by a psychiatrist.

Treatments
Treatment is largely psycho-educational and focuses on combating the ostracism that is experienced by children who have an identity disorder. Separation anxiety is also a problem that is addressed through treatment.

Pathogenesis
The disorder can emerge when the person is a child or it may not present itself until the person is adult.

Prevention
There is no known way of preventing gender identity disorders.

Epidemiology
Because many cases are not reported, in the mistaken belief that a child will grow out of wanting to change gender, it is not known how many people have this condition. It is estimated that transsexualism occurs in 1 in 30,000 genetic males and 1 in 100,000 females.

sexual situation. This dysfunction is usually caused by emotional problems. In women it can result from a previous traumatic incident such as rape or incest. In men it may reflect guilt about sexuality if the individual has a family background in which sexual behavior was considered shameful.

The disorder ranges in intensity from mild to severe. Therapy is aimed at unmasking the cause of the disorder and tailoring therapeutic interventions to extinguish conditioned responses. Without treatment, disorders of desire may persist for a lifetime.

Disorders of arousal

This class of disorders is characterized by an inability to attain the pleasurable sensation and accompanying physiological accommodation that is required for sexual activity. Female sexual arousal disorder is characterized by a lack of adequate vaginal lubrication. Male erectile disorder is the inability to maintain an erection to complete sexual activity. These disorders, which often result from fears about sexual performance or depression, need to be distinguished from those caused by medical problems.

Treatment for arousal disorders begins with a complete sexual history to determine the cause of the disorder. Many cases of infertility occur in marriages where disorders of arousal prevent insemination.

Following normal arousal, some women may be persistently unable to reach orgasm. If this causes personal distress or relationship problems, female orgasmic disorder is diagnosed. This appears to be more prevalent in younger women and may be lifelong. For men, an inability or recurrent delay in reaching orgasm may be situational.

Premature ejaculation refers to orgasm and ejaculation in men that occurs with little sexual stimulation and before the person is ready. It is thought to be caused by both psychological and physiological factors. Some men have this problem early in life but then learn to delay orgasm. Good therapeutic outcomes for premature ejaculation have been reported with certain types of antidepressant medications that target serotonin receptors.

Another category of sexual dysfunction, sexual pain disorder, is characterized by pain that occurs during sexual intercourse. Dyspareunia refers to genital pain, ranging from mild to severe. Little is known about sexual pain disorder or its cause. In men, the cause is usually a physical one, although in rare cases, there can be a psychological cause. If no physical problem can be discovered, such as prostate infection,

then it is presumed to be a symptom of guilt about sexual behavior.

Vaginismus is a condition in which females involuntarily contract the muscles surrounding the vagina, so that they go into painful spasms. This can happen before or after penetration, which, in mild cases, causes tightness and discomfort, and, in severe cases, prevents penetration. The disorder usually has a sudden onset and may follow a sexual trauma (such as abuse or rape) or a first gynecological exam. Vaginal inflammation can lead to vaginismus because intercourse is painful. If not treated by teaching the patient techniques to relax the paravagina muscles, the disorder can persist for a lifetime.

Disorders of sexual desire or sexual arousal can also result from medical conditions, certain prescription drugs, intoxication, or substance abuse.

Paraphilias

Paraphilias are conditions in which a person fantasizes or acts out a sexual desire that is atypical, extreme, or inappropriate. The focus of the paraphilia can be an object, children, or other nonconsenting participants, or the suffering or humiliation of oneself or a partner. The paraphilias cause personal distress, relationship problems, or constitute criminal activity. For some, images of the arousing topic are necessary for sexual activity. Others with paraphilias can sometimes function sexually without the paraphiliac stimulation. The object or stimulus may be very specific. Some people hire prostitutes to act out fantasies, or own collections of objects that they find sexually arousing.

As people generally do not admit to having paraphilias, the disorders are much more prevalent than can be deduced from estimates taken from medical or legal settings. It is not known what causes paraphilias to develop, but they usually begin in early adolescence and tend to be lifelong. Stress may increase the intensity of the paraphilia. These disorders are almost never diagnosed in women. The most common of the paraphilias are listed here.

Exhibitionism describes the exposure of the genitals to an unwitting stranger, typically a female or a child, although no attempt at sexual activity with the stranger is involved. For the exhibitionist, the thought of startling or shocking the observer is sexually arousing. This behavior usually begins in the mid-twenties. Exhibitionists comprise about 30 percent of criminal sex offenders. The behavior is chronic, and many exhibitionists have been arrested multiple times.

Fetishism is a disorder in which a person focuses on

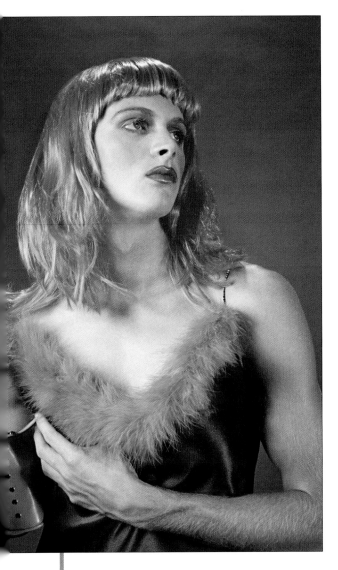

A young man is made up as a woman and dressed in a woman's clothes for his performance on stage as a transvestite artist. Men who entertain in this way at cabarets and discotheques are often called drag queens.

an object in order to generate sexual arousal. The object or "fetish" is typically an item of women's clothing, such as an apron, underpants, shoes, or boots. Men with such fetishes often need a partner to wear the garment in order to engage in sexual activity. Fetishism is chronic, and the object that is the focus has a special meaning to the individual, perhaps dating back to early childhood.

Frotteurism is a paraphilia wherein an individual derives sexual gratification from rubbing against or fondling a stranger. These acts usually occur in crowd-ed places, such as a subway or theater, where a quick escape is possible. This paraphilia typically develops at puberty and wanes in adulthood.

Pedophilia refers to the desire to engage in sexual activity with a child. The pedophile can be attracted to boys or girls, or both, and usually prefers preteens. The range of activities in which the pedophile engages or fantasizes about varies. For some, it may consist of looking at naked children, or exposing themselves, or both, to a child while masturbating. Other pedophiles use force to engage in sexual acts with children. Treatment for this disorder is multifaceted and may involve court-mandated administration of anti-androgenic substances to reduce sexual arousal patterns.

Sexual masochism is a paraphilia in which pain or humiliation and the psychological or physical suffering that ensues create sexual excitement. For some, this may only involve fantasizing about being overpowered during sex. Such fantasies develop early, often in childhood.

However, for others, sexual masochism involves aggressive acts undertaken alone or with a partner. These can include enlisting someone to shock them, whip them, clothe them in diapers, urinate on them, or perform other demeaning or abusive acts. Individuals with this disorder repeat the same masochistic act. Injuries and deaths have occurred as a result of acting out such urges.

Sexual sadism is a chronic disorder that usually begins in early adulthood. With this disorder, a person derives sexual pleasure from inflicting abuse or pain on someone else. In some cases, the partner may be a sexual masochist who consents to the abuse. However, if the partner is nonconsenting, he or she may be injured or killed as a result of the attack. Individuals who attack nonconsenting victims tend to escalate the intensity of the pain they inflict over time, until they are apprehended.

Transvestic fetishism is an urge by a heterosexual male to wear women's clothing and fantasize that he is a female during a sex act. Some men have a cache of clothes that they keep for this purpose; others may use a single item of clothing, such as female undergarments. The behavior usually first appears at puberty and may vary in intensity throughout a lifetime.

For some men, the condition becomes less erotic after puberty, but still creates the desired feeling of tension reduction. Men who cross-dress do not necessarily have other psychiatric problems or seek treatment; they may have spouses who are comfortable with the behavior. For others, however, the feeling may escalate into gender identity disorder, a desire to be a member of the opposite sex.

Voyeurism, often referred to as "peeping," is diagnosed when, in order to create sexual arousal, a man must engage in spying on unsuspecting persons who are either undressing or having sex. Voyeurism usually begins in adolescence or early adulthood. It often results in arrest.

Gender identity disorder

The condition of gender identity disorder is differentiated from gender issues that arise in intersexed persons (who are born with some aspects of both sexes, anatomically or hormonally). Cultures differ in what they deem as appropriate for males and females. Persons who stray from the cultural guidelines are considered gender nonconforming. But gender nonconformity does not constitute gender dysphoria, that is, the belief that one would be better suited as a member of the opposite sex or the feeling that one is "trapped in the wrong body."

Gender identity disorder in children

Children who show distress about being a boy or a girl usually alarm their parents. The first evidence of their gender-variant behavior usually appears between two and four years of age. These children state a wish to be a member of, or the belief that they belong to, the other sex.

For boys, female role-playing and dressing up in girls' clothing is a preferred activity. They avoid rough-and-tumble play, and choose girls as playmates.

Girls with the disorder may state that they will grow a penis. They refuse to wear dresses or engage in any gender-stereotypical activities, such as playing with dolls or playing house.

Gender identity disorder in childhood is rare, and experts do not know how frequently it occurs. Since many parents think the behavior is just a "phase" that the child will outgrow, and few clinics treat this condition, many children with the disorder never come to the attention of professionals. About 75 percent will grow up to have a homosexual orientation but will not have gender identity disorder in adulthood.

Treatment for children who do present to professionals is largely psycho-educational and involves the parents, who can help the child counteract the ostracism that inevitably accompanies this disorder. These children often have other problems, such as separation anxiety. This manifests as feelings of great distress when a child is separated from his or her parents for any reason. The symptoms are holding onto the parent and crying. This behavior is common until the age of about four years, but it diminishes after that. In separation anxiety disorder, the child exhibits clinging behavior that is not usual for the age of the child. Physical symptoms can ensue, such as problems sleeping and headaches. Separation anxiety is addressed during treatment.

Gender identity disorder in adults

With adults, gender identity disorder may have started in childhood. These individuals are preoccupied with changing their appearance to reduce the incongruence between the gender with which they identify and aspire to and the body and sexual gender into which they were born.

Men who want to be women and women who want to be men have existed throughout history and are often referred to as transsexuals. It is estimated that transsexualism occurs in 1 in 30,000 genetic males and 1 in 100,000 females. Some experts believe that the disorder is caused, at least in part, by a neurodevelopmental condition in the prenatal brain.

Psychotherapy alone is not effective in reversing a cross-gender identity. In severe cases of gender identity disorder, a person may be eligible for a program of hormones and genital surgery to reassign the gender.

Some men have a less severe degree of the disorder, wishing to remain male while they occasionally appear as female. These individuals may not be interested in genital surgery, but may desire some feminizing procedures, such as beard removal, to eliminate secondary sex characteristics and avoid detection when appearing in public. Cross-dressers, as such men are called, tend to experience an intensification of the cross-gender longings when they are under stress, or following a major loss or trauma in life. If such urges are accompanied by erotic arousal and masturbation, then a diagnosis of transvestic fetishism is made. If the motive for appearing feminine comes from a desire to express one's sense of a female identity and is not erotically focused, then a diagnosis of gender identity disorder is appropriate.

Randi Ettner

See also
- Childhood disorders • Genetic disorders
- Health care • Hormonal disorders
- Intersexuality • Prostate disorders
- Sleep disorders

Sexually transmitted diseases

Sexually transmitted diseases, or STDs, are a diverse group of infections caused by different pathogens and a major public health issue in the United States and the world. Sometimes called STIs, for "sexually transmitted infections," they are grouped together because of the way they are spread, which is usually through intimate sexual contact. The risk of contracting an STD can be reduced by having fewer sexual partners and adopting safe sex practices.

In some cases, like gonorrhea, sexual transmission is the primary way the infection is spread; in hepatitis B virus and HIV, sexual transmission is just one of the ways the infections can be spread (sharing needles used for intravenous drug use is another way). The Centers for Disease Control and Prevention (CDC) estimates that each year in the United States there are 19 million new STD infections, almost half of them in young people 15 to 24 years of age. Many of these infections are caused by bacteria and can be cured with antibiotics. Other infections, such as genital herpes and HIV (the virus that causes AIDS), are caused by viruses and cannot be cured; they may only be controlled with medication. The overall results in the United States are health and psychological consequences and direct medical costs, which amount to $13 billion every year.

In the United States, some STDs, such as syphilis, gonorrhea, and chlamydia, are "nationally reportable diseases"; health professionals are required to notify designated agencies when a patient has the infection. This information is collected and used to study local and national disease trends and help public health officials decide how to target funds, interventions, and new treatments that may help decrease infection, disease rates, and long-term health consequences.

Other STDs, for example genital herpes, more commonly caused by herpes simplex viruses, and genital warts, caused by human papilloma virus (HPV), are not nationally reportable diseases, but information can be gathered about them through family planning clinics, clinics that specialize in treating STDs, and other health care centers, to help estimate their frequency. Whether diseases are "reportable" or not, many cases go unreported, so the actual number of cases of all STDs is much higher than those reported.

Overview

Worldwide, STDs, including HIV infection, are increasing and have a major impact on health care systems. Women, especially adolescents, are at greater risk for STDs because many women can remain without symptoms while infected. They can unknowingly spread the infection and can develop long-term complications.

STD rates are generally higher in urban areas marked by poverty and low socioeconomic status, where there is more illicit drug use, limited access to health care, and prostitution. Because certain race and ethnic groups are more frequently associated with inner city populations and poverty, some rates of STDs are higher for these groups.

In the United States, African Americans and Hispanics have higher rates of gonorrhea and syphilis than in non-Hispanic whites; and African American women are more likely than white women to develop complications of some diseases, such as pelvic inflammatory disease (PID).

Chlamydia, caused by the bacterium *Chlamydia trachomatis*, and gonorrhea caused by the bacterium *Neisseria gonorrheae*, are the two most commonly reported infections in the United States. More than 900,000 cases of chlamydia are reported, but the CDC estimates that the actual number of cases is about 2.8 million; and 330,000 cases of gonorrhea (CDC estimates the actual number is twice that) were reported in 2004. Both of these bacteria can silently and repeatedly infect the female reproductive tract. Left untreated, these infections can progress to pelvic inflammatory disease, causing inflammation and scarring in the fallopian tubes (tubes through which the egg moves on the way from the ovary to the uterus), infertility, chronic pelvic pain, and ectopic pregnancy (a pregnancy found not in the uterus, but elsewhere, for example in a fallopian tube. In men, untreated chlamydia and gonorrhea can sometimes lead to painful inflammation in the testicles called epididymitis, and in some cases it can cause infertility.

The sexually transmitted infections syphilis, herpes simplex, and chancroid are frequently grouped together and called genital ulcer diseases (GUD), because at some stage of infection they each can cause ulcers, or deep sores, in the genital area. In the United States, herpes simplex virus is the most common cause of genital ulcer disease. Genital sores from syphilis, caused by the very motile bacteria *Treponema pallidum*, are usually painless. Genital sores caused by herpes virus and chancroid, usually a localized infection (although about 50 percent of untreated infections result in a painful infection of lymph glands in the groin) caused by the bacterium *Hemophilus ducreyi* and treatable with antibiotics, are usually painful. In some cases more than one of these microbes can be present in a genital ulcer, so clinical exam and symptoms may not be enough to identify the microbe responsible for the sore. Diagnostic tests for genital ulcer disease include blood test and visual examination (darkfield examination or direct immunofluorescence test) for *Treponema pallidum*; culture or blood test for the antigen to herpes simplex; and culture for *Hemophilus ducreyi*. In all three of these genital ulcer diseases there is also an increased risk of HIV transmission. Left untreated, many STDs

can result in chronic and severe health problems. In syphilis the usually painless sores may be ignored by the infected individual and progress from the primary to the secondary stage. Both stages are highly contagious but easily curable with antibiotics if diagnosed. Untreated, syphilis can cause long-term complications, including nerve and heart damage. *T. pallidum* can be passed from a pregnant woman in utero, causing stillbirth, death of the infant after birth, deformities, and neurological complications in the newborn. Untreated chlamydia and gonorrhea infections can lead to pelvic inflammatory disease (PID). In the case of chronic hepatitis B or hepatitis C infections, the long-term result may be cirrhosis or liver cancer; and in the case of untreated gential warts from human papilloma virus infection, cervical cancer.

Trichomoniasis is the most common curable STD in young sexually active women. It is caused by the single-celled protozoan parasite *Trichomonas vaginalis* and is more common in women than in men. Symptoms in women can range from none to severe vaginal itching and redness with a frothy green vaginal discharge; in men there may be no symptoms or burning while urinating. On pelvic examination the cervix and vaginal walls may have red sores. The infection is commonly diagnosed by collecting a sample from the infected site and examining the sample on a slide under a microscope for the parasite, or sending a sample for culture. It is treatable with medication. Pregnant women with trichomoniasis can have premature or low birth-weight babies.

Preventing STDs

All people who are sexually active are at risk for STDs. The main way to prevent exposure to the pathogens responsible for these diseases is through a strategy called primary prevention. This strategy aims to change high-risk sexual behavior before the infection has the opportunity to be transmitted, so infection never occurs. STD prevention education can be tailored to individuals and their personal risk factors (multiple sex partners, not using latex condoms correctly and consistently, early onset sexual activity in adolescence, living in an area with high STD rates, and use of intravenous and other drugs) and includes practical information. The most reliable way to prevent STDs would be to abstain from sexual intercourse altogether; this includes oral, anal, and vaginal sex. Ways to decrease the likelihood of contracting an STD from another person include not having sex with multiple sex partners, and not having sex with someone who has multiple sex partners; however, this strategy would only decrease the risk, not guarantee prevention. If a sex partner is infected or being treated for an STD, abstinence is recommended until both the individual and the partner have been fully treated and tested. In general, both partners should be tested for STDs and HIV before beginning a sexual relationship. A latex condom provides some, but not complete, protection against STDs and should always be used if a partner's STD status is unknown.

Education can occur at the individual level or through community-based efforts that target large groups. Some of these public health strategies include teaching high-risk groups to use safer sex practices; identifying and treating people infected with an SDT but who have no symptoms; identifying and treating people with symptoms but who are unlikely to seek treatment; locating and treating sex partners of people with STDs; and preventing diseases with vaccines (for example, hepatitis B, hepatitis A, and HPV) before exposure. Male latex condoms, when used effectively and consistently, are effective in preventing transmission of HIV and reducing the

risk of transmission of other STDs, including gonorrhea and chlamydia. However, condoms do not provide complete protection from all STDs because they cover only a limited area of the genitals. If there are sores from syphilis, herpes, or chancroid on parts not covered by the condom, or on the sex partner, microbes can be transmitted and cause infection. Another problem with condoms is the likelihood of breakage during sexual activity. It is estimated that 2 out of every 100 latex condoms break during intercourse. Male condoms made out of materials other than latex have higher slippage and breakage rates, according to the CDC. A new condom should be used with each sexual intercourse. Female condoms, made of a polyurethane sheet, are also an effective barrier to viruses, but effectiveness in preventing STDs is not well studied.

Chemical preparations commonly called spermicides containing nonoxynol-9 (also called N-9) are no longer recommended for preventing HIV or other STDs and may even be associated with genital sores, which can increase transmission of HIV. Women who are not at

This is a greatly magnified pubic or crab louse (Phthirus pubis)*. Lice are transmitted from one person to another by direct sexual contact and infest the pubic hair of adults and the eyelashes of affected children.*

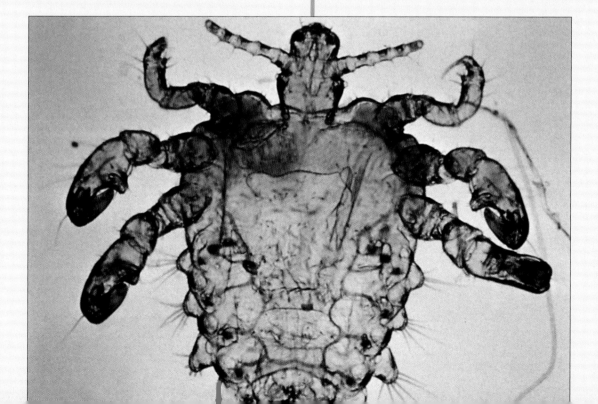

risk for pregnancy because they have been surgically sterilized, use hormonal contraception, have an IUD (intrauterine device) in place, or have had a hysterectomy are still at risk for HIV and other STDs.

Vaccine-preventable STDs

Human papilloma virus (HPV) is the most common sexually transmitted infection in the United States. Almost 50 percent of all people who have had sex will have HPV at some time during their lives. It is passed through sexual contact or skin-to-skin contact. Most people have no signs or symptoms of HPV infection, so it can easily be passed on to others unknowingly. There are different strains of HPV. Some strains of HPV cause genital warts, also known as condylomata acuminata or venereal warts, and some strains cause cervical cancer. A vaccine against strains that cause about 70 percent of cervical cancer and 90 percent of genital warts was approved for use in the United States in 2006.

Another vaccine-preventable STD is hepatitis B. In both cases, these vaccines not only prevent STD infections, they also reduce the risk of developing related cancers. HPV vaccine can prevent many cases of cervical cancer, and hepatitis B vaccine can prevent many cases of chronic HBV infections, which may progress to cirrhosis and liver cancer. In men who have sex with men, hepatitis A vaccine can reduce hepatitis A infection.

The STD-HIV Link

The presence of STDs increases the likelihood of transmitting and acquiring HIV infection, so treating STDs can help reduce the spread of HIV. People infected with an STD are up to five times more likely to become infected with HIV if a sex partner has HIV infection, according to the CDC. An HIV-infected person who also has a sexually transmitted infection is more likely to infect their sex partner with HIV than a person infected with HIV alone.

In genital ulcer diseases (syphilis, herpes, and chancroid), these ulcers, or sores, break down the protective skin or genital tract lining, leaving a portal of entry for HIV to find its way into the body. In STDs like chlamydia, gonorrhea, and trichomoniasis, there is an increased concentration of special cells that can be targets for HIV.

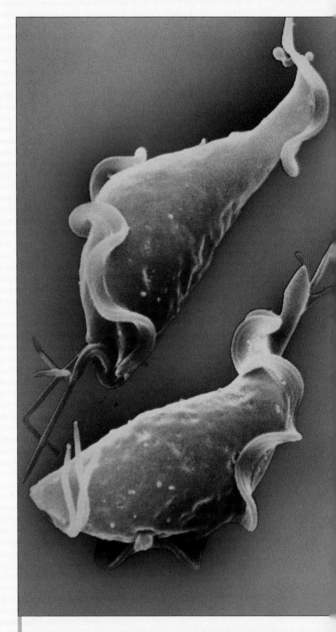

A colored scanning electron micrograph shows two parasitic protozoans of Trichomonas vaginalis. *They can infect the genito-urinary tract of both men and women causing irritation and infection in women; men usually have no symptoms.*

When HIV-infected people also have an STD, they are more likely to have HIV in the secretions in their genital secretions. Men with HIV infection and gonorrhea are twice as likely to have HIV in their genital secretions as men with only HIV infection. Men with HIV also infected with gonorrhea, for example, can have as much as 10 times the amount of HIV in their semen as men with HIV alone.

Partner notification

Partner notification identifies sex partners of those people with HIV and other STDs so that they can be tested, evaluated, and treated for STDs. Also called "contact tracing," partner notification can be used to prevent reinfection of the treated individual and may also be helpful in decreasing the spread of the infection from an untreated partner to other individuals. This can be done by the infected individual, the health care provider, or with the help of designated health agencies.

Pregnant women

The effects of an STD can be serious and even life threatening for a pregnant woman and her baby, with complications that can include early onset of labor, premature rupture of the membranes surrounding the baby in the uterus, and infection of the uterus after the baby is delivered. Infants of women with sexually transmitted infections may suffer from severe health consequences if an STD is transmitted to the developing fetus in utero (inside the uterus) or during delivery. For example, syphilis infection in the mother can cross the placenta and infect the baby in the uterus, leading to congenital syphilis. HIV can also cross the placenta and infect the baby. Chlamydia, gonorrhea, hepatitis B virus, and herpes simplex can infect the infant during the birthing process as the newborn travels through the birth canal. HIV can also infect the baby through breast-feeding.

Some of the health effects from STDs include stillbirth (baby is born dead); low birth weight (less than five pounds); eye infections from chlamydia or gonorrhea; pneumonia; sepsis (severe infection in the baby's blood); blindness; neurological damage; deafness; acute hepatitis; meningitis (infection of the membranes surrounding the brain); and liver disease.

In the United States, STDs infect about 800,000 pregnant women each year, according to the CDC. About 200,000 pregnant women have chlamydial infection, 80,000 have trichomoniasis, 40,000 have gonorrhea, 40,000 hepatitis B, 8,000 have HIV, and 8,000 have syphilis. To identify and treat STDs and reduce health risks for the mother and baby, it is

recommended that at the first prenatal visit, a pregnant woman and her sex partners are counseled on the health dangers associated with STDs. The pregnant woman should be offered a voluntary HIV test, a blood test for syphilis, a blood test for hepatitis B infection, and tests for chlamydia and gonorrhea. If a woman is at risk, she should also have a blood test for hepatitis C infection. She should also have a Pap smear if one has not been done within the preceding year.

Some of these tests may be performed again later in the pregnancy, especially if the woman has multiple sex partners or another risk for HIV or other STDs. Many STDs, like syphilis, gonorrhea, and chlamydia, detected during pregnancy can be treated. Partner notification may also help prevent infections that might be transmitted to newborns, like congenital syphilis, chlamydia eye infection, and chlamydia pneumonia, of untreated female partners.

Adolescents

Rates of some STDs are highest during the adolescent years because young people frequently have unprotected intercourse, are less likely to seek medical attention, and have frequent short relationships. Reported rates of chlamydia, gonorrhea, and HPV rates are highest in young women aged 15 to 19 years. HPV can also be transmitted during the teen years. In recent years, the recommendation has been to vaccinate all children with the hepatitis B vaccine to help prevent the possibility of sexual transmission of the infection during adolescence and later.

In the United States, most adolescents can consent to confidential diagnosis and medical treatment without parental consent or knowledge. In many states, this includes HIV testing.

Men who have sex with men (MSM)

Some of this population is at high risk for HIV and other STDs. Recent data have suggested that increasing numbers of MSM are involved in high-risk behavior that may help transmit HIV as well as other STDs. This population is also at risk for sexual transmission of both hepatitis A and hepatitis B, so the vaccines for both are recommended.

Ramona Jenkin

Shock

Shock is a life-threatening state of an inadequate volume of blood circulating around the body. There is insufficient delivery of oxygen and nutrients to body tissues. There are four major categories of shock: cardiogenic, hypovolemic, distributive, and obstructive.

Cardiogenic shock is caused by the failure of the heart to pump effectively. Hypovolemic shock involves loss of fluid, usually blood. Septic, anaphylactic, and neurogenic shock are types of distributive shock, characterized by insufficient circulating volume due to vasodilation and leaky capillaries. Obstructive shock is caused by conditions that prevent blood flow to or from the heart. Sepsis is caused by overwhelming infection. Anaphylaxis results from severe allergic reactions; neurogenic shock is a consequence of spinal cord damage. In cardiac tamponade, fluid fills the sac around the heart. In tension pneumothorax, air progressively accumulates between the lung and chest wall. A blood clot obstructs lung vessels in pulmonary embolism. Hardening and narrowing of the aortic valve leads to aortic stenosis. Endocrine shock can result from thyroid dysfunction or adrenal insufficiency.

All forms of shock can result in dry mouth, rapid respiration, restlessness, hypothermia, hypotension, unconsciousness, and low urine output. In hypovolemic shock there is a faint, rapid pulse with cool, clammy skin. In cardiogenic and obstructive shock there may be distended neck veins from fluid backup. In septic shock there may be fever and warm extremities. In neurogenic shock there may be a normal or low heart rate and paralysis. In anaphylactic shock there may be rash, breathlessness, and airway swelling.

A careful history and physical exam are essential to recognize the type of shock. Ancillary testing and treatment depend on the causes of shock. Most forms of shock require intravenous fluids, then medications to support blood pressure. A breathing tube may be needed to support respiration. Chest pain, palpitations, and shortness of breath suggest cardiogenic shock. A myocardial infarction needs clot-breaking medication or angioplasty. A cardiac valve may need surgical repair. Profuse bleeding and major trauma suggest hypovolemic shock; blood replacement and surgery are indicated to stop the bleeding. Fever and infection suggest septic shock, requiring antibiotics. An insect sting or allergen exposure with airway swelling indicates anaphylactic shock, calling for antihistamines, steroids, and epinephrine. Paralysis after trauma suggests neurogenic shock. Tension pneumothorax requires needle decompression, then a chest tube. Cardiac tamponade necessitates fluid drainage from the pericardium by a needle or catheter. Massive pulmonary embolism may require clot-breaking medications or surgical clot removal.

There are four stages of shock: initial, compensatory, progressive, and refractory. Initially the lack of oxygen leads to anaerobic metabolism and metabolic acidosis, then hyperventilation and adrenaline release attempt to compensate for the hypoxia and hypotension. Elevated heart rate, low urine output, and cool extremities ensue as the body struggles to maintain blood flow to critical organs. In progressive shock, there is inadequate blood flow to vital organs, acid-base balance is disturbed, and fluid accumulates peripherally. In refractory shock, vital organs fail, and shock is no longer reversible. Brain damage will be present, and death is imminent. The outcome of shock depends on the cause and concurrent problems. Hypovolemic, anaphylactic, neurogenic, obstructive, and endocrine shock respond to treatment in their early stages. Septic shock has a mortality rate of 30 to 50 percent. The prognosis of cardiogenic shock is worse.

Medley O'Keefe Gatewood

KEY FACTS

Description
Hypoperfusion of bodily tissues and organs.

Causes
Cardiogenic, hypovolemic, distributive, obstructive, and endocrine.

Signs
Hypotension, hyperventilation, altered consciousness, low urine output.

Diagnosis
History and clinical exam.

Treatment
Varies with the type of shock.

Pathogenesis
All are treatable early, except for cardiogenic and septic shock, which carry a grave prognosis.

See also
• Brain disorders • Cardiovascular disorders

Sick building syndrome

Sick building syndrome describes a disorder in which individuals experience acute problems with their health or well-being that are associated with the amount of time spent in a particular building, but no specific illness or cause can be identified.

Sick building syndrome is characterized by symptoms that affects clusters of people from the same building. The symptoms will improve or disappear once the affected individuals leave the building. Investigators often believe that inadequate ventilation is the cause of sick building syndrome. This may occur when HVAC (heating, ventilation, and air conditioning) systems do not bring enough fresh air into the building. Designed to conserve energy, some buildings have HVAC systems that introduce only one-third of the recommended amount of fresh air. Another possible cause may be chemical contaminants that come from either indoor or outdoor sources. These may come from adhesives, carpets, furniture, copy machines, pesticides, cleaning agents, and volatile organic compounds. Environmental tobacco smoke and products of combustion (usually from furnaces) may also be part of the problem. Other sources may include motor vehicle exhaust, plumbing vents, and smells from kitchens or shops in the building.

Biological contaminants such as bacteria, mold, pollen, and viruses may also be factors. In many cases, sick building syndrome affects the entire building, but in other locations, it will affect only certain parts of the building.

The World Health Organization states that up to 30 percent of new and remodeled buildings around the world may cause occupants to complain of sick building syndrome. Some studies suggest that psychosocial factors may be equally or more important than the physical factors present in the building. For example, one study showed a relationship between the presence of sick building symptoms and both psychosocial stress at work and the amount of control over one's work environment. This study suggested that such factors as the inability to open the windows or control humidity or temperature lead to an increased incidence of symptoms. There was also a direct correlation between the amount of on-the-job stress and the prevalence of symptoms.

The symptoms of sick building syndrome include: headaches; eye, nose, and throat irritation; dry cough; dry or itchy skin; dizziness; nausea; difficulty in concentrating; fatigue; and sensitivity to odors. These problems usually improve when the person leaves the building. Sick building syndrome can be difficult to resolve, since engineers and building managers must focus on the building and not on the patient. Managers may replace water-damaged carpet and ceilings or eliminate any mold. They may prohibit smoking and improve ventilation where there are adhesives, paint, or solvents. Repairing HVAC systems or increasing ventilation rates will help. Some building owners have added high-performance air cleaners to their HVAC systems. Open communications with the building occupants are needed to educate them about efforts to resolve the situation.

Richard N. Bradley

KEY FACTS

Description
People in buildings are sick for no known reason.

Causes
Unclear, but it may be poor building ventilation, contaminants, or workplace stress.

Risk Factors
Working in large, energy-efficient buildings.

Symptoms
Headache, eye, nose, or throat irritation, cough, dry or itchy skin, dizziness, nausea, difficulty concentrating, fatigue, and sensitivity to odors.

Diagnosis
Elimination of other possible causes of symptoms.

Treatments
Increased ventilation, air cleaning, removal of pollutant source, education, and communication.

Pathogenesis
Unknown.

Prevention
Careful construction of new buildings.

Epidemiology
One in five workers may have some symptoms.

See also
- Allergy and sensitivity • Infections, fungal
- Infections, viral • Throat infections

Sickle-cell anemia

Sickle-cell anemia (SCA) is a severe genetic illness characterized by the production of sickle-shaped blood cells because of an abnormality of hemoglobin (HbS), leading to chronic anemia and vaso-occlusive crises.

SCA follows an autosomal-recessive mode of inheritance. The parents are usually unaffected carriers of the abnormal gene. Couples in which both partners carry the sickle-cell trait have a 25 percent probability of conceiving a child (heterozygote) with SCA.

Risk factors and symptoms

Certain risk factors for SCA have been identified; most important is the percentage contribution of sickle-cell hemoglobin (HbS) in the blood.

Patients with SCA have moderate to severe anemia, although red cell volume is generally normal. Many SCA patients suffer from chronic bone pain. The most common clinical presentation of SCA is a sickle-cell crisis: the blocking of small blood vessels, caused by sickle-shaped red cells clumping together. Occlusion of capillaries leads to painful microinfarcts (obstructions). Common sites include bone, spleen, and lung, the latter resulting in a dramatic acute chest crisis. There is another possible complication in younger children, in which the spleen acutely pools large volumes of blood (splenic sequestration syndrome), causing a drop in hemoglobin levels and circulatory failure. A feared sequel of SCA is stroke, which can occur at any age. Severe systemic infections with encapsulated bacteria, as a result of impaired function of the spleen and salmonella osteomyelitis (favored by dead areas in bone), are a significant problem.

Diagnosis and treatments

The diagnosis is made from a blood sample by hemoglobin (Hb) electrophoresis. In this assay, the different Hb species are separated in a gel based on their electrical charge. Instead of the normal HbA band, SCA patients have HbS. Bone marrow studies show increased erythropoiesis (production of red blood cells).

The mainstay of SCA treatment is pain control and prevention of sickle cell crises and other severe aftereffects of SCA. Behavioral recommendations aim at prevention of hypoxia (lack of oxygen to the body's tissues) by avoidance of cold environments, high altitude and overexertion, and prevention of dehydration, by maintaining high fluid intake, particularly during febrile illnesses, hot weather, or exercise. Parents are taught to check the spleen in their young children for enlargement. Daily folate is recommended for all patients. All patients should receive immunizations against encapsulated bacteria (*Streptococcus pneumoniae*, *Hemophilus influenzae* type B, and *Neisseria meningitides*). Children up to 5 years of age also receive daily

KEY FACTS

Description
Chronic anemia and recurrent painful crises due to inborn defect of hemoglobin.

Causes
Inheritance as an autosomal recessive trait.

Risk factors
The sickle cell mutation is prevalent in equatorial Africa, the Mediterranean, the Middle East, and India. In the U.S., 95 percent of sickle-cell anemia patients are African American.

Symptoms
Chronic anemia and pain, acute painful "sickle cell crises," splenic sequestration syndrome, bacterial sepsis, chronic organ damage (spleen, kidney, heart, eye), leg ulcers, stroke.

Diagnosis
Blood test; hemoglobin electrophoresis.

Treatments
Folate, pain medication, hydroxyurea, prevention of infections and sickle-cell crises, erythrocyte transfusion, bone marrow transplantation, induction of fetal hemoglobin, experimental therapies.

Pathogenesis
Anemia results from decreased life span of sickle-shaped red blood cells, which occlude capillaries and block oxygen and nutrient supply. The result is pain and tissue infarction.

Prevention
Neonatal screening for hemoglobin diseases is performed in most federal states. Prenatal diagnosis is possible. Prevention of crises uses behavioral and pharmacological measures.

Epidemiology
In African Americans in the United States, the frequency is approximately 1 in 600 newborns. More than 70,000 people in the United States are afflicted with sickle-cell disease.

prophylactic penicillin. Low doses of the cancer drug hydroxyurea halve the amount of pain and the frequency of hospitalizations, reduce the number of blood transfusions, and elevate the amount of hemoglobin in the blood, with generally few adverse effects. The mechanism of action is not clear, but induction of fetal hemoglobin may play a role. Sickle-cell clinics address the specific medical needs of these patients.

Acute pain crises require treatment with strong analgesics, generally morphine or derivatives, alone or with anti-inflammatory agents. Oxygen is administered to patients with compromised respiratory function. Bacterial infections can take a more severe course in SCA patients and require aggressive treatment. Antibiotics and intravenous fluids are often required. Patients with severe anemia, with aplastic crises (lack of development of blood cells), and with splenic sequestration syndrome require red blood cell transfusions. Regular transfusions are indicated for individuals at high risk for cerebral stroke.

Bone marrow transplantation is the only cure for SCA. Because of its toxicity, transplantation is currently reserved for high-risk people who have an optimal donor, usually a matched but healthy sibling. Gene therapy is considered a potential emerging cure for SCA; studies are ongoing.

Pathogenesis

Normal hemoglobin is a molecule made up of four protein subunits, two alpha chains and two beta chains. A mutation of the beta globin gene leads to replacement of the amino acid glutamine for valine. This forms hemoglobin S, called HbS rather than the normal HbA. HbS is principally functional, in that it is stable and can carry oxygen. However, HbS molecules form large homopolymers in red cells, and cells containing such HbS aggregates are misshapen. Instead of the normal donut shape, they assume a sickle shape. Some sickle cells are present at all times and are removed by the spleen, leading to decreased erythrocyte survival (10 to 20 days, as opposed to 120 days for normal cells) and anemia. Under conditions of decreased oxygen tension (high altitude, cold, increased oxygen consumption due to exercise or fever) or dehydration, critical numbers of sickle erythrocytes form at the same time, resulting in vaso-occlusive pain crises: the abnormally shaped erythrocytes cannot squeeze through capillary blood vessels. Instead, they clog the capillaries or damage the vessel lining, or both, leading to sticking of inflammatory cells, which contributes to blockage of capillaries. Areas of tissue behind the oc-

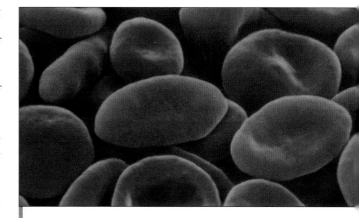

The shape of red blood cells in sickle-cell anemia changes; the normal cells are red and the distorted cells are shown in green. They become fragile and take on a sickle shape.

clusion are deprived of oxygen and nutrients, resulting in tissue death (infarct) and pain. Sickle cells chronically damage kidneys, heart, spleen, bone, skin, eyes, brain, and essentially any other organ in the body.

Prevention and epidemiology

All individuals should be informed about their carrier status prior to making reproductive choices. Genetic counseling is advised for couples in which both partners carry pathological hemoglobin genes. Prenatal diagnostic is possible.

In the United States, 95 percent of SCA patients are African American. In this population, the heterozygote frequency is approximately 1 in 12, and 1 in 600 children is born with SCA. Thus over 70,000 people in the United States are affected by SCA and other, rarer sickle-cell diseases. In some West African countries, more than 1 in 50 children are born with SCA. The high frequency of the mutation may be due to the fact that erythrocytes containing HbS are resistant to malaria. The survival advantage from malaria resistance must have been enormous, since endemic malaria drove Darwinian selection of HbS carriers despite the fact that HbS homozygotes used to die early in infancy. In the United States, which has no malaria, sickle-cell trait is not advantageous, and HbS heterozygote frequency in the United States is decreasing.

Halvard Boenig

See also
- Anemia • Blindness • Blood disorders
- Liver and spleen disorders • Malaria
- Stroke and related disorders • Thalassemia

SIDS

Sudden infant death syndrome (SIDS) is the abrupt and unexpected death of an infant less than one year of age that remains unexplained after a thorough investigation, including performance of a complete autopsy, review of the circumstances of death, and the clinical history. SIDS (also called crib death) is the leading cause of infant mortality between one month and one year of age in the United States. Many factors have been associated with an increased risk of SIDS, including the infant's sleeping position and exposure to tobacco smoke.

Each year, more than 4,500 infants in the United States die suddenly with no evidence of an obvious cause. This sudden and apparently unexplained loss of life in a normal-appearing infant can be difficult for the baby's parents and family to deal with. A great amount of emotional energy is spent trying to find any clue that would suggest a reason for this loss of life, with parents blaming themselves, their partners, or other caregivers, such as baby sitters. Fortunately, the rate of fatal child abuse (filicide) represents only a minority of these cases when fully evaluated.

The current rate of SIDS in the United States is less than 1 in 1,000 live births. This rate represents a significant decrease in the rate of SIDS and is related to lower rates of maternal smoking during pregnancy, but it is mainly a result of the Back-to-Sleep program. In 1992 the American Academy of Pediatrics issued a recommendation that infants always be placed on their back for sleeping. This measure, along with increasing public awareness campaigns, has minimized the incidence of this devastating problem for families.

About 90 percent of SIDS cases occur before 6 months of age. The median age at death is 11 weeks, with a peak incidence between 2 to 4 months. Interestingly, in premature infants, the median age is 4 to 6 weeks sooner than in full-term infants, using postconception dating criteria. This unique distribution suggests that critical stages of development or maturation after birth are more likely to lead to SIDS. A recent multicenter study by National Institute of Child Health and Human Development concluded that there are no strong predictors that would permit screening for infants at high-risk for SIDS. But numerous similarities between infants succumbing to SIDS have been noted.

Causes and risk factors

The association between exposure to tobacco smoke and SIDS has been known since the 1950s. But public awareness campaigns of this fact have been slow until recently. Maternal smoking during pregnancy and tobacco smoke exposure in the home or day care environment increase the risk of SIDS two- to fourfold. This risk of SIDS appears to increase with the amount of tobacco smoke to which the child is exposed. This finding has led many researchers and educators to label tobacco use one of the most current preventable risk factors for SIDS.

Many infants dying of SIDS have been found when they did not wake up, leading researchers to investigate napping and nighttime rest for possible causes. Co-sleeping, the bed and bedding, and clothing have been implicated in numerous studies. Prone (sleeping on the stomach) or side sleeping (particularly in an infant unaccustomed to sleeping on his or her side or stomach) has an increased risk of SIDS. Although babies need to lie on their stomach to strengthen the shoulder girdle, this position should only be allowed when the child is awake and someone is available to watch the baby.

Co-sleeping involves parents or other siblings sleeping in the same space as the infant. The concern is that the larger person would roll on top of or pull bedding over an infant who could not pull them out of the way, leading to suffocation of the infant. Conflicting studies have been noted between parents co-sleeping with the infant in bed, although the risk appears greatest while co-sleeping on a couch or sofa. The risk of SIDS is lower when the infant sleeps in a separate bed in the parent's room, but this reduced risk is not seen when sharing another sibling's room in different beds.

Likewise, the surface the infant sleeps on or clothing has been implicated in SIDS deaths. Soft sleep surfaces, such as soft mattresses, sheepskin, or polystyrene-filled cushions, have all been associated with a twofold increased risk of SIDS. The crib, or cradle, should always be kept clear of soft objects such as pillows and stuffed toys. Overheating the room in which the infant sleeps should be avoided by maintaining the room temperature at a comfortable level for a lightly clothed infant (65°F–68°F; 18.3°C–20°C). Infants should not sleep in the direct sunlight or near a source of heat such as a heater or radiator. A sixfold increased rate of SIDS has been reported in certain Northern Plains Native American communities when two or more layers of clothing are used on sleeping infants.

Other factors that have been associated with SIDS include gestational age, birth weight, and ethnicity. Preterm infants have a three- to fourfold increased risk of SIDS compared to infants born at term. Low birth weight or growth-restricted infants also are noted to have a higher risk of SIDS. African Americans and Native Americans have a two- to threefold higher rate of SIDS compared to Caucasian people in the United States.

The role of genetics in the cause of SIDS is unclear. The risk of SIDS in fellow siblings is noted to represent a five to six times increased incidence (this still totals less than 1 percent using current prevention strategies). The identification of certain gene polymorphisms (different types of the same gene) in certain SIDS cases would suggest a possible genetic role, but the low incidence of SIDS in both twins and the lack of difference in the rate of SIDS between same sex and different sex twins suggest that genetics may play a lesser role as a cause of these unexplained deaths.

Many other factors have been evaluated as risk factors or causes of SIDS. Maternal drug abuse during and after pregnancy has been associated with a fivefold increase in the risk. Sleep apnea—a sleeping disorder in which a person transiently stops breathing—is more commonly seen in premature infants. The Collaborative study from the National Institutes of Health (NIH) on SIDS showed a slightly higher percentage of mothers with infants that died from SIDS recalling an episode of the baby turning blue compared to control infants. Immunizations and pacifier use have not been associated with an increased risk of SIDS and may actually decrease the risks in infants during the first year of life.

Symptoms and diagnosis

SIDS cases need to be differentiated from other causes of infant death that can mimic or are similar to unexpected demise in an otherwise normal and healthy appearing baby. Other causes of death that need to be

KEY FACTS

Description

Sudden infant death syndrome (SIDS) is defined as the sudden, unexpected death of an infant less than one year of age, with onset of a fatal episode apparently occurring during sleep that remains unexplained after a thorough investigation, including a complete autopsy and review of the circumstances of death and the clinical history.

Causes

The current "triple-risk hypothesis" states that SIDS occurs when three events happen in an infant simultaneously: 1) an underlying vulnerability in control (most likely the central nervous system); 2) a critical developmental period (maturation of the nervous system); and 3) a stressor (such as infection or tobacco smoke).

Risk factors

While many factors have been identified as associated with SIDS, common factors including young maternal age, ethnicity (less common in Caucasians), minimal or no prenatal care, preterm birth or low birth weight, and male gender have all been associated with an increased risk of SIDS. Other factors associated with SIDS include tobacco use during pregnancy or after birth around the child, sleeping position (prone), overheating, and sleeping on a soft surface.

Diagnosis

By definition, SIDS can only be diagnosed after no apparent cause of death is found after thorough evaluation of the death scene, review of the clinical history, and careful autopsy in infants less than one year of age.

Treatments

As no treatment is available after infant death, current strategies focus on prevention of SIDS.

Pathogenesis

SIDS occurs in otherwise normal-appearing infants. Delayed maturation of the central nervous system and abnormal development of the arcuate nucleus have been used in the triple-risk hypothesis to help explain why certain infants die of SIDS.

Prevention

Current strategies to prevent SIDS have successfully focused on modifiable risks, including sleeping position (Back-to-Sleep), smoking cessation during pregnancy and around the infant, avoiding overheating, and attention to providing a safe sleeping environment. There is no evidence that the use of home monitors to prevent SIDS in infants with apnea decreases the risk.

Epidemiology

The rate of SIDS in the United States is about 0.56 in 1,000 live births, with a median age at death of 11 weeks.

PREVENTING SIDS

To prevent or minimize the risk of SIDS, the following measures should always be applied. Infants should always be placed on their back (face up) when resting, sleeping, or left alone. Infants who are used to sleeping on their back are more susceptible to SIDS when sleeping on their stomachs for the first or occasional times. Everyone who cares for the child should be aware of the best position, including babysitters, friends, and grandparents. The baby should sleep on a firm surface or on a mattress that fits snugly in the crib's frame. Do not allow soft (pillows, stuffed toys such as teddy bears, or bumpers) or loose bedding in the same area that the baby is sleeping in and do not allow him or her to sleep on chairs, sofas, or waterbeds. Dress the infant in clothes appropriate for the room temperature instead of covering with a blanket. Never smoke or allow others to smoke in a room in which the infant plays, eats, or sleeps. A clean, dry pacifier may be used when placing the infant to sleep.

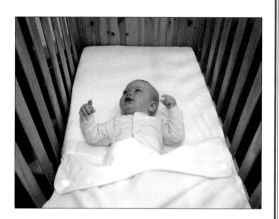

The safest position for a baby in a crib is to lie on his or her back with the feet at the end of the crib so that it is impossible for him or her to move downward and get under the bedcovers.

evaluated include infection, congenital birth defects, congenital metabolic disorders, accidental or intentional suffocation or strangulation, poisoning, obstruction of the respiratory tract, accidental falls, neglect, abandonment, and other maltreatment syndromes, assault and homicide, and other symptoms, signs, and abnormal clinical and laboratory findings. Essential components of this evaluation would include a complete autopsy, assessment of the area of death, and review of the infant and family history. Adjuncts to this evaluation could include a full skeletal survey, assessment of the infant's blood and body fluids for possible infection, metabolic derangement, genetic studies, and toxicology screen. Careful evaluation in the case of apparent SIDS can identify a cause of death in 15 to 20 percent of cases after autopsy in an otherwise normal-appearing but dead infant.

Pathogenesis

The autopsy findings noted in SIDS cases have several common features. None of these features would be considered significant enough by themselves to provide a plausible explanation for the demise of the infant. Infants that die from SIDS are typically normal appearing in size and weight. There is also typically blood-tinged frothy fluid around the child's nostrils. Examination of the internal body on autopsy include congestion of the lungs and small focal areas of bleeding on the inside of the chest.

The triple-risk hypothesis has been proposed to explain the susceptibility of certain infants to SIDS. This triple-risk hypothesis suggests that infants can have a predisposing condition (genetic predisposition or development of the brain tissue), which is triggered by an inciting event such as caused by tobacco-smoke exposure or an infection at a vulnerable time in the development of the infant. Researchers have noted a delay in the maturation of certain portions of the brain, along with a specific change in a portion of the brain called the arcuate nucleus, in infants who have died from SIDS. This area of the brain appears to help in the regulation of the respiratory system. Certain receptors in the ventral portion of the arcuate nucleus are markedly reduced in greater than 50 percent of the SIDS infants.

Interestingly, the peak incidence of SIDS occurs during a period of time when the significant changes are happening in infants' sleeping patterns and the controlling mechanisms for the heart and the lungs. Several recent reports have suggested that cardiac dysfunction or mutations in cardiac channels, a condition called long QT syndrome, may also be seen more frequently in infants who have died from SIDS.

Brian Brost

See also
• Childhood disorders • Sleep disorders
• Smoking-related disorders

Sinusitis

Sinusitis is an infection or inflammation of the paranasal sinuses. Viral, bacterial, and fungal infections, as well as allergic reactions, can cause sinusitis. Conditions that obstruct the sinuses, including infections, allergies, and nasogastric tubes, predispose patients to sinusitis.

Sinuses are hollow air cavities located in the skull or bones surrounding the nose. All the sinuses have an opening into the nose for the free exchange of air and mucus and are lined by a continuous mucous membrane. Acute sinusitis lasts for four weeks or less; chronic sinusitis usually last up to eight weeks, but can continue for months or even years.

Acute sinusitis is caused by *Streptococcus pneumoniae*, *Hemophilus influenzae*, and other organisms and is often precipitated by a common cold or other viral respiratory infection that causes swollen mucous membranes to obstruct the sinuses. Sometimes fungal infection can cause acute sinusitis in people whose immune system is not functioning properly. Allergic rhinitis is another common cause of sinusitis.

Chronic sinusitis is usually caused by inflammation, not infection, although colonizing bacteria can make it worse. Typically, a prolonged inflammatory process such as nasal polyps, thick mucus, allergies, tumor, trauma, or viral upper respiratory infections cause thickened mucous membranes and inflammation and obstruction of the sinuses.

Allergic conditions, a deviated septum, nasal polyps, and immunosuppression increase the risk of contracting sinusitis. People with nasogastric tubes used for feeding, people who are sedated, and patients unable to protect their airways are at extra risk of sinusitis. Drinking alcohol, cocaine abuse, swimming in chlorinated pools, and diving into water all increase the risk. Certain cancers, diabetes, cirrhosis, smoking, kidney failure, and severe burns increase the risk of contracting sinusitis.

Acute and chronic sinusitis have similar signs and symptoms. The area over the sinus is tender and may be swollen. Malaise is frequently present. Other symptoms are fever, fatigue, weakness, running nose, purulent nasal discharge, halitosis, congestion, a cough that is more severe at night, and postnasal drip. Acute sinusitis can last longer than two weeks and causes more symptoms than a cold. Diagnosis is often based on the history of symptoms and physical examination findings. X-ray signs of sinusitis are cloudy (opacified) sinuses, fluid in the sinuses, and thickened mucosa.

Treatment of sinusitis involves antibiotics, decongestants, and pain relievers. Nonprescription decongestants and nose drops or sprays are used for up to 7 days. Antibiotics should be given for 10 to 12 days. Sinusitis that is unresponsive to antibiotics and other measures may require surgery to improve drainage and to remove impacted debris. Some chronic sinusitis may require treatment with oral or topical steroids, or both.

Preventive measures include the early treatment of respiratory infections and avoiding conditions or practices that may increase the risk of sinusitis.

The average adult has two to three colds and influenzalike illnesses yearly; 20 million Americans are affected by sinusitis each year; and 0.5 to 2 percent of colds and flulike illnesses are complicated by acute sinusitis.

Isaac Grate

KEY FACTS

Description
Sinusitis is an infection or inflammation of the paranasal sinuses.

Causes
Streptococcus, hemophilus, and moraxella infections.

Risk factors
Allergic conditions, deviated septum, nasal polyps, immunosuppression, nasogastric tubes for feeding, sedation, alcohol and cocaine abuse.

Symptoms and signs
Tenderness over sinuses, fever, headache, malaise, runny nose, congestion, purulent nasal discharge, cough, and halitosis.

Diagnosis
Symptoms, physical exam. X-rays and CT scans.

Treatments
Decongestants, antibiotics, and pain relievers.

Epidemiology
20 million Americans are affected by sinusitis each year. About 0.5 to 2 percent of colds and flulike illnesses are complicated by acute sinusitis.

See also
- Allergy and sensitivity • Cold, common
- Infections, bacterial • Infections, viral
- Influenza • Smoking-related disorders

Skin disorders

Because skin, the body's largest organ, is so large and exposed, it becomes the target of all kinds of conditions and infections. Many disorders affect the skin, including rashes, parasitic and microbial infections, sweating disorders, benign and cancerous tumors, and pigment and hair disorders. Skin is an indicator of a person's general health.

Skin's most vital function is that of protection. While remaining supple and flexible, skin protects the body from injury, acts as a waterproof shield, and provides a barrier from the sun's rays as well as from foreign invaders such as bacteria. Skin regulates body temperature, maintains water and electrolyte balance, and in its role as a sensory organ, it senses painful and pleasant stimuli. If skin were laid out and pieced together, it would cover about 20 square feet (1.9 sq m) and weigh about 6 pounds (2.7 kg), or about 15 percent of adult body weight.

Skin or the integumentary system

Although skin looks flat, it is composed of three layers: the epidermis, the dermis, and a subcutaneous or fatty layer. The epidermis, which is the outer layer of the skin, is the visible part and is made up of three layers. The outermost layer of the skin, the stratum corneum, is made up of tough and fibrous overlapping dead cells. These cells form a vertical structure, like shingles on a roof, and protect the body from bacteria, viruses, and other foreign substances. Cells on the outer surface are constantly sloughing off; new ones move up to the outer surface and replace the lost cells. It takes about a month for new cells in the living epidermis to become smaller, flatter, and change into a lifeless protein called keratin. The outer layer of keratin is thicker in areas that need the greatest protection. For example, although the average thickness of skin is a fraction of an inch, skin is thin on the eyelids and thick on the palms and soles.

The second layer of the epidermis contains the keratinocytes or squamous cells, which are living cells that provide the skin with protection.

The inner layer of the epidermis contains basal cells, which continually divide to form new keratinocytes to replace the old ones that are shed from the skin's surface. These cells that manufacture skin constitute about 95 percent of the epidermis; the remaining cells contain melanocytes, which are cells that produce melanin to provide the coloring of the skin and protect it from ultraviolet rays. The number of melanocytes is the same in all people at birth, but then genetics determines the rate at which melanin is formed and ultimately the color of the skin.

Another important structure in the epidermis is that of the Langerhans cells, part of the immune system, which detect foreign substances but also play a part in the development of skin allergies.

RELATED ARTICLES

The dermis is the second layer of the skin, the support layer of the skin, which gives the skin flexibility, firmness, and strength. A thick layer of fibrous and elastic protein, made mostly of collagen and fibrillin, the dermis is also home to blood vessels, lymph vessels, hair follicles, and sweat glands. One-third of the blood circulating in the body is used to nourish the skin, so blood vessels in the dermis are very important to health. The nerve endings that sense pain, touch, pressure, and temperature are in this layer. Some areas of the skin have more nerve endings than others. For example, the fingertips and toes have nerve endings that are extremely sensitive to touch.

The fat or cutaneous layer provides insulation, nutrition, and resiliency. Fat is contained in living fat cells held together by fibrous tissue. This layer varies in thickness, from a fraction of an inch on the eyelids to several inches on abdomen and buttocks. Roots of oil and sweat glands are located here. Oil or sebaceous glands are attached to hair follicles and secrete an oily substance called sebum that lubricates the skin. Sweat glands are of two types: eccrine glands, which are distributed throughout the body; and apocrine glands, which secrete perspiration in times of stress or emotion.

Skin and disorders

Skin is an indicator of the person's general health. Because it is so large and exposed, it is also the target of all kinds of infections and disorders. Many disorders can affect the skin: dermatitis, bacterial infections, fungal infections, parasitic infections, hair follicle and sebaceous gland problems, scaling diseases, inflammation reactions, and benign and malignant skin growths.

Itching and noninfectious rashes

Itching and rashes can result from a reaction of the immune system or from an infection or irritation. A large group of rashes are not contagious or life threatening, although their presence can make the individual miserable. These include dermatitis, drug rashes, immune system conditions, and other conditions of unknown origin.

The word *dermatitis* comes from two Greek words, *dermat*, meaning "skin," and the suffix -*itis*, meaning "inflammation of." *Dermatitis* is a broad term covering many different disorders that result in redness, itching, blisters, and often oozing and scabbing. Some of the disorders include drug reactions or contact with certain substances. Contact dermatitis occurs when a person who is sensitive to a particular substance comes in contact with irritants such as acids, alkalis, solvents, strong soaps, natural plants like poison ivy, or latex in rubber. Types of dermatitis include atopic dermatitis of the upper layers of the skin, seborrheic dermatitis of the scalp, nummular dermatitis with coin-shaped spots of tiny blisters, and localized scratch dermatitis that develops from continuous scratching. A dermatologist, a physician who specializes in skin care, evaluates the skin condition on the appearance of the rash.

Certain drugs may cause skin rashes as a side effect. The drug may be taken orally and not even touch the skin. For example, once a person develops an allergy rash to penicillin, he or she cannot take that medication again in any form. Other rashes may not show up until the person has been in the sun. The term *photosensitive* is used to describe reactions that occur in the presence of sunlight. Drugs that may cause photosensitive reactions include antipsychotics, tetracycline, sulfa drugs, and even some artificial sweeteners. Most drug rashes do not itch, and they disappear when the drug is not used.

Itching is a symptom rather than a condition. People react to it by scratching the itch. Many disorders can cause itching: systemic conditions, parasites, hives, allergic reactions, drugs, or an unknown cause. For example, dry skin, or xerosis, a condition resulting from exposure to cold weather, can cause itching; hot baths make the itching worse. Scratching causes more irritation to the skin and leads to more itching. In order to treat the condition, doctors must determine the cause. Sometimes, the cause is obvious, for example, itching caused by poison ivy or insect bites. Systemic diseases may demand blood tests, biopsies, or scrapings.

Psoriasis is a common skin condition in which dry red and patchy silvery scales appear. This disease appears to have genetic and environmental origins. Normally, it takes about a month for new cells to move from the lower layers to the outer layers; in psoriasis, it may take only three or four days, causing a pileup of dead skin. This is a condition of the immune system that affects more than 4.5 million people in the United States. It is considered important in studying other conditions of the immune system. There are many kinds of noncontagious rashes that result from immune system reactions. For example, a reaction to herpes simplex virus may cause a rash called erythema multiforme. This condition is a recurring disorder characterized by patches of red, raised skin that often look like targets and usually are distributed symmetrically over the body. Reactions to bacteria such as streptococcus, fungi, or other viruses may cause erythema nodosum, an inflammatory disorder that produces tender red bumps or nodules under the skin, most often over the shins but also on the arms and other areas. A reaction to a variety of drugs, such as gold, bismuth, or quinine, may cause lichen planus, a recurring itchy disease that starts as small red or purple bumps that become scaly patches. Studies of the rash of psoriasis are providing insight into the treatment of immune reactions.

Other autoimmune reactions may cause blistering. A blister, or bulla, is a bubble of fluid, which forms under a layer of dead skin. When tissue is injured, the mixture of water and protein oozes from the area that is irritated or burned. However, the immune system may mistake certain body reactions as foreign invaders and turn on itself. Three autoimmune blistering diseases are: bullous pemphigoid, which occurs mainly in older people and forms large blistering areas on the skin; dermatitis herpetiformis, which causes small clusters of intensely itchy small blisters and hivelike swellings; and pemphigus, a rare, severe disease in which blisters of varying sizes break out on the skin, the lining of mouth, the genitals, and other mucous membranes.

The origins of some rashes are unknown. Pityriasis rosea is a condition in which small patches of scaly, rose-colored inflamed skin appear. It is common in young adults. Keratosis pilaris is a common disorder, in which dead cells from the upper layer of the skin plug the opening of hair follicles and make the skin feel rough like chicken skin.

Infections caused by microorganisms and parasites

Although the skin provides a good barrier against infections, a break in the skin or a systemic condition such as diabetes may give bacteria, viruses, fungi, and parasites an opening.

The skin is home to many kinds of bacteria. Normally, they do not infect until scratching, sunburn, or cuts damage the skin. The most common types of bacteria that infect the skin are staphylococcus (staph) and streptococcus (strep). For example, *Staphylococcus aureus* or *Streptococcus pyogenes*, or both, cause impetigo, a skin infection characterized by scabby, yellow-crusted sores and small yellow, fluid-filled blisters. Impetigo is very contagious and most often affects the face, arms, and legs of children.

S. aureus also cause skin infections with pus-filled pockets. Skin abscesses are boils or furuncles that are painful to the touch and filled with pockets of infection. These boils may range from an inch to several inches in diameter. Often they come to a point and rupture, spreading bacteria to surrounding tissue. Carbuncles are clusters of abscesses that connect with each other on the skin. Carbuncles are often more common in men and often occur on the back of the neck.

Folliculitis is an inflammation of the hair follicles. Although often resulting from inflammation, folliculitis can also be related to bacterial infection of the follicle; *Staphylococcus aureus* is the most common cause. Hair follicles can also be infected by *Pseudomonas aeruginosa*, commonly acquired in a poorly chlorinated hot tub or whirlpool. Areas of skin covered by a bathing suit, such as the torso and buttocks, are the most common site for *Pseudomonas* folliculitis.

Certain types of staph infections may secrete toxic substances that cause the top layer of the epidermis to split off from the rest of the skin, causing peeling. This is called staphylococcal scaled skin syndrome and may cause skin on the entire body to peel.

Some species of streptococci cause cellulitis, a spreading bacterial infection of the skin and tissues. Bites by humans or animals or injuries in water and dirt may cause cellulitis. Erysipelas is one form of streptococcal cellulitis in which skin becomes bright red and is noticeably swollen.

Many viral infections, such as measles, chickenpox, rubella, and herpes result in rashes, sores, and spots. Two common viruses, which remain in the skin, cause warts and molluscum contagiosum. The poxvirus causes molluscum contagiosum, an infection that results in flesh-colored bumps that are usually

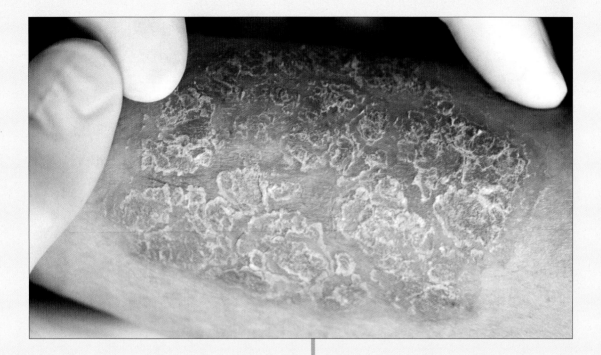

less than ¼ inch (0.6 cm) in diameter. Caused by a contagious virus, these smooth waxy bumps can infect any part of the skin. Most of the lesions of molluscum contagiosum spontaneously disappear in one to two years, and usually no treatment is needed unless they are disfiguring or troublesome.

Fungal skin infections find their ways to surfaces that are moist and hidden, for example, beneath the breasts, between the toes, and genital areas. Obese people, who have more skin folds, are more likely to get these infections. People with diabetes are also very susceptible. Most fungal infections called dermatophytes (literally, "skin plants") invade the stratum corneum and penetrate no deeper.

Under certain circumstances, candida, a normal yeast infection of the mouth, digestive tract, and vagina, can infect mucous membranes and moist areas of the skin, causing a bright red rash with small itchy pustules.

Ringworm is a fungal infection of the skin that causes scaly, red ring-shaped patches. Ringworm appearing on the nail is called tinea unguium; on the scalp it is called tinea capitis, on the body, tinea corporis, and on the beard, tinea barbae. Athlete's foot (tinea pedis) and jock itch (tinea cruris) are common infections that occur frequently in hot weather in tight, warm moist areas.

A doctor examines a patient whose leg has a red, dry flaky rash. By questioning the patient, the doctor will try to ascertain the reason for the dermatitis, which could be caused by an allergy or a reaction to medication.

Common among young adults is tinea versicolor, a fungal infection of the topmost layers that causes scaly, discolored round patches on the chest or back.

Most skin parasites are tiny insects or worms that burrow into the skin and cause itching or burning. Because the larvae dog and cat hookworm cannot penetrate the human circulatory system, the worms stay under the skin and cause larvae migrans or creeping eruption. The larvae weave a winding, threadlike raised pattern with a weepy red rash, which itches intensely.

Lice are tiny wingless insects that infest the skin as three forms: head, body, or pubic. Lice are difficult to see, but their shiny, grayish white eggs or nits are easy to spot. Scabies is a mite that burrows into the skin, producing tiny reddish bumps that itch severely. The mites are easily spread from person to person and difficult to get rid of.

Sweating disorders
The apocrine and eccrine glands create sweat or perspiration that is carried to the surface by ducts.

Composed mostly of water, salt, and other chemicals, sweat helps keep the body cool. However, people who sweat excessively (hyperhydrosis) may sweat under normal conditions. Excessive sweating can affect the entire surface of the body or certain areas, such as palms of the hands, soles of the feet, armpits, or genital area. The condition appears to run in families and may be treated with a variety of drugs or a more drastic measure of surgical cutting of the nerves leading to the sweat glands. In humid climates, trapped sweat may cause prickly heat, an itchy skin rash. The rash occurs when body parts rub each other, for example between the legs or under the arms.

Noncancerous and cancerous skin growths
Skin growths occur when an accumulation of cells of various types appear different from the surrounding skin. Growths may be the same color as the flesh or may be of a different color; growths may be present at birth or appear later. Noncancerous growths that are contained are called benign tumors; cancerous growths that are not contained and spread are called malignant. The cause of many noncancerous growths is puzzling. The most common are moles or nevi, usually dark skin growths that develop from pigment-producing cells in the melanin. They do not itch or hurt, but should be watched to make sure they do not change appearance and become cancerous. Sometimes blood vessels collect in an abnormal dense area and cause red or purple discoloration. If these growths appear at birth, they are called birthmarks. Examples are hemangiomas, port-wine stains, lymphangiomas, and spider angiomas that are overgrowth of blood vessels. More common in middle-aged and older adults, seborrheic keratoses are harmless brown or black growths that range from ¼ inch (0.6 cm) to several inches. Keloids are smooth, shiny, flesh-colored, raised growths of fibrous tissue that form over areas of injury or surgical wounds. They may form in any scar and are more common in blacks than whites. Lipomas are soft deposits of fat under the skin, causing round, raised bumps. More common in women than men, these bumps can grow anywhere on the body. Liposuction—removal of fat by a suction device—may remove the growth.

Skin cancer is the most common form of cancer in the United States. Caused primarily by exposure to the

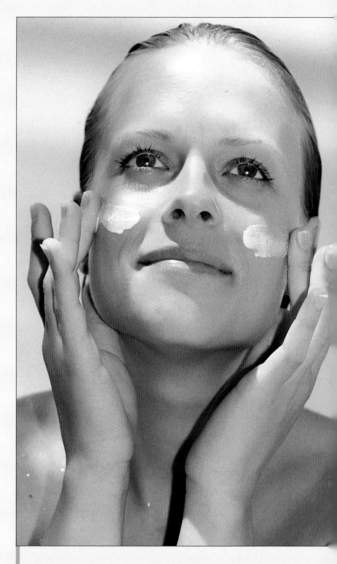

Cleansing and moisturizing are essential to keep skin healthy. Cleansing removes dirt and makeup and moisturizers slow down the rate of moisture evaporation from the skin, and prevent dryness.

sun, the three main types are: basal cell carcinoma, which originates in the epidermis; squamous cell carcinoma; and melanoma, which originates in the pigment-producing cells. Because fair-skinned people produce less melanin, they have less protection against the harmful ultraviolet (UV) rays of the sun. Treated in the early stage, most skin cancers are treatable by surgical removal. Kaposi's sarcoma, a cancer caused by herpes virus type 8, occurs in people of Mediterranean or Jewish heritage, in children from certain parts of Africa, and in people receiving immunosuppressant therapy, such as in treatment for AIDS or after organ transplants. Kaposi's sarcoma appears as flat, pink, brown, or purple patches or bumps on the skin.

Pigment disorders

Melanin produces the various shades of skin color. Fair-skinned people produce little melanin; very dark-skinned people produce a great deal. Albinism is a rare hereditary disorder in which little or no melanin is produced. People with albinism have white hair, pale skin, pink or pale blue eyes, and usually abnormal vision. With no melanin in the skin, people with albinism may get sunburn after only a few minutes of exposure. Melasma is a condition that produces dark brown patches on sun-exposed areas, usually the face. It occurs especially in women who are pregnant or who are taking birth control pills. A condition in which melanocytes are lost, causing white patches in the skin, is called vitiligo. The cause is unknown, but it may involve the attack of the immune system on the melanocytes. It tends to run in families and may occur with other diseases, such as thyroid disease, diabetes, Addison's disease, or pernicious anemia.

Sunburn and overexposure to UV light may damage the skin, through severe burns and blisters. Exposure to sunlight prematurely ages the skin, causing both fine and coarse wrinkles and a higher risk of skin cancers.

Hair disorders

Acne is a common condition that is placed in a separate class because it is caused by an interaction between hormones, skin oils, and bacteria that results in inflammation of the hair follicles. Occurring mostly on the face and neck, acne is a collection of dried oils, dead skin cells, and bacteria that clog the hair follicle and cause a blackhead (open comedome) or white head (closed comedome) to develop. The condition occurs mostly during puberty, when hormone levels stimulate the sebaceous glands. The severity differs with individuals but has no connection to specific foods or sexual activity.

Hair originates in the hair follicles in the dermis and is located on every surface of the body, except lips, palms of hands, and soles of feet. Living cells push the new hair up and outward. Although some people have genetic tendencies for excessive hairiness, the condition may be caused by systemic disorders of the pituitary gland, adrenal glands, or ovaries in women. Certain drugs may also cause the condition. Hair loss usually involves hereditary factors, aging, local skin conditions, certain systemic diseases, or drugs such as chemotherapy. Male-pattern baldness is the most common type of hair loss, affecting about half of all men. Women with the condition may experience thinning hair of the top of the head.

Diagnosis and treatment

Skin infections range from localized superficial infections to widespread life-threatening conditions. Depending on the symptoms, the physician or dermatologist may order blood tests, other laboratory tests, or a biopsy to determine if a systemic disease is causing the problem. A patch test or prick test may determine if an allergy is involved in the problem.

The physician may prescribe topical creams, ointments, lotions, solutions, powders, or gels. Treatments may also include oral antibiotics or, in some cases, surgery.

Psoriasis: Model for drug development

In 1841 Austrian physician Ferdinand von Hebra, who founded the specialty of dermatology, recognized psoriasis as a separate condition, although it probably existed throughout human history. This chronic condition can be mentally and physically disabling. In fact, one study using a quality of life measure found people with psoriasis scored lower on physical and mental dysfunction than any other illness except congestive heart failure.

Scientists now realize that the immune system, especially helper T cells (Type 1), is pivotal in maintaining psoriasis. Recently, drug development in psoriasis has progressed through better understanding of biochemistry and immunology. Several researchers consider psoriasis to be the ideal study condition for drug development for other diseases affecting the T1 cells of the immune system. Patients are usually healthy and can be treated with one drug that can be analyzed for safety and efficacy. Skin is accessible and plaques are visible, so clinical response is easy to assess with relatively short studies.

Evelyn B. Kelly

Sleep disorders

Disruptive patterns of sleep, sleeping too long, difficulty falling and staying asleep, and any unusual associated behavior indicate a sleep disorder. Sleep disorders are classified as primary (disturbances in the amount, quality, or timing of sleep, abnormal events in behavior or physiology during sleep) and secondary (due to general medical condition or substance abuse). There are two stages of sleep: non–rapid eye movement (NREM) and rapid eye movement (REM). Sleep disorders are related to alterations in the sleep-wake cycle of NREM and REM.

Good sleep quality is essential for overall physical and mental health. Inadequate sleep may cause fatigue, changes in mood, impaired performance, and can also negatively affect quality of life, safety, and productivity.

Causes

Certain medical conditions such as pain, metabolic disorders, endocrine disorders, and physical conditions (obesity) may cause sleep disorders. Other causes include: use of stimulants such as caffeine, amphetamines, and cocaine; sedative withdrawal; psychiatric conditions (for example, major depression, bipolar disorders, and anxiety disorders); and neurotransmitters (brain chemicals), for example, elevated levels of dopamine, norepinephrine, acetylcholine, and serotonin. Genetic and environmental factors are also associated with sleep disorders.

Although insomnia is not a disease, it is a chronic problem for about 25 percent of the population. A person with this disorder has difficulty in falling asleep and staying asleep, or they may get no benefit from sleep, resulting in daytime drowsiness and decreased energy and motivation. The condition is diagnosed if disturbance of sleep occurs three or more times per week for at least 1 month. This should not be associated with general medical conditions, substance abuse, or other sleep disorders. For treatment, medications are recommended for short-term use. They include sleeping drugs, antidepressants, and antihistamines. Insomnia can become chronic if untreated; it is exacerbated by stress and other environmental factors. Stress management and sleep hygiene (regular bed-time, no alcohol or caffeine) are forms of prevention. This disorder affects approximately 30 percent of the general population. It is more common in women.

Primary hypersomnia

A person with this disorder experiences excessive or persistent daytime sleepiness that is not relieved by napping. To diagnose the condition, at least one month of the described symptoms should be present. Medications such as stimulants (amphetamines) are first-line treatments. Selective serotonin reuptake inhibitors (SSRIs) may be useful in some patients. Without treatment, hypersomnia may interfere with social and occupational functioning. Environmental stimulation could be helpful as a form of prevention. The course the disorder will take is unknown.

Narcolepsy

A person with this disorder has repeated, sudden attacks of sleep during the daytime with loss of muscle tone (cataplexy), which occurs in 70 percent of patients. Frequent REM sleep with brief paralysis occurs upon awakening (sleep paralysis) in 50 percent of patients. To confirm the diagnosis, the above symptoms must exist for at least 3 months. Treatment involves scheduled daily naps and stimulant drugs (amphetamines and ritalin). In case of sudden loss of muscle power, adjunctive antidepressants may be useful. If untreated, narcolepsy may cause serious occupational and social impairment. Most cases are treated successfully. There is no known prevention for the disorder. The exact prevalence in the population is unknown. Both males and females are equally affected. The onset is usually during adolescence or young adulthood. There may be a genetic predisposition.

Breathing-related disorders

Sleep disruption and daytime sleepiness can be caused by abnormal sleep ventilation from either obstructive or central sleep apnea. Sleep apnea is associated with headaches, depression, and pulmonary hypertension (respiratory problems). These symptoms should be enough to form a diagnosis. Treatment for the condition is nasal continuous positive airway pressure (nCPAP), and weight loss. Nasal surgery or uvuloplasty may treat obstructive sleep apnea. For central sleep apnea, mechanical ventilation (nCPAP) is helpful. These disorders take a chronic course if untreated and cause significant impairment in daily functioning and medical complications. Prevention includes weight reduction by diet and exercise. Approximately 10 percent of adults suffer from this type of sleep disorder. It is more common in men and obese individuals.

Circadian rhythm sleep disorder

This type of sleep disturbance is associated with a mismatch between a person's intrinsic circadian rhythm and external sleep-wake demands. Some of the conditions associated with this disorder include jet lag, shift work, and delayed sleep phase. These symptoms should be enough to make a diagnosis. Jet lag usually resolves spontaneously after 2 to 7 days. Light therapy may be useful for shift workers. The likely progression of the disease is not known. The only way to prevent this disorder is to avoid long travel time and to re-arrange shift work schedules. It is not known how many people suffer from this sleep disorder.

Nightmare disorder

A person may experience repeated episodes of scary dreams with recall during REM sleep causing signifi-

cant distress. The disorder is diagnosed by these symptoms. There is no specific treatment for this type of sleep disorder. Occasionally, tricyclic antidepressants (TCAs) could be used to suppress total REM sleep. The likely outcome of this disorder is also unknown. Stress management is helpful in some cases as a preventive. The onset of this disorder is most often in childhood. It may occur more frequently during stress and illness.

Sleep terror disorder

Repeated episodes of apparent fearfulness during sleep (non-REM stages 3 or 4) with a scream appear. The individual may sit up or cry out and be extremely frightened or anxious. He or she will not awaken and not remember the episode. These symptoms allow diagnosis. There is usually no treatment, but some patients may benefit from small doses of benzodiazepine (valium) or other types of antianxiety medications at bedtime. The likely progression of the disorder is unknown, and there is no known prevention. This disorder usually occurs in children and is more common in boys. Prevalence of the disorder is 1 to 6 percent of children, and it has a familial tendency.

Sleepwalking disorder

Also known as somnambulism, a person with this disorder has repeated episodes of getting out of bed, walking with a blank stare, and is awakened only with difficulty. Other activities during such episodes include getting dressed, talking, or screaming. This behavior usually remits when the patient returns to bed. Some patients appear to be confused for several minutes and are unable to remember the event. It occurs during the non-REM sleep at stages 3 or 4. These symptoms are enough to diagnose the disorder.

Treatment is to provide a safe environment to prevent injury. Sometimes medications such as tricyclic antidepressants can help suppress non-REM sleep at stages 3 or 4. The likely outcome is unknown, and there are no known preventive measures. The onset of the disorder is usually between ages 4 and 8; peak prevalence is at age 12. This disorder is more common in boys and has a familial tendency.

Nurun Shah

KEY FACTS

Description

Disorders associated with disturbances in the amount, quality, and time of sleep, or abnormal events in behavior or physiology during sleep.

Causes and risk factors

Genetic, biochemical, and environmental factors. Secondary sleep disorders are associated with general medical conditions and substance abuse.

Symptoms

Difficulty in falling or staying asleep, excessive sleepiness, sleep attacks during the day with sudden loss of muscle tone, abnormal breathing, sleep disturbances, repeated episodes of frightening dreams, and sleepwalking.

Diagnosis

Evaluation and interview by a psychiatrist.

Treatment

Sleep hygiene, stress management, short-term medications, and breathing treatment.

Pathogenesis

Chronic course.

Epidemiology

10 percent of adults with breathing-related disorder; 1–6 percent have sleep terror disorder. Insomnia is more common in women; breathing-related sleep disorder is more common in men.

See also

- Anxiety disorders • Bipolar disorder
- Depressive disorders • Environmental disorders • Genetic disorders • Metabolic disorders • Obesity

Sleeping sickness

Sleeping sickness, or African trypanosomiasis, is a parasitic illness caused by one of the *Trypanosoma* species. The parasite is a single-cell organism with a flagellum, which is a tail-like structure that helps the organism to move. This parasite exists outside the human cells in the body fluids and multiplies by division. Sleeping sickness is transmitted through a tsetse fly bite; in addition, it can be transmitted from mother to child during pregnancy.

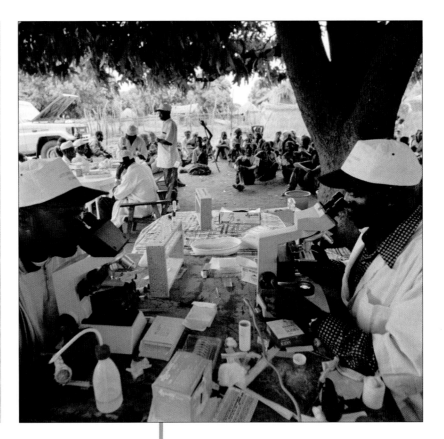

The parasite that causes sleeping sickness has two distinct life-cycle forms called epimastigote and trypomastigote. Tsetse flies feed on an infected human or another mammalian; the trypomastigotes multiply in the fly's gut and transform into epimastogotes. The parasites then travel to the fly's salivary glands so they can be injected by the fly into another human during the bite, so the transmission cycle continues. Once the parasite enters the human body, it transforms again and starts to multiply. Inside the body, the parasite exists in a trypomastigote form, which is distinguished into a long and a short one. Only the short trypomastigote will continue the parasite's life cycle in the fly's body and maintain the transmission.

Causes and epidemiology

The two parasite subtypes have similar structure but cause quite distinct clinical diseases and are transmitted by different species of tsetse fly. They also have a different geographic distribution. *Trypanosoma brucei gambiense*, which causes West African trypanosomiasis

As part of a World Health Organization (WHO) initiative, in 2002 screenings for sleeping sickness were set up in 15 African countries. Around 5 to 9 percent of the population tested during the campaign were infected.

(or gambiense trypanosomiasis), is common in West and Central Africa. *Trypanosoma brucei rhodesiense*, which causes East African trypanosomiasis (or rhodesiense trypanosomiasis), is common in Central and East Africa. Because this disease is transmitted only by a tsetse fly, it is prevalent only on the African continent, where tsetse flies are common. Infection among travelers is rare, unless they travel into rural areas. The actual number of people with sleeping sickness is difficult to establish; this disease is more common in the rural setting, where health resources are frequently scarce. The infection is found in 36 countries of sub-Saharan Africa. According to the World Health Organization (WHO), this infection became very uncommon on the African continent by the 1960s as a result of an aggressive surveillance campaign, but about a decade later the disease reappeared and continues to be a public health issue. West African trypanosomiasis is less commonly reported, while the majority of cases of sleeping sickness are due to East African trypanosomiasis.

Risk factors and pathogenesis

A major risk factor for the illness is contact with the tsetse fly and the presence of environmental factors to support the existence of this vector. Tsetse flies inhabit woody areas along rivers and lakes. People involved in activities such as fishing or hunting in infested areas are at risk for the infection. The parasite causing East African trypanosomiasis can also infect other mammals like cattle and antelopes. Persons traveling to or working at the game parks in East Africa may also be at risk for acquiring this infection.

Pathogenesis of sleeping sickness is defined by the dissemination of the parasite into the blood and lymphatic system. A unique feature of this parasite is the ability to escape the body's immune response. The immune response is determined by the production of antibodies against the antigens contained in the infecting organism. In the case of African trypanosomiasis, the parasite continues to change its antigenic structure, so the antibody response does not become sufficient, and the parasite continues to multiply and spread. Untreated infection will lead to death.

After the tsetse fly bite, a primary skin lesion called chancre can sometimes develop. From the bite area the parasite enters the human body and travels until it reaches the central nervous system. The process of dissemination takes weeks to months. The disease is usually described in two stages. During the first stage, multiplication of the parasite in blood and lymph occurs, followed by a second stage when the parasite enters the central nervous system.

Symptoms

West African (gambiense) trypanosomiasis is comparatively less severe and has a more chronic course. Infection can present as a local skin lesion at the site of a tsetse fly bite one to two weeks later. The first stage of the disease can develop weeks to months after the bite with systemic symptoms such as fever and prominent lymph node enlargement, as well as liver and spleen enlargement. Lymph node enlargement is especially prominent on the back of the neck. The lymph nodes can eventually become firm. Other findings include rash, weight loss, and generalized weakness. During the second stage of the illness, a progressive impairment in the central nervous system would even-

tually lead to coma and death. A major finding in this stage is daytime sleepiness, hence the name of the disease. It is accompanied by insomnia, as well as headache and personality and mood changes. Other impairments, such as loss of speech, movement disorders, or disturbances in coordination, can develop.

East African (rhodesiense) trypanosomiasis frequently presents itself as the more acute illness. Symptoms can develop days after the bite. During the first stage of the East African trypanosomiasis, the swelling of the lymph nodes is much less prominent, but rash and fever are common. Invasion of the heart by the parasite is more common with East African trypanosomiasis and leads to elevated heartbeat (tachycardia) and the development of heart failure. In weeks to months, the infection progresses to the second stage

---

KEY FACTS

Description

Sleeping sickness (or African trypanosomiasis) is a parasitic disease caused by a protozoan.

Causes

Sleeping sickness is caused by *Trypanosoma brucei*, which has two subtypes (subspecies).

Risk factors

The bite of a tsetse fly (vector) that lives only in sub-Saharan Africa. The flies are common in rural areas of tropical Africa.

Symptoms

Tend to develop in two stages: in the first stage, fever, malaise and lymph node enlargement; in the second stage, the organism invades the central nervous system, causing changes in behavior, sleepiness, and weight loss.

Diagnosis

Diagnosis is made by demonstration of a parasite in the body fluids, such as blood or spinal fluid.

Treatments

The disease is fatal if not treated. Treatment is given based on the type and stage of the illness.

Pathogenesis

The organism enters the body through a tsetse fly bite and eventually reaches the central nervous system, where it causes coma and death.

Prevention

The best way to prevent trypanosomiasis is to avoid areas infested with tsetse flies.

Epidemiology

It is estimated that the total number of people with sleeping sickness is somewhere between 50,000 to 70,000, but actual estimates are hard to predict.

LIFE CYCLE OF TRYPANOSOMES

A A tsetse fly feeds on an infected human or other mammal and ingests *Trypanosoma* parasites.

B The parasites reproduce in the fly's gut.

C The parasites travel to the fly's salivary glands; it is there that the parasites become infective.

D A fly with infective parasites in its saliva bites a human, transferring the parasites; the person will then develop sleeping sickness.

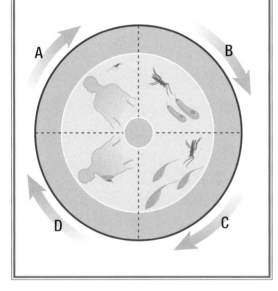

and invades the central nervous system with features similar to West African trypanosomiasis. Persons with East African trypanosomiasis commonly have low blood counts and wasting; coma and death develops in the late stage of the disease if no treatment is given.

Diagnosis and treatments

Demonstration of a parasite in the body fluids or tissue such as the bone marrow or lymph nodes is necessary for definitive diagnosis. The organisms can be found in fluid from chancre, blood, or a small sample of lymph node tissue. These tests may have to be repeated several times to increase the chance of detection. History of tsetse fly exposure in the endemic area of sub-Saharan Africa is also helpful in suspecting this disease. Tests that look for specific antibody response in the blood are available, although they are used for population screening only. If the serological screening is positive, further confirmatory diagnostic tests

should be done. It is important to examine the cerebrospinal fluid in all patients with African trypanosomiasis because it determines the specific treatment course. The typical cerebrospinal fluid abnormalities include elevated amounts of cells and protein.

It is imperative to timely treat the sleeping sickness to avoid progressive damage to the central nervous system. The treatment course is specific to the trypanosome subspecies and the clinical disease stage. The medications for trypanosomiasis are pentamidine, suramin, eflornithine, and melarsoprol. They are effective in clearing the infection but are sometimes not readily available in resource-limited settings. In addition, these medications are difficult to administer (most of them need to be given intravenously) and require monitoring due to toxicities and side effects. For West African trypanosomiasis, pentamidine is used for the first stage and eflornithine is used for the second-stage disease. For East African trypanosomiasis, suramin is used for the first stage and melarsoprol is used for the second-stage disease. The specific suggestions for disease stage and subtype were developed based on the side effect profile, toxicity, and penetration to the central nervous system. Suramin can cause fatal intolerance and kidney damage. Melarsoprol, which is an organic arsenical compound, is associated with a spectrum of side effects and toxicities, including central nervous system damage. It is always given in combination with steroid medication that reduces the inflammation and potential damage.

Prevention

There is no vaccine for this infection. None of the preventive medicines for African trypanosomiasis can be used because of the high risk of toxicity.

The WHO has established a surveillance team to try to eliminate this disease and assist with treatment to those infected. The best prevention method is to avoid areas of heavy tsetse fly infestation or wear neutral colored protective clothing (the flies are attracted to some bright colors). The flies can bite through light fabric, and insect repellants are not usually effective.

Other ways to stop the spread of the infection are tsetse fly control. Fly traps, insecticide use, elimination of breeding sites, or irradiation of the male flies to make them sterile are examples of vector control measures.

Diana Nurutdinova

See also
- Heart disorders • Infections, parasitic
- Nervous system disorders • Sleep disorders

Slipped disk

The spine is made up of bones or vertebrae separated by soft cushion disks. There are disks in the neck (cervical), chest (thoracic), and lower back (lumbar) regions of the spine. The intervertebral disk is interposed between two spinal segments and provides support and height to the motion segment. The disk has two distinct components, a layered outer portion or annulus and an inner "ball bearing" called the nucleus. The nucleus of the disk is gelatinous, with a high water content, and is designed to resist compressive loads, such as gravity and jarring while jumping, and the outer annulus of the disk resists tension when bending and twisting.

The term *slipped disk* describes degeneration of the intervertebral disk of the spine. This term is rarely used clinically; instead, descriptions of disk degneration take into consideration the part of the disk involved and the amount of injury present. A disk protrusion or bulge is used to describe weakness and bowing of the disk wall. Disk herniation or disk extrusion is reserved for movement of the gel-like nucleus from the center of the disk to the edge or out beyond the outer annulus itself. If the gel-like substance squeezes out and becomes separated from the disk, it is called disk sequestration. The annular wall has been called a "tire," a "tire bulge," and "full blow out" to describe the range from herniation to extrusion.

Symptoms and diagnosis

Bulging or herniation of a disk is not directly correlated with pain and dysfunction; it is common to see damage to a disk on an imaging study with no related symptoms. Research has shown that 3 in 10 people have a disk herniation in the lower back and 1 in 10 have a herniation in the neck area, yet the person is unaware of the condition and has no complaints. Finding the injury on an imaging study does not mean that it is the reason for a spinal complaint.

Clinically, it is important that signs and symptoms observed in a person are correlated to the imaging recorded by magnetic resonance imaging (MRI) to ensure that the abnormal findings are actually related to the complaint.

Annular tears can be painful and can relate to central spinal pain. Disk injury becomes a problem when the material pushes on surrounding nerves. If a nerve is compressed, symptoms can be found down the corresponding arm or leg. Evaluation of arm or leg symptoms can give clues of a specific nerve that is probably compromised, and MRI findings can help

KEY FACTS

Description

Slipped disk is a term used to describe stages of disk degeneration in the spine.

Causes

The exact cause of disk herniation remains unknown, although there are factors that contribute to the degenerative process.

Risk factors

Age, environmental physical loading, back injury, and smoking are commonly associated with accelerated disk degeneration, although they do not explain the wide variability seen.

Symptoms

Symptoms can be completely absent in as many as one-third of individuals with lower-back disk disease and one-tenth of those with cervical degeneration. When present, symptoms can comprise central spinal pain; when a nerve is compromised, there may be pain, weakness, or numbness in the arm or leg. Care must be taken to relate the symptoms with the imaging to avoid incorrectly assigning blame to a disk.

Diagnosis

Diagnosis is most often made by imaging; without clinical correlation to signs and symptoms, however, the results may be meaningless.

Treatment

The natural history of spine pain is favorable, and most complaints with or without disk involvement resolve spontaneously or with nonoperative management. Treatment programs consist of activities that reduce pain, resolve symptoms in the arm or leg, and strengthen and train the spinal muscles.

Prevention

The reduction of risk factors is the only available prevention.

Epidemiology

Clear epidemiological rates are difficult to collect because of the challenges in identifying and measuring disk injury and the impact of the disk on the complaints reported.

confirm if a related disk herniation is present and is contributing to the problem.

Treatments and prevention

About 88 percent of cases of recent onset of low back pain will resolve in six weeks, while 98 percent will resolve by 24 weeks. Even in extreme cases in which the patient is unable to stand up straight after an episode of pain, reduced activity coupled with motions that aid in reducing complaints can resolve the problem and return the person to his or her pre-injury activities. Treatment of the condition should be directed at decreasing the person's complaint or radiating symptoms. This often involves exercises and activities that are encouraged or avoided as they relate to improving or worsening of the complaints. Most programs involve some form of stretching, muscle strengthening and education, and gentle aerobic exercise. It is not uncommon to have successful resolution of the symptoms without changing the disk injury or location as seen on the MRI.

In spite of many unknowns about the relationships among the disks, nerves, and the patient's overall complaints, both surgical and nonsurgical options exist. In the case of loss of control of the bowel or bladder, surgery can be immediate; otherwise, surgery is never a first choice.

Surgeons can remove the areas of the extruded disk, remove the disk completely and fuse the two adjacent vertebrae, or increase the space available for the compressed nerve, or both. Consideration for surgery first requires failure of nonsurgical options.

A doctor shows a patient a spinal model to demonstrate the way in which a prolapsed disk can press on a nerve root to cause the painful symptoms called slipped disk.

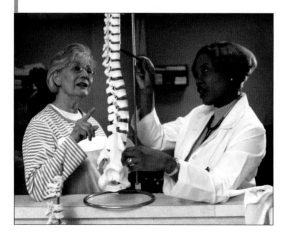

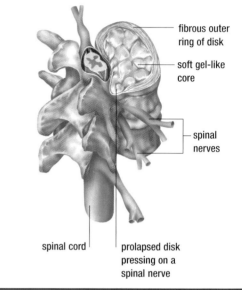

SLIPPED DISK

A slipped disk, or prolapsed disk, is a common occurrence, in which one of the intervertebral disks in the spine ruptures and protrudes, causing pain. If the protruded disk presses on a spinal nerve, loss of sensation can occur in the lower part of the body.

fibrous outer ring of disk

soft gel-like core

spinal nerves

spinal cord

prolapsed disk pressing on a spinal nerve

Prevention and epidemology

Although around 80 percent of the population may experience back pain, disk problems account for less than 2 percent of cases of back pain. Cigarette smoking and obesity have been cited as risk factors for disk disease, although the mechanism remains unknown. Heavy manual labor—including extreme positions of stooping, twisting, pulling, and pushing—and driving or working on vibrating equipment have also been linked to neck and low back disk degeneration. Disk health and water content decrease with age, contributing to a decline in disk health over the life span. Biochemical and genetic factors that may impact the degenerative process are the subject of ongoing research. It is difficult to determine when disk pathology is related to pain and dysfunction, and the area of prevention is still being studied.

Tara Jo Manal

See also
- Aging, disorders of • Backache • Bone and joint disorders • Muscle system disorders • Nervous system disorders • Occupational disorders • Trauma, accident, and injury

Smallpox

Smallpox first appeared more than three thousand years ago. The first cases probably occurred in India or Egypt. Smallpox eventually spread worldwide and became one of the most devastating diseases known to humanity. For centuries, repeated epidemics swept across continents, wiping out populations and changing the course of history. As early as the 1700s, smallpox killed 1 in 10 children born in Sweden and France and 1 in 7 children born in Russia.

In 1798 an English physician named Edward Jenner showed that inoculation with a cowpox virus, which is similar to the smallpox virus, could protect a person against the smallpox virus. The development of the vaccine led to a global eradication program. This effort was completely successful; vaccination eliminated naturally occurring smallpox from the world. The last case was in Somalia in 1977.

Several laboratories maintained stocks of the virus in storage after the eradication of the disease. Eventually, these storage sites consolidated, and by 1984 they had centralized the remaining stocks at the Centers for Disease Control and Prevention (CDC), in Atlanta, and the Research Institute of Viral Preparations, in Moscow. In 1994 the storage site in the Soviet Union was moved to the State Research Center of Virology and Biotechnology (the Vektor Institute), in Novosibirsk, Russia. This center may have been vulnerable when the Soviet Union collapsed in the early 1990s, and many experts are concerned that someone may have misappropriated some of the virus that causes smallpox during this time.

If this happened, smallpox could pose a significant bioterrorism threat. The virus is easy to grow, and experts could probably modify it in a way that protects it from heat. It can survive in aerosol form and thus someone could load it into weapons or deliver it from a spray device. Today many countries are preparing to deal with a potential attack that uses smallpox.

Causes and risk factors

The variola virus causes smallpox. It affects only humans and is very contagious. It usually spreads from person to person by tiny droplets created when an infected person coughs. Contaminated clothes and bedding can also spread the disease, but the risk of infection from these sources is much lower. Although direct face-to-face contact is usually required for smallpox to spread from person to person, the disease does spread relatively easily.

Before 1970 almost everyone in the world had some immunity against smallpox. Either they had been infected and survived, which gave them natural immunity, or they had received a vaccination that gave them artificial immunity. These people may have some protection in the event of a future smallpox outbreak, but no one knows how long protection lasts after a smallpox vaccination. Some experts recommended revaccination every ten years. Health officials, however, discontinued all of the routine vaccination programs after they eradicated the disease. Only a very few people have received a vaccination against smallpox since 1980. Therefore, almost no one in the world has any immunity that would provide protection in a

KEY FACTS

Description
Viral infection of the human respiratory tract.

Causes
Infection by variola virus.

Risk factors
Contact with an infected person; exposure to a biological weapon.

Symptoms
Fever, cough, and body aches, followed by a spotted, bumpy rash.

Diagnosis
Confirmed by testing blood or the fluid from the blisters.

Treatments
None currently approved, but experts are testing some medications.

Pathogenesis
The virus enters and multiplies in the respiratory passages.

Prevention
Avoiding those with the disease. During an outbreak, a vaccine is available that will prevent the disease or lessen its severity.

Epidemiology
Completely eradicated from nature but could be a potential biological weapon.

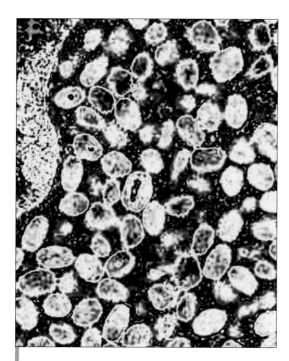

In this colored and magnified photomicrograph, the variola virus can be seen (yellow) against a blue background. The virus causes smallpox, but the disease has been eradicated since the late 1970s.

appears, first on the face, hands, and forearms, and then after a few days moving to the chest, abdomen, and back. The rash starts as pink bumps. The name *smallpox* comes from the Latin word for "spotted" and refers to these bumps. The bumps eventually become blisters and then fill with pus. After several days, they dry up and form scabs.

Complications of smallpox
Smallpox can lead to blindness, and brain inflammation has also been reported. Other disorders are eye infections, bacterial skin infections at the site of the lesions, pneumonia, arthritis, and bone infections. People who have recovered from the disease usually have severe scars on the face, legs, and arms.

Treatment
There is no effective treatment for smallpox, although many different medications are under investigation. Since there is no cure for smallpox, medical treatment is limited to caring for complications of the disease, such as shock or respiratory failure.

Prevention
People who have been around smallpox but have not yet started to have any symptoms can receive the smallpox vaccination. If it is given early enough, it can prevent the disease or reduce its severity.

In the event of an outbreak, many governments have stockpiles of the smallpox vaccine that they could use in an emergency. The governments of both the United Kingdom and the United States, for example, have enough to vaccinate the entire population of their countries, if necessary. Another important step to stop the spread of a future outbreak will be to ensure that healthy people stay away from those who are sick. Those with smallpox must be isolated until the last scab comes off the body. In a large outbreak, infected individuals would be encouraged to stay at home to help reduce the spread of the disease. Public health authorities may recommend "social distancing," which involves requesting people to avoid crowded places, in order to reduce the spread of smallpox. In the event of a smallpox outbreak, it is important that the public stays informed.

Richard N. Bradley

future smallpox outbreak. During previous decades when smallpox was occurring, about 3 in 10 cases of smallpox among individuals without immunity were fatal. Even though most people in the world probably do not have any immunity today, advances in modern health care might moderate the relatively high fatality rate.

Symptoms and signs
Smallpox, like many infectious diseases, has an incubation period. During this time, the virus is multiplying in the person's body, but he or she looks and feels healthy and cannot infect others. The incubation period for smallpox is from seven to seventeen days, but for most people, it will be between 12 and 14 days.

After the incubation period, the infected person will quickly become very ill with flulike symptoms. The symptoms include fever, weakness, headache, and muscle and joint pain. Two to three days later, the fever improves and the patient feels somewhat better. At this point, sores develop in the person's nose and mouth. These become raw and release large amounts of virus. Each cough propels large numbers of these virus particles into the air. Next, the characteristic rash

See also
- Blindness • Infections • Infections, viral
- Influenza • Kidney disorders • Pneumonia
- Skin disorders

Smoking-related disorders

Cigarette smoking affects nearly every organ in the body. The adverse health effects of cigarette smoking account for approximately 440,000 deaths, or nearly 1 in every 5 deaths each year in the United States. Smoking-related disorders include lung cancer, chronic obstructive pulmonary disease (COPD), emphysema, bronchitis, coronary artery disease, mouth cancer, and many others.

Smoking remains the leading cause of preventable death and has negative health impacts on people at all stages of life. It harms unborn babies, infants, children, adolescents, adults, and seniors. An estimated 21 percent of all adults smoke cigarettes in the United States. Prevalence is highest among young adults and lowest in older people: 18 to 24 years, 23.6 percent; 25 to 44 years, 23.8 percent; 45 to 64 years, 22.4 percent; and 65 years or older, 8.8 percent. Cigarette smoking is more common among adult men (23.4 percent) than women (18.5 percent). There are significant differences by race and ethnicity: American Indians and Alaska Natives, 33.4 percent; followed by whites, 22.2 percent; African Americans, 20.2 percent; Hispanics, 15 percent; and Asians, 11.3 percent.

Among youth, 23 percent of high school students in the United States are current smokers (23 percent of females and 22.9 percent of males). African Americans in high school have the lowest smoking prevalence (13 percent), followed by Hispanics (22 percent), and whites (26 percent). In the United States each day, approximately 3,900 adolescents between the ages of 12 and 17 years initiate cigarette smoking. Furthermore, an estimated 2,000 adolescents become daily cigarette smokers in the United States.

Lung cancer

Lung cancer remains the leading cause of cancer-related deaths in both men and women worldwide as well as in the United States, with 174,470 estimated newly diagnosed cases and 162,460 deaths occurring in the United States in 2006. The risk of dying from lung cancer is more than 22 times higher among men who smoke cigarettes, and about 12 times higher among women who smoke cigarettes, compared with those who have never smoked. Eighty to ninety percent of lung cancer mortality is attributable to cigarette smoking, and the relative risks for lung cancer increase with the number of cigarettes smoked each day and the duration of smoking.

There are two major types of lung cancer: non–small cell lung cancer and small cell lung cancer. The most common type is non–small cell lung cancer. It usually spreads to different parts of the body more slowly than small cell lung cancer. Squamous cell carcinoma, adenocarcinoma, and large cell carcinoma are three types of non–small cell lung cancer. Small cell lung cancer, also called oat cell cancer, accounts for about 20 percent of all lung cancers. Lung cancer kills three times as many men as prostate cancer, nearly twice as many women as breast cancer, and more than twice as many men and women as colorectal cancer. Only 15 percent of those people diagnosed with lung cancer live longer than five years. One of the reasons for this low survival rate is that so many of the lung cancers are diagnosed at later stages. Approximately 70 percent of all lung cancers diagnosed are late stage. There has been little improvement in the five-year survival rate for lung cancer since 1971. By comparison, the five-year survival rate for breast cancer is now 88 percent and prostate cancer is 99 percent. The federal government does not support early screening for lung cancer, but it does for other major cancers such as breast cancer, prostate cancer, and colorectal cancer.

How is lung cancer detected?

In its early stages, lung cancer usually does not cause symptoms. When symptoms occur, the cancer is often advanced. Symptoms of lung cancer include chronic cough, hoarseness, coughing up blood, weight loss, loss of appetite, shortness of breath, fever without a known reason, wheezing, repeated bouts of bronchitis or pneumonia, and chest pain.

These conditions are also symptomatic of many other lung problems, so a person who has any of these symptoms should see a doctor to find out the cause. When a person goes for an exam, the doctor asks many questions about the person's medical history, including questions about the patient's exposure to hazardous substances. The doctor will also give the patient a physical exam. If the patient has a cough that produces sputum (mucus), it may be examined for cancer cells. The doctor will order a chest X-ray or

THE EFFECTS OF NICOTINE

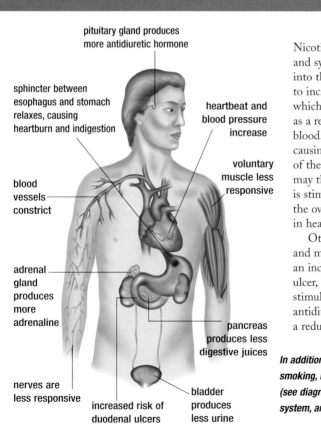

pituitary gland produces more antidiuretic hormone

sphincter between esophagus and stomach relaxes, causing heartburn and indigestion

heartbeat and blood pressure increase

voluntary muscle less responsive

blood vessels constrict

adrenal gland produces more adrenaline

pancreas produces less digestive juices

nerves are less responsive

increased risk of duodenal ulcers

bladder produces less urine

Nicotine has an effect on many of the organs and systems of the body. Nicotine passes rapidly into the bloodstream and causes the heart rate to increase and the blood vessels to constrict, which can lead to the early stages of thrombosis as a result of an increase of fatty acids in the blood. The acids have an effect on platelets, causing them to stick together in the walls of the blood vessels. The clumping of platelets may then block the vessel. The adrenal gland is stimulated to produced more adrenaline; the overall effect is to cause an increase in heartbeat and blood pressure.

Other changes that can occur are: nerves and muscles become less responsive, there is an increased chance of developing a stomach ulcer, and digestion can be affected. Nicotine stimulates the pituitary to produce more antidiuretic hormone; as a result, there is a reduced urine output.

In addition to the damage to the lungs caused by smoking, nicotine affects the body in many other ways (see diagram at left). It can stimulate the central nervous system, and large doses of nicotine have a sedative effect.

specialized X-ray such as a computed tomography (CT) scan, which helps to locate any abnormal spots in the lungs. The doctor may insert a small tube called a bronchoscope through the nose or mouth and down the throat, to look inside the airways and lungs and take a sample, or biopsy, of the tumor. This is just one of a number of ways in which a doctor may take a biopsy sample. A growing number of doctors are using a form of CT scan in smokers to spot small lung cancers, which are more likely than large tumors to be cured. The technique, called helical low-dose CT scan, is much more sensitive than a regular X-ray and can detect tumors when they are small. More studies on this type of screening will show whether routine screening will save lives of smokers and others at risk for lung cancer.

Lung cancer treatments

Treatment of lung cancer is dependent on many factors, such as the type of lung cancer, the size, location, and extent of the tumor (whether or not it has spread), and general health. There are many treatments, which may be used alone or in combination.

Surgery may cure lung cancer, and surgery is used in limited stages of the disease. The type of surgery used depends on where the tumor is located in the lung. Some tumors cannot be removed safely because of their size or location.

Radiation therapy is a form of high-energy X-ray that kills cancer cells. It is used in combination with chemotherapy and sometimes with surgery to offer relief from pain or to alleviate blockage of the airways.

Chemotherapy is the use of drugs that are effective against cancer cells. Chemotherapy may be injected directly into a vein or given through a catheter, which is a thin tube that is placed into a large vein and kept there until it is no longer needed. Some chemotherapy drugs are taken in pill form. Chemotherapy may be used in conjunction with surgery or in more advanced stages of the disease to relieve symptoms; and it may be used in all stages of small cell cancer.

Chronic obstructive pulmonary disease

Chronic obstructive pulmonary disease (COPD) is a term that refers to a large group of lung diseases

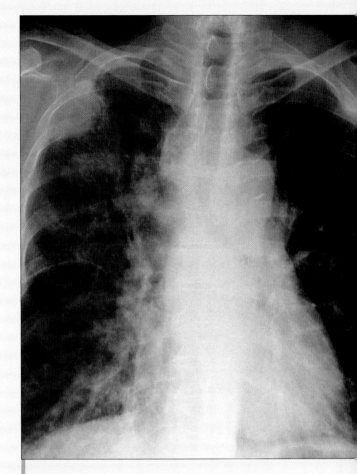

This X-ray of the frontal view of a man's chest shows lung cancer. The man was aged 58 and was a smoker. For a man who smokes, the risk of dying of lung cancer is 22 times greater than that of a nonsmoker.

characterized by obstruction to air flow that interferes with normal breathing.

Emphysema and chronic bronchitis are the most major conditions that compose COPD, and they frequently coexist. Smoking damages airways and alveoli of the lung, eventually leading to COPD.

In COPD, the airways and air sacs lose their shape and become floppy. Less air gets in and less air goes out; the airways and air sacs lose their elasticity, the walls between many of the air sacs are destroyed, the walls of the airways become thick and inflamed, and cells in the airways will make more mucus than usual, which tends to clog the airways.

COPD is the fourth leading cause of death in the United States, claiming approximately 123,000 lives, with more women dying from COPD than men. Approximately 11.4 million adults are estimated to have COPD. Cigarette smoking is associated with a tenfold increased risk of dying from COPD. Approximately 90 percent of all deaths from COPD are attributable to cigarette smoking.

Female smokers are nearly 13 times as likely to die from COPD as women who have never smoked. Male smokers are nearly 12 times as likely to die from COPD as men who have never smoked. There is no cure for COPD. The damage to the airways and lungs is irrevocable and cannot be reversed.

How is COPD detected?

The signs and symptoms of COPD include cough, sputum (mucous) production, shortness of breath (especially when exercising), wheezing, and tightness of the chest.

A breathing test called spirometry is used to confirm a diagnosis of COPD. This test is easy and painless and shows how well the lungs work for an individual. The person breathes hard into a large hose connected to a machine called a spirometer. The spirometer measures how much air the lungs can hold and how fast the air is blown out of the lungs after taking a deep breath. Spirometry is the most sensitive and commonly used test of lung function and can detect COPD long before symptoms develop.

Treatment for COPD is to quit smoking. Not smoking is the single most important thing a person can do to reduce the risk of developing COPD and slow the progress of the disease.

None of the existing medications for COPD has been shown to modify the long-term decline in lung function that is the hallmark of this disease. Therefore, the goal of pharmacotherapy for COPD is to provide relief of symptoms and prevent complications or progression of the disease, or both, with minimum side effects. COPD cannot be cured. The goals of COPD treatment are to relieve symptoms with no or minimal side effects of treatment; slow the progress of the disease; improve exercise tolerance; prevent and treat complications and sudden onset of problems; and improve overall health.

Bronchodilator medications (prescription drugs that relax and open air passages in the lungs) are central to the symptomatic management of COPD. Bronchodilators can be either short acting or long acting.

Short-acting bronchodilators last about four to six hours and are used only when needed. Long-acting bronchodilators last about 12 hours or more and are used every day. Most bronchodilator medicines are delivered by inhalation, so the medication goes directly into the lungs, where it is most needed.

For people with severe COPD and low levels of oxygen in the blood, oxygen therapy may be indicated. Surgery may be recommended for some people who have severe symptoms, have not had improvement from taking medicines, or have great difficulty breathing most of the time.

The two types of surgeries considered in the treatment of severe COPD are bullectomy and lung volume reduction surgery (LVRS). Bullectomy involves the removal of one or more very large bullae from the lungs of people who have emphysema. Bullae are air spaces that are formed when the walls of the air sacs break. The air spaces can become so large that they interfere with breathing. Lung volume reduction surgery involves the removal of sections of damaged tissue from the lungs of patients with emphysema. Finally, a lung transplant may also be performed for some people with very severe COPD. A transplant involves removing the lung of a person with COPD and replacing it with a healthy lung from a donor.

Chronic bronchitis

Chronic bronchitis is the inflammation and eventual scarring of the lining of the bronchial tubes. When the bronchi are inflamed or infected, or both, less air is able to flow to and from the lungs, and heavy mucus or phlegm is coughed up. The condition is defined by the presence of a mucus-producing cough most days of the month for three months of a year for two successive years, without other underlying disease to explain the cough. This inflammation eventually leads to scarring of the lining of the bronchial tubes.

Once the bronchial tubes have been irritated over a long period of time, excessive mucus is produced constantly, the lining of the bronchial tubes becomes thickened, and an irritating cough develops. Air flow may be hampered and the lungs become scarred. The bronchial tubes then make an ideal breeding place for bacterial infections within the airways, which eventually impedes airflow.

An estimated 9 million people in the United

NICOTINE ADDICTION AND DEPENDENCE

The main definition of nicotine dependence or addiction is based on the definitions in the *Diagnostic and Statistical Manual of Mental Disorders*, fourth edition (DSM-IV), of the American Psychiatric Association. According to DSM-IV, there are seven dependence criteria associated with smoking behavior. The criteria are tolerance; withdrawal or smoking to reduce withdrawal; smoking in larger amounts or longer than intended; persistent desire or unsuccessful efforts to cut down; great deal of time spent to obtain cigarettes, smoking cigarettes, or recovering from smoking; activities given up or reduced; and smoking despite physical or psychological problems caused or exacerbated by smoking. An individual is classified as dependent or addicted to nicotine if they experience at least three of the seven dependence criteria.

CRITERIA

1. Tolerance is defined by either of the following:
a) A need for markedly increased amounts to achieve intoxication or the desired effect.
b) A markedly diminished effect with continued use of the same amount of nicotine.

2. Withdrawal, as manifested by either of the following (a) or (b):
a) Characteristic withdrawal syndrome; both (c) and (d)

b) The same or closely related substance taken to relieve or avoid withdrawal symptoms.
c) Daily use of nicotine for at least several weeks.
d) Abrupt cessation or reduction in the amount of nicotine use, followed within 24 hours by four or more of the following signs: dysphoric or depressed mood, insomnia, irritability, frustration or anger, anxiety, difficulty concentrating, restlessness, decreased heart rate, increased appetite or weight gain.

3. The substance is often taken in larger amounts or over a longer period than was intended.

4. There is a persistent desire or unsuccessful attempts to cut down or control substance use.

5. A great deal of time is spent in activities necessary to obtain the substance or recover from its effects.

6. Social, occupational, or recreational activities are given up or reduced because of substance use.

7. The substance use is continued despite knowledge of having a persistent or recurrent physical or psychological problem that is likely to have been caused or exacerbated by the substance.

States report that a physician has diagnosed their condition as chronic bronchitis. Chronic bronchitis affects people of all ages, but is higher in those who are more than 45 years old.

Emphysema

Emphysema begins with the destruction of air sacs (alveoli) in the lungs, where oxygen from the air is exchanged for carbon dioxide in the blood. The walls of the air sacs are thin and fragile. Damage to the air sacs is irreversible and results in permanent holes in the tissues of the lower lungs.

As air sacs are destroyed, the lungs are able to transfer less and less oxygen to the bloodstream, causing shortness of breath. The lungs also lose their elasticity, which is needed to keep airways open.

Emphysema develops very gradually, and years of exposure to the irritation of cigarette smoke usually precedes the development of emphysema. Of the estimated 3.6 million adults ever diagnosed with emphysema, 91 percent were 45 years or older. Symptoms of emphysema include cough, shortness of breath, and a limited exercise tolerance. Diagnosis of emphysema is made by pulmonary function tests, along with the person's history, examination, and other respiratory tests.

Coronary artery disease

Coronary artery disease (CAD) occurs when the arteries that supply blood to the heart muscle (the coronary arteries) become hardened and narrowed. The arteries harden and narrow due to buildup of a material called plaque on their inner walls. The buildup of plaque is known as atherosclerosis. As the plaque increases in size, the space in the coronary arteries becomes narrower, with the result that less blood can flow through them. Eventually, blood flow to the heart muscle is reduced, and, because blood carries much-needed oxygen, the heart muscle is not able to receive the amount of oxygen it needs to function normally. Reduced or cut-off blood flow and oxygen supply to the heart muscle can result in angina and heart attacks. CAD is the most common type of heart disease. It is the leading cause of death in the United States in both men and women.

Toxins in the blood from smoking cigarettes contribute to the development of atherosclerosis. Atherosclerosis is a progressive hardening of the arteries caused by the deposit of fatty plaques and the scarring and thickening of the artery wall. Inflammation of the artery wall and the development of blood clots can obstruct blood flow and cause heart attacks or strokes.

Cigarette smokers are two to four times more likely to develop coronary artery disease than nonsmokers.

How is coronary artery disease diagnosed? There is no single test to diagnose coronary artery disease. Several factors, including a medical history, family history, physical exam, and several other tests are conducted to determine the risk for coronary artery disease. Specific tests that may be used include the electrocardiogram (ECG), which measures the rate and regularity of a person's heartbeat.

The echocardiogram is another test, which uses sound waves to create a moving picture of the heart. The echocardiogram provides information about the size and shape of the heart and how well the heart chambers and valves are functioning. This test can also identify areas of poor blood flow to the heart, areas of heart muscle that are not contracting normally, and previous injury to the heart muscle caused by poor blood flow.

Stress tests involve exercising to make the heart work harder and beat faster while heart tests are performed. During exercise stress testing, the blood pressure and ECG readings are monitored while the person walks or runs on a treadmill or pedals a bicycle.

Newer tests currently being used along with stress testing include magnetic resonance imaging (MRI) and positron emission tomography (PET). MRI shows detailed images of the structures and beating of the heart, which may assist in identifying areas of the heart that are weak or damaged. PET scanning shows the level of chemical activity in different areas of the heart. This test helps doctors determine if enough blood is flowing to different areas of the heart. A PET scan can show decreased blood flow caused by disease or damaged muscles that may not be detected by other scanning methods.

Treatment of coronary artery disease. Treatment for coronary artery disease includes lifestyle changes, medicines, and special procedures. Changes in lifestyle can help treat coronary artery disease. These changes include eating a healthy diet to prevent or reduce high blood pressure and high blood cholesterol and to maintain a healthy weight; quitting smoking for current smokers; exercising; losing weight if overweight or obese; and reducing stress.

Several types of medicines are commonly used to treat coronary artery disease. Cholesterol-lowering medicines, such as statins, help reduce cholesterol to recommended levels.

Anticoagulants help to prevent clots from forming in the arteries and blocking blood flow. Aspirin and other antiplatelet medicines help to prevent clots from forming in the arteries and blocking blood flow. Angiotensin-converting enzyme inhibitors (ACEs) help lower blood pressure and reduce strain on the heart.

Beta blockers slow the heart rate and lower the blood pressure to decrease the workload on the heart. Calcium channel blockers are prescribed to relax blood vessels (arteries and veins), and they also lower the blood pressure.

Angioplasty and coronary artery bypass surgery are two special procedures used to treat CAD when medicines and lifestyle changes have not improved symptoms or when a person's symptoms are getting worse. Angioplasty is a procedure that opens blocked or narrowed coronary arteries.

Sometimes a device called a stent is placed in the artery to keep the artery propped open after the procedure. Coronary artery bypass surgery involves taking arteries and veins from other areas of the body to bypass the narrowed coronary arteries.

Won Choi

Spina bifida

Spina bifida is one of the most common birth defects in the world, and it is also one of the easiest to prevent. Simply adding folic acid to a mother's diet before pregnancy can dramatically reduce the number of cases of spina bifida each year, though the actual cause remains a mystery.

Spina bifida is a birth defect that can occur before a woman even knows she is pregnant. Preventive measures therefore focus on the general population. In the United States, breads, cereals, and other grain products have been fortified with extra folic acid, a nutrient that appears essential to normal embryonic development. In this way, most women of childbearing age will have sufficient folic acid in their diets well before a pregnancy begins.

Causes

Just 18 days after a sperm fertilizes an egg, a critical developmental milestone occurs. The neural tube begins to close up around the developing brain and spinal cord. By the fourth week of pregnancy, the process is complete. If the mother is at risk or suffers from a nutritional deficiency, the neural tube may not close properly. When the gap occurs along the spine, the result is spina bifida, which means "split spine."

Different forms and different outcomes

There are multiple forms of spina bifida. The two major forms are spina bifida occulta, which means "hidden," and spina bifida manifesta, in which the spinal defects are obvious. Spina bifida manifesta can be subdivided into two types: meningocele and myelomeningocele. These names describe the specific type of damage caused by the disorder.

Spina bifida occulta is a common condition, and some health professionals estimate that it may occur in up to 20 percent of apparently healthy people. There might be a slight dimple along the spine, unusual pigmentation, or a hairy patch over the area. This disorder rarely causes symptoms or problems for the patient unless there is an associated fatty deposit that can press on the spinal cord and spinal nerves.

The meningocele form of spina bifida is the least common form. In this disorder, only the meninges, which are the protective membranes around the spinal cord, extrude from the spinal column. Nerve damage can result, and these patients might suffer minor disabilities or neurological problems later in life.

The most severe form of spina bifida is myelomeningocele, and this is the form most people recognize as spina bifida. In this case, the opening extends along several vertebrae, and both the meninges and spinal cord itself are pushed out of the opening. It is quite common for these patients to experience some degree of paralysis or weakness in their legs and lower back. Nerve damage can affect both bladder and bowel functions. In addition, 70 to 90 percent of patients with this form of spina bifida will also have hydrocephalus, or "water on the brain." This condition can lead to problems with learning and memory, behavior, and decision making.

One of the most important factors in determining how severe the damage will be is the actual location of the lesion. Lesions higher on the spinal column are more likely to result in paralysis and severe disabilities. Patients with lower lesions can often lead normal lives and even raise families of their own.

Risk factors

The cause of spina bifida remains unknown, but several risk factors have been identified. The most important risk factor is insufficient folic acid in the diet before and during early pregnancy. Other risk factors include certain drugs used to treat epilepsy, kidney dialysis, alcohol abuse, obesity, diabetes, and fevers or high temperatures during early pregnancy. Although whites and Hispanics are at higher risk overall, socioeconomic factors that lead to poor nutrition can raise the risk for other racial groups. Parents who have had one child with spina bifida are at higher risk of having a second child with the disease. Spina bifida patients also have a higher risk. However, scientists have not located a specific gene associated with the disorder.

Since 1997, the U.S. government has officially recognized exposure to Agent Orange as an additional risk factor for spina bifida. Agent Orange was a defoliant used during the Vietnam War, and many veterans were exposed. Veterans who have children with spina bifida can receive up to $1,200 a month in disability payments and assistance with vocational training and rehabilitation. No benefits are provided to patients with spina bifida occulta.

Symptoms and diagnosis

Most cases of spina bifida can be identified by routine prenatal blood tests during the second trimester of pregnancy. A triple screen test looks for the presence of alpha-fetoprotein (AFP) and measures levels of two important hormones. If the AFP levels are abnormally high, an ultrasound scan will be used to look for defects along the spinal column. The test is not definitive, because not all cases of spina bifida will produce high levels of AFP.

In the more severe forms of spina bifida, the physical defects are obvious at birth. A fluid-filled sac protrudes from the back, and there may be an opening in the skin around the lesion. In less severe cases, symptoms such as weakness in the legs and lower back pain may develop later in life. Spina bifida occulta may never be diagnosed unless the patient happens to need a spinal X-ray at some point.

Treatments

There is no cure for spina bifida. Damaged nerves can never be repaired or replaced. Therefore, the most important treatment for spina bifida is surgery to prevent additional nerve damage by repairing the hole in the spinal column. This surgery is normally performed within the first 24 hours of life, although some doctors are experimenting with prenatal surgery. For patients with hydrocephalus, a shunt is normally implanted to help drain cerebrospinal fluid. Without the shunt, pressure can build up and damage the brain and central nervous system. Patients may need additional surgery later in life. A common complication is a condition called "tethered spinal cord." As the patient grows, the spinal cord becomes stuck and must be surgically freed to allow proper movement and fluid flow around the cord. If the spinal cord remains tethered and stretched, additional nerve damage can occur.

Other treatments focus on keeping a patient active, healthy, and mentally fit. Even patients confined to wheelchairs will get special exercise programs to keep their weight under control, to prevent pressure sores, and to maximize their fitness. Good hygiene is also important to avoid infections and skin sores. Many patients have very poor sensation in their lower limbs, so it is important to check frequently for skin damage and bruises. Patients are also more likely to have latex allergies, so it is important to avoid all latex products, such as balloons.

Social impact

It is estimated that 70,000 people in the United States are living with spina bifida. The highest rates of the disease are in the southeastern part of the country. Worldwide, the highest rates are found in China. Differences in nutritional status and the availability of medical care can greatly affect the quality of life for these patients.

Patients with myleomeningocele spina bifida are often confined to wheelchairs or require braces to walk. Problems with learning and memory are common; however, most patients will have average IQs. Advocacy groups have been established to help patients with spina bifida lead normal productive lives. Special training or educational programs can help patients cope with learning disabilities, poor hand-eye

---

KEY FACTS

Description
A developmental disorder that can lead to paralysis in severe cases.

Cause
Unknown, but both genetics and environmental factors probably play a role.

Risk factors
Insufficient folic acid in the mother's diet before and during pregnancy; anti-epileptic medicines; obesity; and diabetes.

Symptoms
Congenital deformities of the spine, lower back pain, and weakness in the back or legs.

Diagnosis
Prenatal blood tests and ultrasound can be used to diagnose most cases in utero. Spinal deformities are obvious at birth.

Treatments
Severe cases require surgery in the first days of life. Mild cases may need no treatment at all.

Pathogenesis
The course of the disease varies considerably and depends on both the location and severity of the malformation. About 90 percent of babies born with spina bifida will survive to adulthood.

Prevention
Adequate consumption of folic acid before and during pregnancy.

Epidemiology
Hispanics and whites of European descent are at highest risk. In the United States, the current rate is about 1 in 5,000 live births.

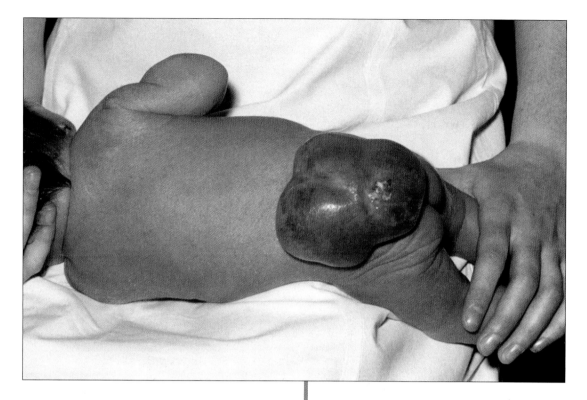

coordination, and behavioral disorders associated with spina bifida and hydrocephalus. Mental health professionals can help patients deal with the stress and depression that often occur in people who have chronic illnesses.

Pathogenesis

Comprehensive care is required throughout life, which makes spina bifida a very expensive disorder. The lifetime cost can be as high as $1 million per patient in the United States. With proper care, however, the majority of patients will survive to adulthood and some are able to raise families of their own. These patients do face an increased risk of having a child with the disorder, however.

Patients with spina bifida occulta may not experience serious health problems, but they might discover they have difficulty getting health insurance or getting hired. To avoid these potential difficulties, many health professionals do not use the term *spina bifida occulta*. They will report the defect as a "vertebral fusion defect" instead.

Prevention and epidemiology

Spina bifida cases dropped 28 percent from 1995 to 2003 after the U.S. government mandated the addition of folic acid to grain products such as bread and

A newborn baby has spina bifida, in which part of the spinal cord and its coverings are exposed through a gap in the backbone. Symptoms can include paralysis, incontinence, and mental retardation.

cereal. Studies indicate that one-half to three-quarters of all cases of spina bifida can be prevented by folic acid supplementation.

However, scientists still cannot determine exactly how folic acid prevents birth defects. They do know that it is essential for cells to make RNA and DNA, for the production of new red blood cells, and for the breakdown of homocysteine, a metabolite that can damage tissue when present in high concentrations. Foods high in folic acid include leafy green vegetables, orange juice, eggs, and enriched grain products.

According to the Centers for Disease Control and Prevention (CDC), approximately 20 cases of spina bifida occur in every 100,000 live births in the United States.

Chris Curran

See also
- Alcohol-related disorders • Birth defects
- Diabetes • Kidney disorders • Mental retardation • Neural tube defects • Obesity
- Vitamin deficiency

Spinal curvature

The human spine, or backbone, has natural gentle curves. However, poor posture or inheritance can result in misaligned curves, pain, and impaired respiration.

The normal vertebral column forms a straight line down the center of the back. Viewed from the side, the vertebral column displays a curvature that develops with growth and age. The infant spine is flexible and forms a C curve (viewed from the side) as infants curl their head toward the center of their body. This early curve is a kyophotic curvature because the spinal convexity is directed backward. As infants grow and develop muscle control, they begin to lift their heads against gravity when they are lying on their stomachs. The neck muscles bring the cervical spine into a reverse curvature, with the convexity directed toward the body's front. A curvature with an forward-directed convexity is called a lordotic curvature. When a baby learns to sit up, a second lordotic curvature forms in the lumbar region of the lower back. The result is alternating curvatures: lordotic curvatures in the cervical and lumbar regions and kyphotic curvatures in the thoracic and sacrococcygeal regions. The spine continues to change throughout adolescence until growth is completed.

Types of spinal curvatures

The vertebrae are connected individually and as segments by an intricate array of muscles and ligaments. Column segments are so interdependent that shifting or injury associated with any vertebra can alter the alignment of articulating vertebrae. It is inevitable that a cascade effect will alter the mechanics and alignment of the vertebral column as a whole. An idiopathic curvature is inherited. A postural curvature is due to poor posture. Individuals may choose to sit or stand with a postural curvature to protect themselves from pain.

Kyphosis

Kyphosis is a posterior curvature normal to the thoracic and sacrococcygeal areas. Excessive thoracic kyphosis appears as a "humped" area in the shoulders and mid-back. Postural kyphosis is flexible and is the result of poor posture. Individuals with a "flat" lower back often slump in the shoulders to optimize their center of gravity, resulting in a kyphotic stance. The hump of idiopathic kyphosis is called a "gibbus" and is often the result of a fracture, tumor, or bone disease that altered the shape of some thoracic vertebrae. Postmenopausal women may have a so-called dowager's hump as a result of osteoporosis of the upper and mid-thoracic vertebrae. Severe and persistent kyphosis related to changes in the vertebral column can lead to painful nerve root impingements and muscle discomfort.

Lordosis

Lordosis is a forward-directed convexity. Excessive lordosis is a condition of the lumbar spine and often

---

KEY FACTS: SCOLIOSIS

Description

A lateral shift and rotation of the spinal vertebrae. The spine forms an S or a C shape.

Causes

Postural or idiopathic, which may be due to vertebral abnormalities or abnormal muscle control in the trunk.

Risk factors

A strong genetic component to idiopathic scoliosis.

Symptoms

Usually asymptomatic at adolescence. Severe curve progression and rib cage rotation can lead to impaired respiration. Large lumbar deviations may lead to painful osteoarthritis.

Diagnosis

Physical examination and X-ray.

Treatments

A mild scoliotic curvature (less than 30 degrees deviation) is generally monitored. Moderate curvatures (30–45 degrees deviation) may need bracing; severe curvatures may require surgery.

Pathogenesis

Predispositions include heredity, connective tissue disorders, and neuromuscular disorders. Progression of scoliotic curve can lead to pain, restricted movement in the trunk and arms, and impaired respiration.

Prevention

Bracing may prevent curve progression, but there is disagreement about the success of bracing. Early intervention offers best results.

Epidemiology

Thoracic curvatures of greater than 60 degrees deviation are associated with reduced life span. Adolescent girls are affected by scoliosis at least five times more often than boys.

accompanies scoliosis. Lordosis is often the result of an anteriorly tilted pelvis and shortened hip flexor muscles. Individuals with weak trunk and hip muscles, such as those with muscular dystrophy, often compensate for their weakness by assuming a lordotic stance.

Scoliosis

Lateral shifting occurs when the spinal column does not form a straight line or deviates from the vertical center of the back. Lateral spinal column deviation is referred to as scoliosis. These lateral deformities usually occur in either the thoracic or lumbar spine, or both coincidentally. The spinal column shifts laterally as a result of rotational forces on the vertebrae. Because the vertebrae articulate directly with the rib cage, severe scoliosis alters the rib cage and impairs the lungs' ability to expand. Impaired respiratory function is a very serious consequence of severe scoliosis. A rib hump is often apparent at the most severe rotational point.

A scoliotic curvature may form a C curve, with one lateral convexity (to the left or to the right), or an S curve, with two convexities directed in opposite directions. Scoliosis can be mild and nearly unidentifiable, or severe. Postural scoliosis is flexible and often the result of body posturing. It can be corrected by pressure at the lateral convexities or with conscientious effort to improve posture. Often, postural scoliosis is the result of a posture that protects a painful back.

Individuals with one leg longer than the other may also display postural scoliosis as they shift their posture in standing to keep their field of vision level and centered.

Girls are at least five times more likely than boys to be affected by idiopathic scoliosis. It is usually painless and asymptomatic; however, severe curvatures may cause respiratory limitations and pain in adult years. Idiopathic scoliosis is often the result of a vertebral abnormality that changes the structural alignment of the spinal column.

Scoliosis is common in individuals with neuromuscular disorders such as cerebral palsy and poliomyelitis. An imbalance in muscle "pull" on either side of the spinal column results in a lateral shift and vertebral rotation toward the stronger side of the back. Neuromuscular disorders that result in weakness and poor trunk control, such as muscular dystrophy, spina bifida, or spinal cord injury are also at risk for scoliosis. Since trunk muscles help enhance breathing, individuals with weak trunk muscles due to neuromuscular disorders may be at higher risk of respiratory compromise if they also have severe scoliosis.

Diagnosis

A diagnosis of kyphosis or lordosis is generally made through observation and measurement. Idiopathic causes of these spinal curvatures, such as vertebral wedging or other abnormalities, can be confirmed through X-ray. Osteoporosis, a potential cause of kyphosis, can be confirmed with a bone density scan.

A plumb line centered at vertical midline of the back can help identify both subtle and obvious scoliosis. Idiopathic scoliosis may also be detected when an individual with scoliosis bends forward with hands joined and arms hanging down. Individuals with scoliosis show asymmetries in the two sides of the back when bending forward. An X-ray can confirm scoliosis and help monitor its progression. An MRI may be necessary if the individual presents with neurological signs.

Practicing good posture is the best way to prevent postural disorders of the spinal column. Postural scoliosis related to back pain is best resolved by treating the source of back pain, possibly nerve root impingement or other inflammatory conditions. Postural thoracic kyphosis can often be treated with posture reeducation and focused strengthening exercises.

Idiopathic thoracic kyphosis due to vertebral wedging, fractures, or vertebral abnormalities is more difficult to manage, since assuming a correct posture may not be possible with structural changes in the vertebrae. Children who have not completed their growth may show long-lasting improvements with bracing. Exercises may be prescribed to alleviate discomfort associated with overstretched back muscles. A variety of gravity-assisted positions or gentle traction can minimize pain associated with nerve root impingement. Surgery may be recommended for severe idiopathic kyphosis.

Treatment for idiopathic scoliosis depends upon the severity of the curvature, the spine's potential for further growth, and the risk that the curvature will progress. Mild scoliosis (less than 30 degrees deviation) may simply be monitored and treated with exercise. Moderately severe scoliosis (30–45 degrees) in a child who is still growing may require bracing. Severe curvatures that rapidly progress may be treated surgically with spinal rod placement. Bracing may prevent a progressive curvature, but evidence is not strong in favor of correction with brace wear. In all cases, early intervention offers the best results.

Patti Berg

See also
• Bone and joint disorders • Muscle system disorders • Osteoporosis • Spinal disorders

Spinal disorders

In vertebrates, the spinal column serves to protect the spinal cord, to allow for a wide range of movement and to support the weight of the body. For most animals, the weight of the body is spread among all the vertebrae. But the spines of humans, who primarily walk on their "hind" legs, have to act as a flexible column, with all the weight resting upon the base. As a result, humans face a host of unique challenges when the health of their spine is impaired.

Spinal problems result from a host of causes: primarily trauma, improper curvature, infection, malnutrition, wear and tear, and genetics. Signs and symptoms can range from the acute, such as temporary back pain, to debilitating, such as paralysis.

Trauma

With the numerous bones, muscles, and nerves that compose, connect to, or run through the spinal column, it is especially vulnerable to many kinds of traumatic injuries. Trauma can range from mild strains of the muscles connected to the vertebrae to more severe injuries, such as fractures of the bones and severing of the nerves.

A common cause of spinal trauma is failure to maintain proper posture when picking up or moving heavy objects. Muscles are easily strained, ligaments can stretch or tear, and, in more severe cases, disks can slip or rupture (herniate), leading to pinched nerves or erosion of the cartilaginous cushion between vertebrae. Something as simple as a muscle spasm can trigger other symptoms if the muscle puts excessive pressure on spinal nerves.

More severe trauma results from accidents and falls. Fractures or dislocations of the spine, in addition to damaging the bones involved, can trigger inflammation that puts excessive pressure on the nerves, thus impairing their function, or the pressure can sever the nerves outright.

One common type of spinal injury is a whiplash—extreme backward bending (hyperextension) of the head, followed by extreme forward bending (hyperflexion) of the head. Whiplashes are a common result of automobile accidents in which one vehicle is rear-ended by another. Injuries associated with whiplashes include strained or torn muscles and ligaments, vertebral fractures, and herniated disks.

Improper curvature

Abnormal spinal curvature can trigger a number of problems. The most common curvature disorder is scoliosis, in which the spine bends to the right or left. An obvious sign of scoliosis is one shoulder higher than the other. Scoliosis, which is more common in

SPINAL CURVATURE

The bones of the spinal column are part of the axial skeleton, the bones that lie around the longitudinal (head to toe) axis of the body, along with the skull, ear bones, hyoid bone, sternum, and ribs. The spinal column encloses and protects the spinal cord. The spinal column also serves as an attachment point for the ribs and the bones of the pelvis, as well as the muscles of the trunk.

The spine consists of a series of connected bones called vertebrae (singular: vertebra). Each vertebra consists of a thick portion in front called the body. A series of processes off the back of the body form the vertebral arch. The arch and body form a hollow space, the vertebral foramen, through which runs the spinal cord (the transmission line between the brain and the nerves that run through the rest of the body). Off the vertebral arch are seven processes or structures. The three larger ones—the spinous process that extends toward the back and two spinous processes that extend toward either side—serve as attachment points for muscles. Four smaller processes, called articular processes, form joints with other vertebrae. When connected, the processes leave openings, intervertebral foramen, for passage of spinal nerves.

Between each pair of vertebrae are intervertebral discs made of tough, fibrous cartilage outside (the annulus pulposus) and a spongy elastic material inside (the nucleus pulposus). The discs are an integral part of the intervertebral joints, with an especially important role in providing a cushion against shock and the grinding of adjacent vertebrae.

The interlocking nature of the vertebrae allows for a wide range of movement (forward, backward, sideways, and rotation) and provides a sturdy base of support for the weight of the trunk and head. Especially important in this supporting role are the first two vertebra, which are significantly different from the others. The first vertebra, or atlas (named for the mythological Titan who bore the weight of the world on his shoulders), supports the skull. It is essentially a ring of bone, without the body characteristic of other vertebrae, that articulates with the skull in such a fashion to allow a fore-and-aft nodding motion of the head. The second vertebra, the axis, has a vertical process that extends up from the body, called the dens. The dens creates a pivot upon which the atlas and skull can rotate, allowing a side-to-side motion of the head.

When looking through the body from front to back (or vice versa) the spine should appear straight.

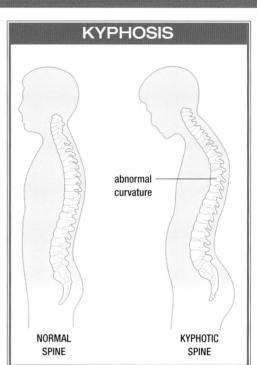

KYPHOSIS

abnormal curvature

NORMAL SPINE

KYPHOTIC SPINE

The kyphotic spine is abnormally curved in the thoracic area of the spine, creating a stooped appearance.

However, when looking though the body from side to side, the spine should have a series of curves toward the front and back. The curvature begins with the cervical curve, in which the vertebral bodies bulge slightly forward, through the thoracic curve, a more pronounced curve in which the vertebral bodies bulge backward. In the lumbar curve, the vertebral bodies bulge slightly forward again. The fused sacral and coccygeal vertebrae form the sacral curve, which, like the thoracic curve, bulges backward so that the tip of the coccyx points slightly forward. Proper curvature is important for spinal function, since it reduces wear and tear on the vertebrae and disks.

Early in their development, humans have 33 vertebrae, but some in the lower part of the spinal column fuse, so that adults have only 26: 7 in the cervical region (neck); 12 in the thoracic region (chest and upper back); five in the lumbar region (abdomen and lower back); one consisting of 5 fused vertebrae in the sacral region (pelvis); and one consisting of 4 fused vertebrae in the coccygeal region (essentially the tail).

females, primarily affects the thoracic vertebrae and has a number of causes, from congenital defects to infections (such as polio), poor posture, or unequal leg length. Severe cases may progress to the point at which breathing is impaired.

Kyphosis is an exaggeration of the thoracic curve, with affected persons developing a stoop-shouldered appearance. Like scoliosis, it has a number of causes. Tuberculosis of the spine causes partial collapse of vertebral bodies. Degeneration of disks, osteoporosis leading to microfractures of the vertebrae, rickets, and poor posture can also lead to kyphosis.

Lordosis is an exaggeration of the lumbar curve. Increased weight gain, such as during pregnancy, can cause it, but tuberculosis, rickets, osteoporosis, and poor posture can contribute to it as well.

Infection

As with polio and tuberculosis, infections can cause a number of spinal problems. Viruses, bacteria, and fungi are all capable of infecting vertebrae, nerves, or supporting tissues of the spine. Spinal infections can result from person-to-person contact or can result from abuse of intravenous drugs, from spinal injuries, or as a result of spinal surgery.

Tuberculosis of the spine, which is known from mummies from ancient Egypt, is caused by *Mycobacterium tuberculosis* and other *Mycobacterium* species. It most often occurs in people who contracted tuberculosis as a child, before the ends of most bones have calcified. Bacteria enter the bones through the ends, or epiphyses. As the bacterial colonies grow, they damage the surrounding bones and adjacent joints. In time, the vertebrae can collapse and paralysis may result. Other bacteria, such as *Staphylococcus*, *Brucella*, *Salmonella*, and *Francisella*, may similarly damage the spine.

Bones and joints are not the only spinal components vulnerable to infection. The nerves may also be affected. Polio, caused by a virus, damages cells of the central nervous system, such as those of the anterior horn portion of the spinal cord, where many motor neurons of spinal nerves originate. As the cells are destroyed, the nerves fail to function, and paralysis of the affected muscles ensues.

Meningitis, an infection of the fluid and membranes that surround the spinal cord, can be caused by either bacteria or viruses. Initial symptoms include pain, fever, and nausea, but when treatment is delayed, death may result. Fungal infections of the spine are rare, and are most commonly seen in patients with compromised immune systems.

Malnutrition

Malnutrition, which is caused by a diet lacking essential nutrients, causes a number of spinal disorders. A common disorder is spina bifida. Spina bifida is congenital disorder often related to a lack of folic acid, a B vitamin, in the mother's diet. The spinal cord and vertebrae originate as a fold of skin down the back of a developing fetus. The edges of the fold fuse to form a neural tube, which in turn develops into the components of the central nervous system (brain and spinal cord) and bones of the spine. When folic acid in the mother's diet is lacking, the tube fails to close properly, leaving portions of the baby's spinal cord exposed to the outside.

Other nutritional disorders of the spine include rickets and osteoporosis. Both rickets and osteoporosis are caused by a vitamin D deficiency. The vitamin promotes mineralization (incorporation of calcium and phosphorus into the bone tissue), which in turn promotes strength of the bones. When the vitamin is lacking, the mineral levels become too low and the bones eventually weaken, leading to an increased risk of fracture.

Rickets is commonly found in children, in whom the lack of vitamin D leads to developmental defects during growth. Osteoporosis typically affects postmenopausal women or women who are underweight. A number of factors contribute to increased risk of osteoporosis, such as a lack of vitamin D, which promotes calcium absorption, or a lack of calcium, which leads to loss of bone mass.

Wear and tear

Bones and joints take a beating over a lifetime; thus it is inevitable that parts of the body that are worked hard begin to wear out with time. Among the spinal disorders caused by wear and tear are degenerative disk disease and arthritis.

Degenerative disk disease can result in a number of other disorders, including spinal stenosis (narrowing of

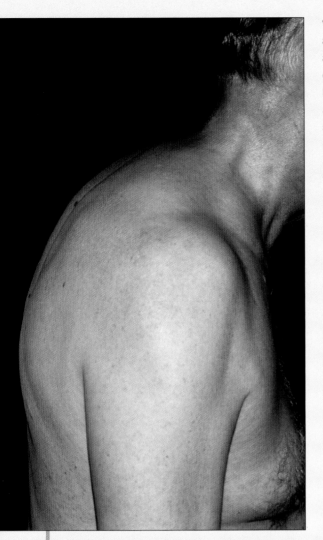

vertebrae, lower parts of the body are most often affected. Both rheumatoid arthritis and osteoarthritis affect the spine. In osteoarthritis, the cartilaginous cushion between bones wears away, and when bone contacts other bone, the portions of the bones along the interface begin to be worn down. Bone spurs may form. This may or may not be accompanied by degenerative disk disease. Rheumatoid arthritis may give rise to inflammation of the joints between vertebrae. The inflammation may in turn trigger degeneration of the affected joints. Rheumatoid arthritis strikes younger patients; osteoarthritis affects older people.

Genetics

Ankylosing spondylitis is another degenerative disorder of the spine that has a strong genetic link. Most people with the disease share a genetic marker called HLA-B27. Ankylosing spondylitis features inflammation of the intervertebral joints, as well as the joints between the sacrum and the bones of the pelvis, leading to pain and stiffness of joints. Calcium may be deposited in the soft tissues of the joints, which leads to eventual fusion of the bones on either side of the joint. Other parts of the body may also be affected.

Genetics increase the risk of a number of spinal disorders, among them scoliosis, spina bifida, rheumatoid arthritis, and some forms of degenerative disk disease.

The outward curvature of the spine (kyphosis) is apparent on this 68-year-old man who has ankylosing spondylitis. This is an inflammatory disease that affects the joints between the spinal vertebrae. The condition worsens until eventually there is a curvature and increasing immobility.

the spinal canal), spondylolisthensis (slipping of disks or vertebrae forward, or both), and retrolisthensis (slipping of disks or vertebrae backward, or both). Bone spurs may grow near the intervertebral joints. In all of these cases, the spinal cord or spinal nerves may be constricted, which puts pressure on nerves and leads to nerve damage, with ensuing impairment of organs supplied by the nerves.

Since degenerative disk disease most commonly affects the lower vertebrae, such as the lumbar

Tumors and cancer

Tumors of the spine may occur, but they are rare. Vertebral tumors usually spread to the spine from other areas of the body. Tumors are more likely to originate in the spinal cord and associated tissues. A relatively common type of spinal tumor is a meningioma, or tumor (usually benign) of the meninges, which is the layer that protects the nerve cord. While the tumors are usually benign, they are often difficult to remove. Tumors also arise in the cells that support the nerve cells. These intermedullary tumors can be either benign or malignant. The risk of spinal cord lymphomas, which are cancers of white blood cells, is increased in patients who have weakened immune systems.

David M. Lawrence

Spirochete infections

Spirochete infections are caused by slender, fragile spiral organisms that belong to the order *Spirochaetales*, which includes the families *Spirochaetaceae* and *Treponemataceae*. Conditions caused by spirochetes include syphilis, endemic syphilis, yaws, pinta, relapsing fever, leptospirosis, Lyme disease, and spirillary rat-bite fever, or soduko.

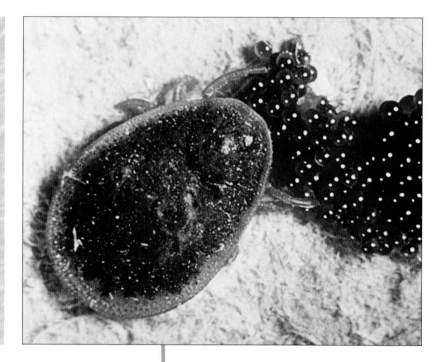

Appearing like a group of corkscrews under the microscope, spirochetes can cause a variety of conditions. The spirochetes are fragile and are tightly coiled with flagella on the end that allow them to burrow into skin tissue. The most well known and infamous spirochete is *Treponema pallidum*, which causes the sexually transmitted disease syphilis. These diseases have some factors in common: they are caused by a spirochete, are found in places where hygiene is lacking, and can be treated with antibiotics. Otherwise, their symptoms, treatment, pathogenesis, and epidemiology are different and vary with the disease. Spirochete infections can be grouped as endemic syphilis, tick-borne and louse-borne infections, relapsing fever, leptospirosis, and rat-bite fever.

Endemic spirochetes

Unlike syphilis, endemic spirochetes or treponematoses are not caused by sexual contact but are chronic within a population and are spread by bodily contact. Diagnosis is made by appearance of the lesions, but in laboratory tests it is difficult to distinguish these parasites from the ones that cause syphilis. The following conditions are caused by endemic spirochetes.

Endemic syphilis, nonvenereal syphilis, or Bejal is a condition found in Arab countries of the eastern

This soft tick lives in North America and is a member of the Argasidae family. The tick is female and has laid a batch of eggs (on the right of the picture). Over a period of years, after each blood meal, she will lay one batch after another. Some soft ticks are known to be a vector for the spirochetes that cause relapsing fever.

Mediterranean and North Africa. Transmission is from mouth-to-mouth contact, such as sharing eating or drinking utensils. The symptoms begin in childhood as mucuslike patches, usually in the mouth. In later stages, lesions appear on the trunk and extremities, inflammation forms around the bones, and large sores develop in the soft palate and nose. This condition is caused by *Treponema pallidum II*.

Diagnosis is made from the typical appearance of the lesions in persons from endemic areas. It is difficult in laboratories to distinguish from the venereal syphilis. The International Task Force for Disease Eradication has determined that eradication is not a feasible goal; rather, they believe that education about transmission is the only possible course of action.

Yaws, or frambesia, is found in humid equatorial countries. Yaws begins when the spirochete *Treponema pertenue* penetrates an opening in the skin, and a painless bump arises within two to eight weeks and grows at the entrance of the site. The initial site may heal, and then recurring secondary crops of bumps with swollen glands occur, with lesions on the face, extremities, and buttocks. These painless bumps become filled with pus and burst. The child feels extremely unwell and loses appetite. In its late stage, it can destroy skin, bones, and joints and cause tender lesions on the soles of the feet called dry crab yaws.

Scanty clothing, poor hygiene, and skin trauma favor the transmission of yaws. The term *yaws* comes from a Caribbean word *yaya*, meaning "sore." This common disease of children is found in the tropics and is a particular problem in overcrowded conditions where there is poor hygiene. Yaws can be simply cured with a single shot of penicillin.

Pinta is a condition that is found among the Indians of Mexico, Central America, and northern South America. This infection is caused by *Treponema carateum*. Beginning with small sores at the site of entrance, it soon changes, and large red sores appear on the face and extremities after several months. Like the condition vitiligo, the skin pigment may disappear, and calloused skin develops on the soles of the feet and palms of the hands. The lesions are confined in the dermis, the second layer of skin, and treponema does not get into other body systems. However, the destructive lesions do leave scars. In fact, all these endemic conditions may leave scars. The infections are usually easily treated with penicillin or other antibiotics. Currently, transmission of these conditions is not well understood.

Tick-borne and louse-borne infections

The spirochete *Borrelia burgodorferi* is the agent for Lyme disease, the most frequently reported human tick-transmitted disease in the United States. The tick *Ixodes scapularis* is the most common vector; the tick usually lives on deer. Lyme disease produces fever, headache, muscle aches, fatigue, and other neurological and cardiac problems. If Lyme disease is not treated promptly, other complications, such as meningitis, can develop. However, diagnosis is not always straightforward because other spirochete infections produce similar symptoms and are transmitted by a variety of organisms.

Relapsing fever

Relapsing fever, called also tick, recurrent, or famine fever, can be of two types. Endemic relapsing fever is caused by at least 15 different species of *Borrelia spirochetes*. The insect vector may be different species of the soft tick of the genus *Ornithodoros*. Tick-borne diseases are seen in the Americas, Africa, Asia, Europe, and the western part of the United States. When the tick attaches to the skin, infection takes place within minutes; this is different from Lyme disease, in which the tick must be attached for several hours before the organism gets into the body.

Epidemic relapsing fever is caused by the head and body louse and tends to be more severe than the tick-borne variety. Louse infections are endemic in parts of Africa where civil wars and refugee camps provide fertile grounds for transmission. When an infected louse feeds on an uninfected human, the organism *Borrelia recurrentis* gains access when the victim crushes the louse or scratches the area where the louse is feeding. The organism goes into the skin and then quickly enters the bloodstream.

An ingenious mechanism causes the prevalent symptom: relapsing. Relapses occur when *Borrelia* produces genetic clones that destroy antibodies against the original spirochete. The patient improves until the new clone multiplies sufficiently to cause another relapse. Tick-borne disease tends to have more relapses,

---

KEY FACTS

Description
Diseases caused by a group of bacteria called spirochetes.

Causes
Direct skin contact with others who have the condition or with animal carriers such as ticks or rats.

Risk factors
Unsanitary conditions or inhabiting areas where the carriers are present.

Symptoms
Flulike symptoms in the early stages but then different symptoms according to the disease.

Diagnosis
Examination by experienced medical personnel who find the spirochete in laboratory tests.

Treatments
Antibiotics.

Pathogenesis
If left untreated, organisms invade many organs of the body.

Prevention
Avoiding contact with people who have the condition, contaminated water, and animals that may carry the spirochete.

an average of three compared to the louse-borne variety, which has only one relapse.

Symptoms include high fever, rigors, severe headache, muscle pains, weakness, anorexia, weight loss, and cough. The first fever ends about three to six days after onset, then about seven to ten days later, the relapse occurs. Other symptoms include an enlarged spleen and liver, jaundice, rash, respiratory problems, and nervous system involvement.

Diagnosis includes finding the spirochetes in the blood during the fever periods. *Borrelia* are delicate, threadlike organisms, with pointed ends and four to ten large, irregular coils. However, many cases probably occur that are misdiagnosed or unreported.

Treatment with antibiotics is usually quickly effective. Prevention includes insecticide treatment, rodent control, and improved hygiene.

Leptospirosis

Leptospirosis is an inclusive term for infections from any of the 130 different species of the genus *Leptospira*. Names for the condition include Weil's disease or syndrome, infectious spirochetal jaundice, and canicola fever. Weil's disease is the most severe form of leptospirosis. Regardless of the type, the disease is a zoonosis, that is, it is carried by animals. *Leptospira* organisms have been found in cattle, pigs, horses, dogs, rodents, and wild animals. However, the condition may exist in many animals that show few signs and symptoms.

Humans get the infection through contact with water, food, or soil containing urine from these infected animals. The person may swallow the contaminated food or water, or organisms may enter through the skin, eyes, nose, or any place the skin is broken. The disease does not appear to be spread from person to person. Infection can occur at any age, but 75 percent of patients are males. It may be an occupational hazard of farm workers, veterinarians, pet shop owners, slaughterhouse workers, coal miners, and workers in the fishing industry. Some people may get exposure in recreational waters.

It takes about two days to four weeks from the time exposure occurs to the contaminated source until symptoms begin to appear. The illness usually begins with an abrupt fever and may occur in two phases.

During the first phase the person has fever, chills, headache, muscle aches, vomiting, or diarrhea and then recovers for a time.

Called Weil's disease, the second phase is more severe, and the person may have widespread internal bleeding, kidney or liver failure, or meningitis. The illness may last from a few days to three weeks or longer, and without treatment, recovery may take several months. Although antibiotic treatment is effective if given promptly, kidney and liver function can take a long time to restore. The condition can be fatal.

Leptospirosis exists worldwide, especially in temperate to tropical zones. The incidence in the United States has steadily increased, but it is generally underdiagnosed and unreported.

Laboratory studies are essential for diagnosis. Culturing the organism, then finding the corkscrew organisms indicates their presence, but the condition may be difficult to determine in certain phases of the disease. Special laboratories carry out other tests that include the ELISA, a test for a reactive antigen, urinalysis, and examination of cerebrospinal fluid.

Treatment is with antibiotics, such as doxycycline or penicillin, which should be given early in the course of the disease. After the first stages, intravenous antibiotics are required.

Prevention of the disease is by not swimming or wading in water that might be contaminated with animal urine. Workers should wear protective clothing and footwear to prevent them from coming into contact with the organisms.

Rat-bite fever

Spirillum minus is one of the two causes of rat-bite fever, a hazard to those living in socially deprived areas. This spirochete is acquired through a rat or mouse bite. The wound heals promptly, but inflammation occurs at the site of the bite after about four to 28 days. The person has a relapsing fever, inflammation of lymph nodes in the surrounding areas, and sometimes the joints may be inflamed and painful. A rash may also accompany the symptoms.

Diagnosis is made when the spirochete is found in blood smears or tissues from the lesions in the lymph nodes. The diagnosis may be difficult because the physician may not be aware of the rat bite. Penicillin or other antibiotics are effective treatments.

Evelyn B. Kelly

See also
• Environmental disorders • Infections, animal-to-human • Infections, bacterial • Infections, parasitic • Kidney disorders • Lice infestation • Liver and spleen disorders • Lyme disease • Meningitis • Syphilis

Sports injury

All bones, joints, muscles, and tissues are susceptible to injury, which can occur in both athletes and non-athletes. The most common injuries are caused by carelessness, lack of training, biomechanical factors, accident, and overuse of muscles. More than 10 million sports injuries are treated each year in the United States; just under half of these are in children under 15.

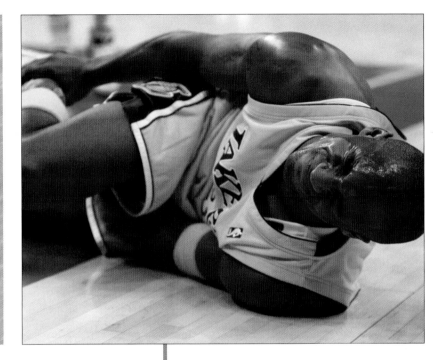

Athletes are prone to muscle and tendon injuries. They can be caused by insufficient warm-up, tiredness, and using excessive force, such as pushing or pulling, during games. Ligament sprains and strains are also common sports injuries.

Improving physical performance was essential for ancient man to stay alive to fight. Egyptian hieroglyphics depict running, swimming, rowing, archery, and wrestling competitions. The first sports-related medical text was the Kahun Papyrus, dated around 1700 B.C.E. For the Olympic Games in 776 B.C.E., Greek athletes were given specialized training under the supervision of specialists in the gymnasium. Sports medicine developed early in history and has become a major specialty within orthopedic surgery during the twenty-first century.

With the increase in physical activity as a remedy for the problem of obesity, more sports-related injuries are being reported, primarily related to carelessness, poor training, and the improper use of equipment. Everyone has tissues that are susceptible to injury because of inherent body weakness or biomechanical factors. For example, people who have a deep curvature of the spine (lumbar lordosis) are at risk for back pain when they swing a baseball bat; people with flat feet whose feet turn out (pronation) are at risk for knee pain when they run long distances. In all sports, specific motions must be repeated. When the activity is stopped, pain usually stops until the activity is tried again.

Whether an athlete experiences the thrill of success or the distress of defeat, physical pain may occur, injuring bones, joints, ligaments, or muscles. Some injuries require no treatment other than rest; others require immediate attention.

Sports injuries to bone

The thrills of the school playground come with a price: fractures. A fracture is a broken bone. Bones are hard because they contain mineral, notably calcium, but surrounding the calcium are living bone cells and blood vessels. Usually bones absorb shocks by bending, then returning to their normal rigid position, but if bones are weakened or if the force is too great, bones will break.

There are four types of fractures that are more common in sports injuries. For a simple fracture, a clean break occurs, but the skin is not broken. Surrounding muscle and blood vessels are not damaged. In a compound fracture, broken bone penetrates the skin and is visible; considerable damage may occur to surrounding tissue. Greenstick fractures are usually seen in children; bone cracks and bends as if it were a green stick.

A comminuted fracture is when the bone is broken in two or more places or is crushed.

Children with broken bones heal much faster than adults. However, injuries to children are so common that most children have seen an orthopedic surgeon (a doctor who specializes in bone repair) before they reach the age of five.

Recognizing an open or compound fracture is obvious when a piece of the bone is visible, but the following symptoms indicate a closed or simple fracture: a break or snap is heard; a grating sensation is felt with movement; swelling, bruising, or reddening may occur; limbs may look deformed with different lengths, sizes, or shapes; an improper angle may be noted; when the person moves, there is intense pain; numbness or tingling may occur in the extremities; or unusual pain in the rib cage occurs when one breathes or coughs. Breaking a bone is a shock to the entire body. Some people may feel sick or dizzy, and others feel no pain because of shock.

A concussion is a hairline fracture to the skull. It is the most common head injury and results in temporary brain disturbance due to trauma. Concussion may be caused by a sudden or violent movement of the head, which may occur in a tackle or collision, or spinning of the head caused by a blow to the side of the head. The player may have a concussion and be conscious or may have a vacant stare with slow responses, slurred or incoherent speech, or may forget events after the impact. The following signs indicate a concussion: bruising around the eye or ear; bleeding from the nose; pupils unequal in size; and swelling of the skull.

If there is any risk of neck or head injury, the player should be stabilized and taken from the field on a stretcher. No player with a concussion should return to the sport unless checked by a medical practitioner.

Metatarsals are the long bones of the foot. A march fracture is a type of injury usually found in walkers or runners, resulting from repeated periods of excessive stress on the metatarsals. Runners often push off from their toes and place great stress on the first two metatarsal heads. There, the bones are thin, and a fracture may occur. Resting and strapping the foot with adhesive plaster for a few weeks helps healing.

Ligaments and sprains

Although the word *sprain* is used to describe a variety of medical conditions, a true sprain is an injury to a ligament, the tough elastic band that connects bone to bone at a joint. A violent twist can damage any ligament. Following are three types of sprains:

In a simple stretch (grade I sprain), ligament fibers are overstretched with minor pain and some tenderness and swelling. X-rays are normal and the person can put weight on the area without too much pain.

In a partial tear (grade II sprain), a ligament tears but does not rupture. Movement is moderately painful with some swelling and discoloration.

A complete tear (grade III sprain) is a severe injury because the joint is completely misaligned. The whole area is swollen and discolored.

Sports injuries to the ankle and knee joints are the most common. An ankle sprain results in overstretching or tearing of one or more ankle ligaments. Sprains usually occur on the outside, making the foot turn inward and causing excess tension on the outer ankle ligaments. When a sprain occurs the "RICED" procedure can be used (see box on page 813). Rehabilitation and exercise are necessary to restore function.

KEY FACTS

Description
Injuries that occur when participating in a variety of sports activities; injuries can involve bone, cartilage, joints and ligaments, tendons, and muscles.

Causes
Carelessness, lack of training, overuse of muscles, improper use of equipment; intrinsic factors, or the way the body is constructed, and extrinsic factors, may cause injuries.

Symptoms
Pain; severity depends on the injury.

Diagnosis
After physical examination and taking of medical history, the person may be referred to specialists for carefully selected tests such as X-rays, computed tomography scans, bone scans, and magnetic resonance imaging scans.

Treatments
First aid treatment includes rest, ice, compression, elevation (RICE); depending on the injury, the person may be recommended to a specialist in sports medicine.

Pathogenesis
If treatment is followed, recovery is usually good.

Prevention
Warming up, stretching, cooling down; focusing or paying attention.

Epidemiology
More than 10 million sports injuries are treated each year in the United States; around 3.5 million of these are in children under the age of 15.

Sprained knees occur when a tear or complete rupture occurs of one or more of the knee ligaments, most commonly the anterior cruciate ligament (ACL). When a runner makes a sudden movement (for example, when tackling or twisting in football or rugby), the knee is suddenly rotated. A blow to the outer knee when the leg or foot is firmly planted damages the medial collateral ligament (MCL), the large ligament supporting the inside of the knee. Posterior cruciate ligament (PCL) injuries occur when a force hits the front of a bent knee. Using the RICED procedure is important to lessen the impact of such injuries. Some charts add "P" in front of "RICED" for "protect." Prevention involves two important factors: warm-up and cool-down exercise. Many amateur participants are eager to jump into the activity and forget important procedures, such as use of devices that tape, brace, or wrap knees, ankles, wrists, and elbows. "Train, don't sprain" should be the motto of all athletes.

Dislocations occur when a bone is moved out of place at the joint. Usually a blow has enough force to tear the ligaments, and in addition, damage may occur to the surrounding muscles, blood vessels, and bone. Shoulder dislocations happen when a force moves the ball-and-socket joint in one of four directions: forward, backward, up, or down. Dislocations are common in sports that use a large range of motion of the shoulder, such as swimming, gymnastics, or collision sports. The recommended procedure here is "RICD"; elevation is left out because of the normal position of the shoulder. If someone has a dislocation, it is difficult to move the joint; medical help should be sought as soon as possible.

Tendons and tendinitis

Tendons are strong fibrous bands that attach muscle to bones. Sports injuries of tearing and inflammation of tendons are common in the shoulder, elbow, wrist, and lower leg or ankle.

The rotator cuff holds the head of the humerus, or bone of the upper arm, into the scapula or shoulder blade. Certain sports that require the arm to be moved over the head repeatedly often tear or inflame tendons in this area. Examples are baseball, swimming freestyle, backstroke, butterfly, weight lifting, and racket sports. Chronic irritation can cause bursitis or inflammation of the bursae, small fluid-filled sacs that cushion areas where muscles cross bones or other muscles. The sacs lubricate the area for smooth movement of muscle.

Many repetitive movement disorders are common in sports. Tennis elbow is known also as lateral

RICED

For sports injuries, follow this procedure:
REST No weight should be put on the injured part.
ICE Applied as packs, massage, or immersion. Ice cools the tissue and reduces pain, swelling, and bleeding, by slowing metabolism in the cells and allowing tissue to survive a temporary lack of oxygen. The ice must not be applied directly to the skin; it should be first wrapped in a cloth.
COMPRESSION Firm bandaging helps to reduce bleeding and swelling.
ELEVATION This helps to stop bleeding and reduce swelling.
DIAGNOSIS A medical professional should be consulted if pain or swelling does not go down within 48 hours.

humerus tendonitis epicondylitis and is caused by repetitive strenuous pushing of the wrist against resistance when hitting a ball. A tear or inflammation of the tendon that links muscle to bone may become a chronic condition if the area is not rested. Tennis elbow can also be caused by frisbee throwing and other activities that tighten the muscles in the hand or forearm. Often reconstructive surgery is necessary.

When running, the calf muscles lower the forefoot to the ground after the heels strikes the ground and raise the heel when the toe lifts off. Although most tendons have a sheath that surrounds them, the Achilles tendon located at the back of the lower leg has only the lining or fatty tissue that separates the tendon from the sheath. Early pain of Achilles tendonitis is due to injury to this covering; if the pain is ignored, inflammation spreads to the tendon and causes degeneration. The athlete must stop running and reduce tension on the area by placing a heel lift in the shoes and stretching the hamstring muscles.

Muscles and strain

Pulled muscles can occur anywhere, but certain muscles appear more at risk in sports injuries. The hamstrings are a group of three muscles at the back of the thigh. A strain is caused when an overstretch results in a tear or complete rupture of one or more of these muscles. Hamstring strains are common in sports that require explosive stop-start running motions, such as football or rugby, volleyball, and athletic sprinting events. The injuries often occur at the beginning of a game or training session due to inadequate warm-up or near the end of a game when fatigue becomes a factor. For hamstring injuries, the RICED procedure is used.

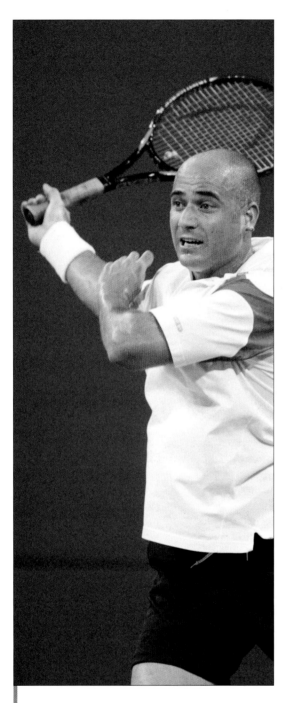

Tennis players, such as U.S. player Andre Agassi, are vulnerable to many muscle, bone, and joint injuries because playing in one tournament after another often does not give them time to recover fully from injuries. Tennis elbow is a common injury in tennis players.

Any great force can tear the muscles and tendons of the lower back. Lumbar strain occurs in sports that require pushing or pulling against great resistance, such as weight lifting, football, basketball, baseball, or golf. The person should be treated with RICD (because elevation is not essential); once healing has begun, the person can benefit from exercises that strengthen the abdominal muscles and stretch the back muscles to restore flexibility.

Shin splints, known as anterior compartment syndrome, are probably the most common overuse problem. Resulting from the repeated straining of muscles between the shinbones, shin splints cause pain in the lower leg between the ankle and knee. The swollen muscles press on blood vessels, thus transferring stress to the bones, causing tiny cracks. Shin splints may occur, for example, when a tennis player shifts from a soft to a hard surface, or a basketball player suddenly has to play extra time. These microfractures are so fine that they do not show up in X-rays. Treatments include rest, proper diet rich in calcium, and training in the proper use of equipment.

Drug abuse in sports

When an athlete exercises, the nervous system produces hormones, such as adrenaline, that in turn increase the amount of blood for muscles and glucose to provide muscle energy. Some athletes illegally take drugs that will give them an unfair advantage over other athletes. The problem is international; it involves both amateur and professional athletes in a wide range of sports and includes the use of anabolic steroids, ephedrine and its derivatives, stimulant drugs, painkillers, nerve relaxants, growth hormone, diuretics to lose weight quickly, and corticosteroids. The U.S. Olympic Committee and the International Olympic Committee bans the use of these enhancers and stimulants.

Anabolic steroids are chemically related to natural hormones and mimic the effects of the male hormone testosterone. The athlete gains weight, muscle mass, and strength. However, use of these steroids has been linked to liver failure, heart damage, reproductive system damage, and extreme aggressiveness.

Evelyn B. Kelly

See also
• Aging, disorders of • Backache • Bone and joint disorders • Fracture • Head injury • Muscle system disorders • Repetitive strain injury • Slipped disk • Substance abuse and addiction • Trauma, accident, and injury

Stomach disorders

The stomach is a segment of the gastrointestinal tract that participates in the digestion of food and other important physiological responses to food. It is a muscular sac linking the esophagus and the first portion of the small intestine, known as the duodenum. Anatomically, it lies just below the diaphragm in the abdominal cavity. The stomach is not required for normal digestion and absorption of nutrients to occur, but its dysfunction can result in several disease states.

The primary functions of the stomach are to begin the process of digestion, and to serve as a reservoir for ingested food so that it can be delivered at a controlled rate to segments of the intestine. This results in an optimal rate of digestion and absorption of ingested nutrients, so that the capacity of the small intestine for these processes is not overwhelmed.

The stomach is also an important portal for the absorption of certain classes of drugs. Finally, the stomach functions under normal circumstances to reduce the risk of infections that take place via the oral route. In healthy individuals, clinically significant gastrointestinal infections are relatively unusual, despite the large numbers of bacteria that are ingested every day.

The stomach is continuous with the tubular segments of the intestine that both precede (esophagus) and follow it (duodenum) but is an outpouching of the intestinal tract into a muscular bag, or sac. Normal stomach (or gastric) functions can broadly be divided into those that relate to its secretory functions and those that arise from contraction of the smooth muscle layers that surround it.

The stomach secretes a number of characteristic products from cells that line its interior. Perhaps the best known of these is hydrochloric acid, secreted by so-called parietal cells located in glands that drain into the central portion of the stomach. Gastric acid is secreted in response to cues that a meal is about to, or has entered the stomach. The acidity begins the process of breaking down the large molecules present in a meal. The acid is highly toxic to ingested bacteria and thus serves as a host defense mechanism. The parietal cells also secrete a substance called intrinsic factor, which is vital for the absorption of vitamin B_{12} (also known as cobalamin). Also within the gastric glands, cells known as chief cells secrete pepsinogen, which is an inactive form of the digestive enzyme pepsin. When pepsinogen encounters acid, it becomes active and can break down proteins derived from the diet. Acid and pepsin can harm cells, raising the question of how the stomach avoids digesting itself. To accomplish this, cells above the glands secrete mucus and bicarbonate. These blanket the inner surface of the stomach, protecting it from acid or peptic injury, or both. These cells also secrete substances that stabilize this mucus-bicarbonate layer, known as trefoil factors.

The physiological function of the stomach as a reservoir that controls the delivery of nutrients to the

RELATED ARTICLES

small intestine is provided by its motility patterns. The stomach has a remarkable property known as "receptive relaxation." As the stomach's volume is increased by the entry of meal components, the muscles in its wall relax so that the increased volume can be accommodated without an increase in pressure. This minimizes the risk of backflow of gastric contents into the esophagus as well as allowing for control of exit from the stomach. While in the stomach, the contents are churned around to ensure optimal mixing of the meal with the gastric secretions. The motion also breaks the meal into small particles in a similar action to a blender. This increases the total surface area of the food particles, further increasing their ability to be digested. When the particles are small enough (less than 1 to 2 mm in diameter), they are expelled from the stomach into the duodenum through a small opening known as the pylorus. The rate at which the stomach empties is regulated by signals coming from the small intestine (emptying is inhibited when nutrients are in this segment) and also by the physical and chemical characteristics of the meal (for example, liquid or solid; protein, carbohydrate, or fat).

Even during fasting, the stomach is not completely quiet. A pacemaker in the stomach serves as the origination point for a strong wave of contractions that sweep across the stomach and on into the small intestine through a fully relaxed pylorus. The contraction is thought to be a "housekeeper" to ensure that any remnants of the meal that remain in the stomach are swept out before the next meal. This is the reason that coins and other small objects that cannot be digested may eventually appear in the stool if swallowed.

Diseases associated with gastric dysfunction

Based on the foregoing, it is perhaps not surprising that several disease states can result when gastric function is abnormal. Many such diseases reflect alterations in gastric secretion or motility, or both.

Stomach disorders related to secretory dysfunction can arise due to both the over- and underexpression of gastric secretory function, or depend on the presence of a specific gastric secretory product. For example, stomach ulcers, which are described in greater detail elsewhere, only occur in the presence of gastric acid and pepsin that serve to injure the cells lining the

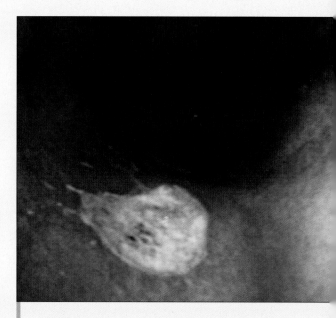

This endoscopic view of a stomach shows the presence of a stomach ulcer (white). Ulcers develop when the lining of the stomach is attacked by digestive juices.

stomach, so that the lining is no longer continuous and hemorrhage can result. This accounts for the utility of medications designed to suppress gastric acid secretion in relieving the symptoms of ulcer disease. However, many cases of stomach ulcers are now known to be caused by chronic infection with a particular bacteria (see box, page 818) and can thus be more definitively treated with antibiotics that eradicate the infection. Gastric ulceration is also a frequent complication of nonsteroidal anti-inflammatory drugs (NSAIDs) that are taken over long periods of time by patients with other chronic diseases, such as arthritis. Indeed, NSAID ulcers are an increasing health problem as the population ages.

Gastric acid is also thought to be the culprit in the very common condition known as gastroesophageal reflux disease, or GERD (known more commonly as heartburn). In this condition, the barrier to backflow of gastric contents into the vulnerable esophagus does not function properly, and acid and pepsin damage the esophageal lining and activate pain receptors. If left untreated for a long period of time, GERD can also predispose someone to the development of esophageal cancer, and it is one of the most common reasons patients seek the assistance of a gastroenterologist.

Gastric acid secretion can also be increased abnormally in the setting of tumors, located in the stomach or elsewhere, that secrete excessive quantities of the chemical messengers normally responsible for the control of secretory function. The most classical example of this is a condition called Zollinger-Ellison syndrome, in which patients suffer from a tumor that secretes large amounts of the hormone gastrin. Patients with this condition display high levels of gastric acid secretion even when fasting, and this can result in abdominal discomfort, poor digestion of fats, and gastric and duodenal ulceration. Similarly, carcinoid tumors synthesize excessive quantities of a neurotransmitter, serotonin (also known as 5-hydroxytryptamine), which can increase gastric secretion as well as having effects throughout the body, such as causing itching and flushing of the skin.

Dysfunction of the stomach can also arise when its secretory function is inhibited. The best-known example of this is a disease caused pernicious anemia, in which patients develop auto-antibodies that damage the parietal cells in the gastric glands. This results in a profound suppression of gastric acid secretion, which is associated with an increased risk for infections acquired via the oral route. Similarly, because parietal cells are also the source of intrinsic factor, patients suffering from this condition can become deficient in cobalamin, which can manifest as iron-deficiency anemia and may also be accompanied by numbness in the extremities and generalized weakness. Of note, there is a natural decline in parietal cell numbers with aging; very elderly patients can display increased susceptibility to oral infections and signs of anemia attributable to cobalamin malabsorption. Similarly, secretory function of the stomach can decline if the lining is injured as a result of inflammation, most commonly occurring in response to chronic infection.

Stomach disorders related to abnormal motility

Diseases also occur if the normal motility functions of the stomach are disrupted. In general, these diseases fall into two categories. The first are caused by an inability of the pylorus to relax, so that the stomach retains the gastric contents. The second are caused by inadequate contractions of the body of the stomach, impairing or delaying gastric emptying without actual evidence of an obstruction. Gastric emptying can also be impaired if the stomach or its opening are physically obstructed, for example, by a large tumor or the development of scar tissue after an ulceration. Ironically, impaired gastric motility itself may lead to obstructions, since in the absence of "housekeeper" contractions during fasting, the non-digestible residues of meals may accumulate in the stomach and become stuck together with gastric mucus. Eventually, a large ball of such debris, called a bezoar, can fill the entire cavity of the stomach.

Pyloric stenosis is a congenital condition, more commonly seen in boys, that manifests shortly after birth with regurgitation of milk and projectile vomiting. Such infants will also suffer from malnutrition if left untreated. The disease results because the pylorus is not able to relax to allow meal particles to exit into the duodenum appropriately, although the precise cause is unknown. Patients with pyloric stenosis are treated by performing an operation in which the muscles around the pylorus are severed. This operation is the most common reason for surgery in the first six months of life. Pyloric stenosis can recur in adulthood, or can newly arise if the function of the pylorus is impaired by a tumor or by scarring.

With respect to abnormal gastric emptying, gastroparesis refers to a collection of conditions in which the normal controls that regulate contractions of the stomach walls are lost. The symptoms include nausea, vomiting, bloating, and abdominal discomfort, with patients often vomiting partially or even undigested food some time after they have eaten. In such individuals, liquid meals may be tolerated more readily since they are easier to empty from the stomach. There are many possible causes for gastroparesis, but often no underlying cause is found. However, perhaps the most common form of gastroparesis is that seen in patients with long-standing diabetes, which results in damage to the nervous system, including the nerves that control the muscle layers of the stomach.

Diagnosis and treatment of stomach disorders

The initial approach to diagnosing stomach disorders is to obtain a careful history from the patient about the nature and duration of the symptoms, including when they occur in relation to eating meals. Many patients with serious gastric symptoms that do not

HELICOBACTER PYLORI: THE STOMACH BUG

Gastric and duodenal ulcers were once thought to be caused by stress, diet, lifestyle or other unknown factors. However, Robin Warren and Barry Marshall, a pathologist and a gastroenterologist working in Australia, were intrigued by the frequency with which they observed a strange bacterium in gastric biopsies obtained from patients with ulcer disease. These spiral-shaped bacteria were called *Helicobacter pylori* and were highly adapted to live in the hostile environment of the stomach, where they colonized the mucus layer.

Warren and Marshall's hypothesis that ulcers had an infectious basis encountered spirited opposition, even when Marshall drank a culture of *Helicobacter* himself and developed gastric injury shortly there-after. However, we now know that many individuals worldwide, particularly in developing countries, are chronically infected with *Helicobacter* and that some of these individuals will develop ulcer disease as a result. If the bacteria are eradicated, the ulcer disease resolves and does not recur.

Infection with *Helicobacter pylori* also increases the risk of various forms of gastric cancer, and the World Health Organization has categorized this microorganism as a carcinogen. Warren and Marshall's discovery revolutionized the treatment of many patients with ulcer disease. They were amply vindicated for the initial skepticism their work encountered when they were awarded the 2005 Nobel Prize in Medicine for their discoveries.

respond promptly to medical treatments will also be scheduled for an upper endoscopy, in which, under light sedation, a thin, fiber-optic tube with a camera is passed through the throat and esophagus and into the stomach to inspect its lining. This enables the gastroenterologist to visualize ulcers, tumors, sources of recent or ongoing bleeding, and evidence that the stomach lining is inflamed. These visual impressions can be confirmed by taking small biopsies of the gastric lining from regions of interest, which are later examined under the microscope. Such biopsies may reveal infection with microorganisms (especially *Helicobacter pylori*), alterations in the structure of gastric glands, the presence of cancerous cells, and other abnormalities. *Helicobacter pylori* infection can also be diagnosed by a breath test based on the ability of the bacteria to convert urea to ammonia. Patients are given a solution of radioactive urea, and the presence of radioactive ammonia in their breath is suggestive of infection.

Tests of secretory and motility function can also be conducted. Gastric secretions can be suctioned from the stomach, both under fasting conditions and following injection of an analogue of gastrin, and their acidity determined. Blood tests are also carried out for levels of various gastrointestinal hormones. Similarly, the motility of the stomach can be monitored by asking the patient to drink a radioactive suspension, and then imaging how quickly it leaves the stomach. However, these "scintigraphic" tests are more commonly used in research studies than in clinical practice since their value in the diagnosis of gastroparesis may not be as useful as information about the patient's history.

The treatment of stomach disorders obviously depends on the underlying cause but may also be dictated by the patient's age and symptoms. In a young individual complaining of indigestion, but without so-called "alarm signs" such as recurrent vomiting, weight loss, or evidence of bleeding, the physician may first elect to try a course of acid-suppressive medication such as antihistamine drugs or a proton pump inhibitor that blocks the enzymatic machinery necessary for the secretion of gastric acid. If there is evidence of infection with *Helicobacter pylori*, antibiotics are also given to eradicate the microorganism. For patients with symptoms consistent with a motility disorder, a trial of a drug capable of promoting gastric emptying (a prokinetic) may be undertaken. However, if symptoms persist, or are more serious, endoscopic evaluation is critical and may guide further therapy. Certainly, any sign of active bleeding from the stomach is a medical emergency that requires prompt intervention. Sometimes, it is possible to stop the bleeding by cautery via the endoscope, but in other cases surgical intervention is necessary. Surgery is also the treatment of choice for gastric tumors, pyloric stenosis, and obstructions.

Kim E. Barrett

Stomach ulcer

Stomach ulcers are small holes or sores in the lining of either the stomach or the duodenum. Most often the result of a bacterial infection, ulcers cause a burning feeling in the upper abdomen, and in severe cases may cause bleeding, vomiting, or weight loss. Every year, more than 500,000 new cases of peptic ulcer disease are diagnosed in the United States.

Stomach ulcers, more accurately called peptic ulcers, are small, painful sores that can develop in the lining of the stomach or the duodenum, the upper part of the small intestine. Long ascribed to stress and dietary factors, most ulcers are now believed to be caused by infection with *Helicobacter pylori*, a common bacterium that weakens the protective mucous coating of the stomach and duodenum, allowing acid to penetrate to the sensitive lining beneath. Left untreated, severe ulcers may eventually eat a hole through the wall of the stomach and cause infection of the abdominal cavity.

Causes and risk factors

A definitive link between ulcers and the *Helicobacter pylori* bacterium was established only in 1982. Though acceptance of this connection has been slow to spread, the majority of peptic ulcers are now treated as bacterial infections, spread from person to person primarily via the gastro-oral route, or through contaminated water sources. Long-term use of anti-inflammatory drugs such as aspirin or ibuprofen may also irritate the lining of the stomach, while stress and the use of tobacco and alcohol can worsen the symptoms.

Signs and symptoms

Symptoms are a burning sensation in the abdomen, which is worse when the stomach is empty and may last several hours. Less common symptoms include nausea, vomiting, or loss of appetite. Blood from severe ulcers may appear in vomit or bowel movements.

Diagnosis and treatments

Ulcers may be seen directly through endoscopy, in which a tiny camera is threaded down the esophagus into the stomach. If an ulcer is seen, a tissue sample may be taken to identify the presence of *H. pylori*, which may also be detected by blood, breath, or stool tests.

Treatment for *H. pylori*–related ulcers typically involves a short course of antibiotics, combined with the use of drugs that reduce or neutralize acid production in the stomach. Ulcers that fail to respond to such treatment may be due to antibiotic-resistant *H. pylori*, or, in rare cases, to diseases and syndromes that affect the digestive system. Surgery is necessary only when the ulcer does not respond to aggressive drug treatment.

Prevention

Recommendations for avoiding *H. pylori* infection involve washing hands thoroughly, eating food that has been properly prepared, and drinking water from a clean source.

Jonathon Cross

KEY FACTS

Description
Sores or holes in the lining of the stomach or duodenum.

Causes
Infection by *Helicobacter pylori* bacterium.

Risk factors
Use of nonsteroidal anti-inflammatories, smoking, and alcohol use.

Symptoms
Burning sensation in the upper abdomen.

Diagnosis
By endoscopy, biopsy, breath, blood, or stool tests.

Treatments
Antibiotics in combination with acid-reducing drugs.

Pathogenesis
Left untreated, ulcers may eventually penetrate the stomach or intestinal wall.

Prevention
Basic hygiene methods to prevent oral-oral or fecal-oral transmission.

Epidemiology
H. pylori affects up to 70 percent of people worldwide. Up to 15 percent of these will develop peptic ulcers.

See also
• Alcohol-related disorders • Infections, bacterial • Smoking-related disorders

Stroke and related disorders

Strokes occur when the blood supply to part of the brain is suddenly stopped or when a blood vessel bursts, spilling blood into the area vessels surrounding the brain cells. A stroke is often referred to as a "brain attack." Strokes are the leading cause of adult disability. Each year about 760,000 people have symptomatic strokes; more than 11 million suffer silent strokes.

The Greek physician Hippocrates (460–377 B.C.E.) observed a condition in which people suddenly became unable to speak or walk. The Roman physician Galen (129–216) continued these studies and called the condition *apoplexy*. He theorized that women had these attacks because of the female menstrual cycle. Centuries later, a Swiss doctor Johann Wepfer (b. 1620) performed autopsies of humans and connected the postmortem signs of bleeding in the brain with persons who died from apoplexy. He also observed the blockage of the carotid and vertebral arteries that supply blood to the brain.

Like Galen and Wepfer, physicians throughout the centuries had no power over the condition. However, stroke medicine is changing rapidly, and scientists of the twenty-first century are garnering better therapies each day.

Description of stroke

The medical term for stroke is *cerebrovascular disease*, and it is sometimes referred to as a cerebrovascular accident, or CVA. The word *cerebrovascular* comes from the Latin word *cerebro*, which means "brain," and *vasa*, which means "vessel."

The brain requires about 20 percent of the heart's output of fresh blood to supply its requirements for oxygen and glucose. Two artery systems, the carotid arteries, carry blood through the neck to the brain.

Anything that disturbs the blood flow, even for a few seconds, affects the brain's function. Depending on the area of the brain, a variety of following symptoms may occur: sudden numbness, weakness, or paralysis on one side of the body, such as the face, arm, or leg; sudden nausea, fever, or vomiting; sudden difficulty speaking or understanding speech (aphasia); sudden blurred vision, double vision, or decreased vision in one or both eyes; sudden dizziness, loss of balance, or loss of coordination; sudden loss of consciousness; sudden confu-

sion or memory problems, loss of spatial orientation or perception; sudden headache, as a bolt out of the blue. The key word for each of these symptoms is sudden. There will frequently be more than one sign. Any of these symptoms signal a medical emergency. Every minute the brain cells are deprived of oxygen increases the risk of damage. Chances for recovery are much better when the right treatment is begun within the first few hours of noticing stroke symptoms.

Two major types of cerebrovascular events are ischemic stroke, in which blood does not get to part of the brain due to a disturbance in blood flow; and cerebral hemorrhage, during which blood vessels in the brain bleed and the released (hemorrhagic) blood damages brain tissue. The term *stroke* is commonly applied to the clinical symptoms and not to a specific condition.

Ischemic stroke

The word *ischemia* literally means "to hold back blood." This type of stroke occurs when an artery suddenly becomes blocked and decreases or stops the flow of blood to the brain. Cells may begin to die within minutes. This type is responsible for 80 percent of all strokes. There are two conditions that cause this type of stroke. The first is embolic stroke, which is a type of ischemia, in which a clot forms in another part of the body, travels through blood vessels, and becomes wedged in a brain artery. The free-roaming clot or embolus often forms in the heart. The type of clot is often caused by irregular beating in the two upper chambers of the heart. This irregular beating is called atrial fibrillation, which leads to poor blood flow and the formation of a clot.

The second type is thrombotic stroke, in which a blood clot forms in one of the cerebral arteries and grows until it is large enough to block the blood flow. Buildup of plaques (a mixture of fatty substances including cholesterol and other lipids) causes stenosis or narrowing of the artery as a result of these fatty deposits in the artery wall. When a stroke occurs as a result of small vessel disease, an infarction occurs. An infarction is the deprivation of blood supply of part of a tissue or organ in which an area of dead tissue (infarct) forms. Infarcted tissue swells and becomes firm, blood vessels around the infarct widen, and plasma and blood may flow into the infarct, thus increasing the swelling. The infarct then shrinks and is replaced by fibrous scar tissue, and function is lost.

Transient ischemic attacks (TIAs) may indicate that a stroke is coming. These are minor attacks in which the person may have a sudden onset of weakness, vertigo, or imbalance that lasts only a few minutes. These attacks have the same origin as ischemic stroke. Attacks are probably due to atherosclerosis, when plaque fragments break off and travel to a site in the brain. Major risk factors are high blood pressure, smoking, diabetes, and advanced age. The most significant factor is that the symptoms and signs last no more than 24 hours. If the symptom recurs, it often is a warning that a stroke may follow. One of the most common treatments for this condition is aspirin. Aspirin inhibits the way in which platelets clump together. Too many platelets gathered in a constricted area may block the flow to the brain.

Hemorrhagic stroke

Hemorrhage is the medical word for bleeding. A hemorrhagic stroke occurs when an artery in the brain bursts, sending blood into surrounding tissue. Symptoms include severe headache, drowsiness, seizures, or confusion after a head injury, paralysis on one side of the body, or changes in personality. This type of stroke accounts for about 20 percent of all strokes and happens in two ways. First, it can happen as an aneurysm; a thin or weak spot on the artery wall balloons out and ruptures, spilling blood into spaces surrounding the brain tissue. The ruptured brain arteries bleed into the brain itself or into spaces surrounding the brain.

Second, the stroke can occur as an intracerebral hemorrhage, when the vessel in the brain leaks blood into the brain itself. In this case, brain cells beyond the leak are deprived of blood and are also damaged.

High blood pressure is the most common cause of hemorrhagic stroke. High blood pressure causes small arteries in the brain to become stiff and subject to cracking or rupture. A subarachnoid hemorrhage is bleeding under the meninges into the outer covering of the brain, which contaminates the cerebrospinal fluid (CSF). Because the CSF circulates through the cranium, this type of stroke can lead to extensive damage and is the most deadly of all strokes.

A head injury or blow to the head, such as a car accident or simply bumping the head, may cause a hemorrhage (this type of hemorrhage is never classified as a stroke). Subdural hemorrhages occur when an injury results in bleeding between the brain and the dura matter (the outer covering of the spinal cord and brain). Blood accumulates and produces a mass called a hematoma, which is literally a blood tumor. If the hematoma forms between the skull and the brain, it is called an extradural hematoma. Both these conditions put pressure on the brain and require immediate

---

KEY FACTS

Description

A stroke is a condition that occurs when the blood supply to part of the brain is suddenly stopped or when a blood vessel bursts, then spills blood into the vessels surrounding the brain cells.

Risk factors

Family history, hypertension (high blood pressure), atherosclerosis (hardening of the arteries), high levels of lipids or fat in bloodstream, sleep disorders, high homocysteine levels, age, and certain lifestyle behaviors.

Symptoms

Sudden numbness, weakness or paralysis on one side of the body, loss of speech, sudden nausea, dizziness, blurred vision, loss of balance, sudden headache, person has difficulty swallowing and talking.

Diagnosis

Suddenness of the attack and symptoms; physician will study blood vessels using a variety of imaging techniques.

Treatments

Drugs to improve blood flow and also neuroprotective agents.

Pathogenesis

Getting the victim to a physician who can quickly treat and determine the type of stroke. The stroke may be disabling or lethal.

Prevention

Lifestyle changes in eating and exercise, drugs to keep channels open, and neuroprotective agents

Epidemiology

The leading cause of adult disability; each year about 760,000 people have symptomatic strokes; more than 11 million suffer silent strokes.

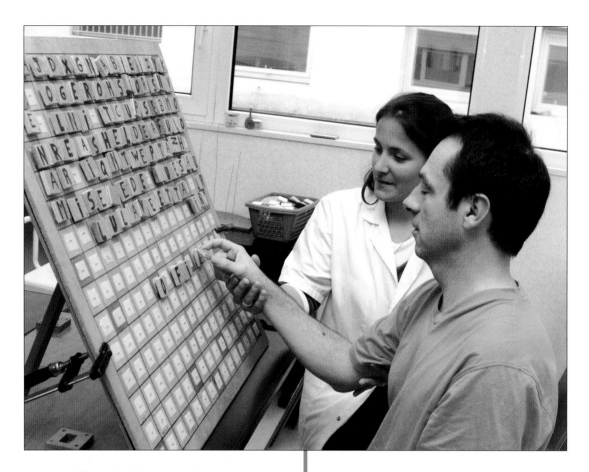

attention. The risk of dying is substantial with this type of injury and hemorrhage.

Risk factors

Several red flags for stroke include hypertension, hyperlipidemia, obesity, sleep disorders, homocysteine levels, and certain lifestyle behaviors. The chance of risk is slightly higher if one of the parents or brother or sister has had a stroke or TIA; age is also a risk factor. High blood pressure (HBP), also called hypertension, is highly correlated to stroke. Blood pressure is measured on a device called a sphygmomanometer, which reads the pressure during the relaxing phase (diastolic pressure) and also the peak pressure reached during the pumping contraction (systolic pressure). People who have abdominal fat (apple shapes) tend to have elevated blood pressure. For example, obese adults ages 20 to 45 are six times more likely to have high blood pressure than normal adults of the same age. Obese people who are 20 percent above standard weight show a 10 percent risk of stroke. A 2001 study by the North Manhattan Group found that doctors were prescribing few medications for

An occupational therapist helps a patient who is recovering from a stroke to construct words on a board. This exercise is part of a rehabilitation program designed to improve the patient's coordination and help with muscle control.

hypertension but were encouraging more attention to blood pressure control.

Hyperlipidemia or elevated levels of serum triglycerides (fats) are linked to stroke. Healthy arteries have a thin and smooth inner surface that allows blood to flow freely to deliver oxygen to the cells, including the 20 percent payload that the brain demands. In a diseased artery, the inner layer consists of a pool of fat that becomes covered with a hard crust called plaque, which forms inside the artery. Smooth muscle cells migrate to the built-up area, and a small crack appears in the lining, where a blood clot forms.

The buildup can be in any artery in the body, including the carotid artery in the neck that leads to the brain. As the abnormal deposits of fats and cholesterol grow and develop, the internal bore (lumen) of the artery gets narrower and narrower. Also, some of the plaque may break away and circulate in the bloodstream to the brain. According to several studies, TIA strokes appear closely related to hyperlipidemia.

People who sleep more than eight hours a night, who snore, or who experience daytime drowsiness have increased risk for stroke. Obstructive sleep apnea (OSA) is a sleep disorder characterized by episodes of not breathing, called apnea. This condition results from a collapse of the upper airway at the area of the back of the throat called the pharnyx. During an episode of apnea, the person tries to breathe against the closed airway, but he or she is not getting oxygen, and a condition called hypoxia occurs. The brain senses the lack of oxygen, and the person wakes up briefly to restore the upper-airway passage. The cycle may be repeated a hundred times during the night, disrupting normal sleep. The person rarely remembers. OSA can lead to stroke by reducing the amount of oxygen that reaches the brain.

Several lifestyle behavioral factors correlate with stroke. One study found that 28 percent of strokes follow alcohol use and 8 percent after heavy exertion. Other examples were lifting more than 50 pounds, 10 percent; straining during urination or defecation, 4 percent; anger outbursts, 4 percent; and sexual intercourse, 2 percent. Another lifestyle condition is metabolic syndrome, or Syndrome X, in which a cluster of major risk factors of life habits such as alcohol abuse, improper nutrition, inadequate physical activity, and increased body weight all converge to create cardiovascular problems and risk of stroke. Other factors include gender (women tend to die more with strokes), cigarette smoking, diabetes, and use of birth control bills, and hormone therapy.

Certain medications have been related to stroke. In October 2000 the U.S. Food and Drug Administration (FDA) removed phenylpropanolamine (PPA) from over 400 over-the-counter cold, cough, and some diet medications. The FDA found PPA caused 200 to 500 strokes in people under 50, who were mostly women.

Epidemiology

Accurate reporting techniques are being developed and refined. A 2001 study reported that rates of the first ischemic stroke, intracerebral hemorrhage, and subarachnoid hemorrhage were 25 to 50 percent higher among people of African American descent than among Caucasians. The study found that the general U.S. population will suffer 760,000 strokes each year, and more than 11 million suffer silent strokes or TIAs. Historically, the Southeast, especially Alabama and Mississippi, has been referred to as the stroke belt because the area had more strokes than other sections of the country. However, there are indications that the western states of Oregon, Washington, and Arizona may, in the future, have the highest incidence of strokes.

Figures from the National Stroke Foundation have revealed a startling number of young adults who have had strokes. About 225,000 Americans under the age of 45, including young and middle-aged women, have had strokes. One stroke victim of a brain aneurysm was 13; she was fortunate the aneurysm had only ballooned out, and it was caught before it burst. Drug abuse has led to 85 to 90 percent of hemorrhagic strokes occurring in people in their 20s and 30s. In 2002 around 275,000 people in the United States died after having a stroke; stroke accounted for 1 in 15 deaths in the United States. Stroke is the third leading cause of death after heart disease and cancer.

Diagnosis and treatments

When the rapid development of symptoms of stroke occur, emergency facilities should be contacted immediately, but first aid care must be taken in the meantime. Timely first aid is of vital importance for the patient. If breathing stops, cardiopulmonary resuscitation (CPR) should be administered. For minor breathing difficulties, the head should be elevated by positioning the head and shoulders on a pillow. The affected person should not be given anything to eat or drink, and the paralyzed parts must be protected. Depending on circumstances, emergency personnel may begin to administer anti-clotting medications, such as aspirin and ticlopidine, and anticoagulants, such as heparin or warfarin.

In order for the doctor to pinpoint treatments, an image of the brain is necessary. One type of image is called cerebral arteriography or angiography, which is an X-ray that shows the fluid in the arteries to the brain. This image allows the physician to see blood circulating through the brain and to note exactly where there are abnormalities, such as narrowing of the arteries or escape of blood from an artery. The patient is conscious during the procedure. A long flexible catheter is inserted through an artery in the groin, then is passed through the trunk and into the carotid artery or vertebral artery. Dye is injected through the catheter to reveal abnormalities or obstructions. This type of procedure lasts from one to three hours and can be very tiring for the patient.

Many advances in imaging have occurred in the past

few years. Computerized tomography (CT) scans image brain anatomy and blood movement in a series of scans. A new generation of CT scanner applies noncontrast CT, perfusion (the way in which the blood passes through the brain), and CT angiography, all in a scanning time of 23 minutes. Magnetic resonance imaging (MRI) uses a strong magnetic field to generate a three-dimensional view of the brain. This test is sensitive for detecting brain tissue damaged by ischemic stroke. Also, MRI techniques have improved. A technique called fluid-attenuated inversion recovery, or FLAIR, suppresses bright signal images from the cerebrospinal fluid that interfere with reading. Echocardiography is an ultrasound technology that creates images of the heart. A new procedure called neurosonology applies transcranial Doppler (TCD) ultrasound to monitor therapy.

Drugs for acute therapy treatment fall into two categories: medication to improve blood flow and neuroprotective agents.

Improving blood flow. At present, treatment with intravenous thrombolytic tissue plasminogen activator (t-PA) continues to be the first choice for acute stroke within the first three hours. Genetech, a biotechnology firm, developed the clot dissolving Activase (r), a genetically engineered version of naturally occurring t-PA. Since approval in 1996, more than one million people have benefited from the drug.

Other anti-thrombotic drugs include heparin, aspirin, and abciximab. A seven-year study of 2,206 patients at 48 centers compared aspirin to warfarin for recurrent stroke prevention and found that aspirin works as well as warfarin in helping to prevent strokes in most patients. Aspirin affects blood platelets and clotting and has been used for over one hundred years. However, its beneficial effects to prevent stroke and heart attack were only recognized in the 1970s. A large group of new thrombolytics is being investigated. Another new strategy is the use of the laser-based endovascular photo acoustic recanalization (EPAR) system, which combines laser "clotbusters" with pharmaceuticals.

Neuroprotective agents. It is now known that substantial amounts of neuronal tissue damage may be reversible. These strategies consider how to preserve or even reverse neuronal areas. Many of these drugs are in trials. Hypothermia or reducing body temperature as a neuroprotective in animal models continues to be explored in adults. An experiment compared patients who had been wrapped in cooling blankets with water baths at 90°F (32°C) to those without the blankets. The study

found that the patients treated with hypothermia had less disability three months after the stroke.

Surgical procedures are sometimes necessary to remove blood that has been leaking into the tissue from a cerebral hemorrhage. An operation called a carotid endarterectomy may be used to clean arterial plaque deposits as a preventive measure. Sometimes this is used to prevent a minor stroke from recurring. If there has been a subarachnoid hemorrhage, surgical treatment of the aneurysm is often needed.

Rehabilitation

Over 500,000 people survive strokes each year. Half of these patients live over five years, and 10 to 13 percent live ten years. There are an estimated 2.5 million disabled stroke survivors in the United States. Some have only minor disabilities. It is hopeful that many of these patients will walk again and be able to care for themselves. However, about two out of ten will require extended care in a long-term care facility.

Rehabilitation for people who have had strokes is very important for their livelihood and morale. Living at home, if possible, is a great booster. Ingenious adaptive devices and modifications can help the person at home, to allow them to be more independent and to remain a useful part of society. In 1990 the Americans with Disabilities Act (ADA) prohibits discrimination on the basis of disability. Public facilities must accommodate those who have some type of disability to enable them to do things that other people can do. Ramps, special chairs, and bathroom accommodations must be available. Recovery and rehabilitation depend on the area of the brain involved and the amount of tissue damaged. If the speech area is affected, the person may need speech therapy.

Prevention

Prevention of stroke by a healthy lifestyle and avoiding risk factors makes good common sense. A number of strategies include taking preventive drugs that keep open channels and act as neuroprotective agents. Some doctors recommend routinely taking a low-level dose of aspirin (75 mg) as a routine protective against heart disease and stroke. The aspirin keeps the blood flowing and attacks the clotting mechanism of the blood platelets. Other anti-platelet agents are estradiol and vitamins.

For those who have had strokes or TIAs, one of the most hopeful areas of research is that of stem cell transplants to enhance recovery from cerebrovascular damage. Adult stem cells found in the bone marrow or

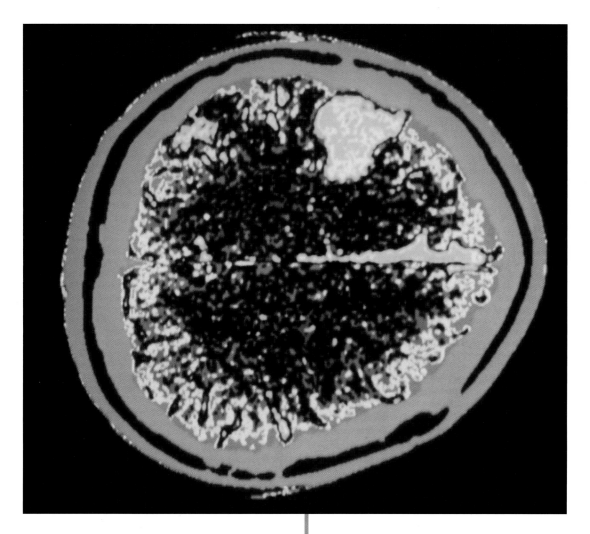

This computed tomography scan is a transverse cross section of the brain of a person after a vascular accident. A cerebrovascular accident or stroke is caused by hemorrhage and results in the destruction of brain tissue (green patch at top center right of picture).

embryonic tissue can develop into brain cells. In rat models of stroke, stem cells have grown in the area of the damage and formed connections with adjacent cells. A study showed that human umbilical cord blood cells injected into rat's tails migrated to the brain within hours and began repairing damage. The umbilical cord is a rich source of immature stem and progenitor cells.

Other new medical procedures are currently under investigation. Putting stroke victims in a hyperbaric oxygen chamber, in which oxygen is at greater pressure than in the normal atmosphere, has proved helpful to some stroke victims.

Stroke may have a genetic element. A 2001 study found a genetic link to hemorrhagic strokes in young white women. The investigators focused on genetic variations in factor XIII, a protein involved in blood clotting. Although few data exist, gene therapy may offer promise for stroke recovery.

Research has come a long way in offering hope to stroke victims. Studies have shown that brain injury occurs within minutes and can continue for days afterward. Timing is critical; educating the public for the signs, symptoms, and necessary action is essential.

Evelyn B. Kelly

See also
- Aging, disorders of • Alcohol-related disorders • Arteries, disorders of
- Cardiovascular disorders • Genetic disorders • Head injury • Heart disorders
- Paralysis • Prevention • Thrombosis and embolism • Treatment

Substance abuse and addiction

Many people have had some contact with substances that have a potential for abuse. For the majority, this exposure is limited to a first try of a cigarette, a prescribed course of painkillers, or a few beers at the end of the week. However, for some people, the use of substances can lead to a profound change in how they live their lives, often with detrimental effects on their health.

The types of substances generally abused range from seemingly innocuous household products, such as coffee, paint, or glue, to high-strength pharmaceuticals and illegally manufactured drugs. These substances are abused for the psychoactive (mood-altering) effects they have on the brain. Most produce a euphoria caused by the substance's effect on the pleasure centers of the brain. Others have a stimulatory or calming effect, depending on the mood the user is trying to induce. Typically, all substance use produces a response that the user finds rewarding, which encourages the user to repeat the behavior.

Not all substance use results in addiction. Many people limit their intake to an amount that fits their commitments and lifestyle. This type of use is sometimes described as habitual or recreational use

and may include having a drink after work or occasionally smoking marijuana. However, because such substance use is not a main focus of the individual's life, the person usually maintains that it can be discontinued at will.

Social and cultural traditions also play a significant part in restricting use to ritualized occasions or limiting the amount consumed. For example, a wedding represents an occasion at which alcohol is expected to be consumed in the form of toasts and as an accompaniment to a meal. While a certain amount of mild drunkenness may be regarded as a natural part of the celebration, extreme or socially embarrassing intoxication is not. In particular, the use of "hard" drugs, such as heroin, would not be tolerated at such an event. Other practices, such as glue sniffing, are considered unacceptable in public. Thus, most misuse of substances tends to occur in isolation or among groups of like-minded people.

Substance use becomes abuse when it develops into a pattern of repeated use that is causing or has caused actual physical or mental damage to health. Among the adverse consequences that define substance abuse are impaired performance at work or school, recurrent social or interpersonal problems, recurrent use that puts the user or others in danger

RELATED ARTICLES

(for example, driving when drunk), and recurrent legal problems. If any one of these criteria is met, then the substance use is defined as abuse.

The path to addiction

Addiction is an acquired condition that develops as a result of the repeated pursuit of a substance or behavior. Contrary to popular belief, no drug causes instant addiction, although the desire to repeat the intense but short-lived "high" of drugs like crack cocaine may reduce the intervals between episodes of drug taking and speed up the time it takes to become addicted.

The term *addiction* comes from the Latin *addicere*, meaning "to enslave." The American Psychiatric Association (APA) distinguishes substance abuse from addiction through the component of motivation, which becomes so disrupted in addicts that getting a drug and taking it becomes a dominant force in the addict's life. This need overrides normal motivations, such as family, career, and self-care.

Addiction can begin as a response to a pleasurable feeling or "buzz" that results from taking the substance. This process is described as positive reinforcement by psychiatrists. While the drug remains in the brain, it produces a variety of effects that include changes in attention, memory, perception, or mood that the user finds rewarding. The drug may also have physical effects on other parts of the body, such as heart rate, movement, or blood pressure.

Negative reinforcement occurs when an individual takes a drug to relieve uncomfortable symptoms or a negative stimulus, such as the relief of pain. It also happens when a drug is being eliminated from the system and produces a loss or reversal of the pleasurable effects, a process called withdrawal. An addict in withdrawal will often take more of the drug or another drug to prevent the unpleasant effects that he or she is experiencing.

Both positive and negative reinforcement are thought to contribute to the development of addiction. The relevant contributions vary according to how far the addiction has progressed and how tolerant and sensitized to the drug the addict has become. *Tolerance* is the term used to describe the process in which the body gradually adapts to the presence of a drug. The process and function of tolerance are not well understood, but it is believed to be an important mechanism in maintaining bodily systems at an optimum level. Over time, the body becomes less responsive to the drug, and the user has to take larger or more frequent doses to reproduce its initial effect. As the addiction progresses, more and larger doses fail to produce the same level of euphoria, suggesting that positive reinforcement has less importance in maintaining drug use. However, not all drug effects involve tolerance, and other effects may work in opposite ways. This process is called sensitization or reverse tolerance. Sensitization to a drug produces an increase in some of its effects at lower and lower doses. As these effects are often encountered in withdrawal, the addict becomes averse to the process of withdrawal, suggesting that negative reinforcement becomes more important in maintaining addiction. Sensitization is also thought to play a key role in craving for drugs as well as relapse when attempting to come off drugs.

Diagnosing addiction

Physicians and psychiatrists working in the field of substance abuse prefer to use the term *dependence* rather than *addiction* when making a diagnosis. Dependence can be split into two categories: physical or physiological dependence, in which the user has acquired tolerance to a drug or suffers withdrawal symptoms; and psychological dependence, in which the user is motivated to continue to take the drug for its psychological effects and not simply to avoid withdrawal symptoms. An individual can develop one or both forms of dependence according to the type of substance being abused. For example, alcoholism can be diagnosed as psychological dependence with or without physiological dependence, while users of LSD can only be described as psychologically dependent because it is impossible to develop tolerance to hallucinogenic substances.

In making a diagnosis, clinicians refer to criteria set out in the *Diagnostic and Statistical Manual of Mental Disorders*, fourth edition, often abbreviated to DSM-IV, produced by the APA. These criteria are listed in the table on page 828. To be diagnosed as dependent, an individual must meet three of the criteria within the same twelve-month period. The manual also provides for a diagnosis of polysubstance abuse, in which an

DSM-IV CRITERIA OF SUBSTANCE USE

CRITERIA OF SUBSTANCE ABUSE

A. A pattern of substance use leading to significant impairment or distress as manifested by one or more of the following in the same one-year period:
1. Recurrent substance use that impairs performance at work, school, or home
2. Recurrent use in physically dangerous situations (for example, driving while intoxicated)
3. Recurrent legal problems resulting from substance use
4. Continued substance use despite social problems related to substance use

B. Has never met criteria for substance dependence for this particular substance

CRITERIA OF SUBSTANCE DEPENDENCE

A pattern of substance use leading to significant impairment or distress as manifested by three or more of the following in the same one-year period:
1. Tolerance (physiological dependence)
2. Withdrawal (physiological dependence)
3. More substance taken than intended
4. Persistent desire or unsuccessful efforts to cut down or control use
5. Large time expenditure on substance-related activity
6. Important social, work, or leisure activities reduced or replaced by substance use
7. Continued substance use despite knowing that physical or psychological problems are caused or worsened by use

individual is using three or more substances (other than nicotine). In such cases the individual may not be dependent on any one substance but does meet the criteria when the combination of drugs is considered as a whole.

Clinicians take a detailed history of the patient's substance use that includes the times of first and last use, patterns of use, tolerance and withdrawal symptoms, any adverse reactions to the drug, psychological and social consequences of use, and attempts to change the pattern or control use. They also physically examine the patient and order tests, such as analysis of urine and blood or liver function tests, to screen for evidence of recent drug use and any other health impacts. Often, after obtaining the permission of the patient, clinicians will interview family members, partners, employers, teachers, work colleagues, or friends. This is useful in determining the true pattern of use, as a drug user will frequently try to minimize or deny the extent of his or her habit. A psychological assessment is also made to determine whether the patient has any mental issues that may confirm a diagnosis, such as anxiety, depression, suicidal thoughts, or panic attacks.

Once all the information has been gathered, the clinician decides whether the diagnosis is abuse or dependence. This assessment has relevance for future treatment, as the loss of control associated with dependence requires different handling from abuse. If the patient is diagnosed with substance dependence, the clinician has to determine whether physiological dependence is present, since treatment may require medication or supervised withdrawal. The substances involved also require consideration in polysubstance abuse, since different types of drugs may need different medications.

A further complication arises if the patient is diagnosed with a psychiatric illness as well as substance dependence, which is termed *dual diagnosis*. The two disorders may have no relation to each other and require assessment as to how the individual should be treated for each disorder. If one of the disorders is causing or maintaining the other, clinicians must take into account how the disorders affect each other. Scientists have found that substance use has a definite effect on the severity of psychiatric symptoms and often involves more hospitalizations, relapses, and noncompliance with treatment regimes.

Similarly, co-occurring psychiatric illnesses have been shown to push up levels of substance use, hospitalizations, and relapses back to abuse.

Treatment

The majority of substance users never receive any form of medical treatment and are able to stop by themselves or through the support of groups such as Alcoholics Anonymous. Others need a package of care tailored to their individual needs. The key to starting recovery is that the individual recognizes that he or she needs help. This process may be instigated by the user, prompted by the intervention of family or friends, or may be the result of a legal mandate by a court.

Detoxification. This is often a preliminary step in treating severe addictions, when withdrawal is an issue or when there are significant medical or psychiatric problems. A hospital stay of two to five days is usually necessary for doctors to monitor withdrawal and administer medication. Its purpose is to get the patient to a state at which recent drug use has been eliminated from the body so that the patient is more receptive to counseling services. In less severe cases, detoxification takes place at home under the supervision of a doctor or nurse.

Counseling. Counseling can take place at an outpatient clinic or under a partial hospitalization program. It can take various forms: one-on-one sessions, in groups, or with members of the family present. Individual counseling sessions last up to an hour, with the therapist helping the drug user to recognize the factors that drive the addiction, how to make personal changes to support abstinence, to be aware of triggers that might cause a relapse, and how to deal with problems that have arisen as a result of substance use. Group counseling involves six to ten substance abusers and one or two counselors who share experiences and help each other to stay abstinent. Family therapy also seeks to resolve any issues or conflicts that have arisen because of substance use and provide support to both the individual and family members. Partial hospital programs are designed for more severe addictions and provide an intensive inpatient regime over a period of weeks.

Behavioral therapies. There is a wide range of treatments available to help the individual manage addiction and develop the motivation to change his or her drug behavior. The most common are cognitive

A group of young people take part in an informal group counseling session to share their experiences of drug using. The support and encouragement of a group are often helpful to people who are trying to overcome an addiction.

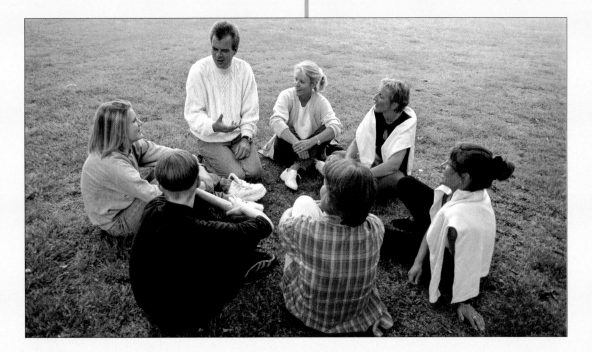

behavior therapy, in which the focus is on helping the individual to change beliefs and learn ways to avoid drug use behaviors; and step programs such as Alcoholics Anonymous, which take the individual through a sequential program of recovery through group support and the help of a sponsor. Other treatments aim to reduce the risk of relapse, identify risk factors, provide social skills training, or deal with upsetting emotions. These strategies often take place as part of counseling or in residential rehabilitation facilities and therapeutic communities.

Medication. Medication is often given to people going through withdrawal from alcohol, opiates, and sedatives. Buprenorphine and naltrexone are commonly administered to withdrawing opiate addicts and are also used as a maintenance therapy to prevent addicts from getting high if they take an opiate while undergoing treatment. Methadone is prescribed under license to opiate addicts who wish to avoid withdrawal. It is long-acting and reduces cravings for other opiates. However, users can develop tolerance in the long term and may undergo withdrawal if the dose is reduced too quickly.

Alcoholics are also treated with naltrexone to reduce cravings. Some are prescribed disulfiram (in the form of tablets or an implant), which makes the alcoholic vomit if he or she has a drink. Withdrawal from severe alcoholism should always be undertaken in a hospital as there is a risk of life-threatening complications.

Smokers can use nicotine replacement therapies to help them give up cigarettes. Nicotine is not particularly harmful when compared with other ingredients in a cigarette, but it is addictive and produces strong cravings in people attempting to quit. By taking nicotine in the form of sprays, patches, or gum, the smoker can relieve withdrawal symptoms while gradually reducing the dose until the desire to smoke is gone. Buproprion is another drug that is sometimes prescribed to relieve nicotine cravings.

Health effects of drugs

Aside from their addictive qualities, the use of substances can have significant impacts on physical and mental health. Once drugs enter the body, they are distributed by the blood. They can then work directly on the organs themselves or can affect systems in the brain that regulate bodily functions. Drugs that are normally used therapeutically may not have the risks of illegal street drugs that have been badly prepared or cut with other substances, but they often have side effects or unexpected reactions when combined with other substances. The method of ingestion, such as smoking or injection, can also cause localized problems at the site.

Smoking. Inhaling drugs through the mouth can cause damage to the soft tissues of the mouth and the throat. Tobacco smoke is hot, particularly if the cigarette has no filter, and that of marijuana, crack cocaine, and heroin is hotter still. This smoke may burn the tissues, causing soreness and lesions that can become infected. With marijuana there is a tendency to inhale more deeply, increasing the intensity of the exposure. Other chemicals in the smoke may have an irritant effect on any lesions or may be carcinogenic. The gums can shrink and teeth rot with prolonged exposure and lack of dental care.

The smoke travels down the windpipe into the bronchial tubes and the lungs. The bronchial tubes are covered in very fine hairlike cells called cilia, which become clogged with particulates and tar from smoke, reducing their efficiency in clearing the tubes. Particulates and irritants in the smoke may trigger asthma or coughing fits through contraction of the airways. They can also cause the airways to become inflamed and infected, leading to bronchitis, which can become chronic with repeated exposure. When it reaches the lungs, chemicals in the smoke attack the alveoli so they can no longer absorb oxygen efficiently, and breathing becomes difficult. This condition is called emphysema. If it occurs with bronchitis, the condition is known as chronic obstructive pulmonary disease, or COPD. COPD is a leading cause of death in the United States, with around 120,000 fatalities per year out of a total of 10 million sufferers.

Pulmonary edema is a buildup of fluid in the lungs that can result from direct injury to the lungs by heat and toxins in smoke. Sufferers have difficulty breathing, feel like they are drowning, and cough up blood in their sputum.

Lung cancer arises when a group of malignant cells grow into a tumor. Cigarette smoke contains a number of known carcinogens, and lung cancer is the second leading cause of death in the United States.

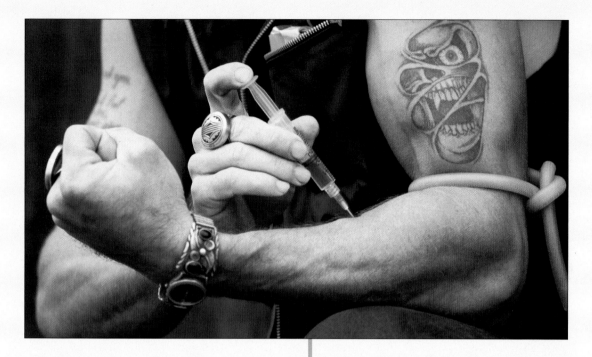

Inhalation. A number of commonly abused substances are inhaled through the mouth or nose, a process known as snorting for illegal drugs, or huffing or bagging in glue sniffing and solvent abuse. As well as the problems they cause to the respiratory system, solvents also cause crusty red lesions to form around the mouth and nose. Direct inhalation from canisters can cause freeze injuries to the back of the throat and can rupture the lining of the lung and collapse it. Suffocation is another danger if the abuser places a bag over the head to inhale the substance and then passes out. More worrying is the potential that inhalants have for causing the heart to stop suddenly, which is called sudden sniffing death syndrome. Solvents also affect the liver and kidneys, cause nerve damage, reproductive complications, and dermatitis, and interfere with heart rhythms.

Snorting powdered drugs through the nose can affect its structure, causing the cartilaginous septum that divides the nostrils to erode and collapse. Less well known is that snorting can also form holes through the roof of the mouth, affecting breathing and eating. Plastic surgery may be necessary to correct the damage. Rubbing powder on the gums can erode the tissue and loosen teeth.

Injection. Injecting drugs presents a number of risks to health that do not occur with other methods of

A man injects a drug into a vein. The dangers associated with intravenous injection are the possibility of a pulmonary embolism and the transmission of viruses such as hepatitis and HIV. Other risks are blood poisoning and abscesses.

ingestion. Regular injection causes veins to collapse and become scarred through overuse. Veins can also become blocked if drugs have been cut with an insoluble substance or the drug user is crushing pills. Insoluble substances can clump to form emboli in the lungs, leading to pulmonary hypertension. Lack of hygiene when injecting may cause abcesses around the injection site and blood poisoning. Infective endocarditis is an infection that usually affects the heart valves, causing major complications and death in a quarter of cases. It is caught by using nonsterile needles or unusual injection practices such as "rebooting," in which a small amount of blood is drawn out of the vein and reinjected. Injecting into the groin can lead to deep vein thromboses (blood clots) that can block arteries and cause a stroke or heart attack. Polyenteritis is an inflammation of the arteries that occurs when amphetamines are injected. The arteries become necrotic, which leads to tissue loss. If this condition occurs in the brain, it may cause a stroke. Injecting drug users also run the risk of contracting blood-borne diseases, such as HIV and hepatitis B and C, through sharing dirty needles. Contaminants can also cause immune system disorders, including arthritis and rheumatic problems. The generally poor health of injecting drug users leaves them vulnerable to colds and flu and longer-term conditions such as pneumonia and tuberculosis.

Heart and circulatory problems

Most drugs have an effect on the heart rate and blood pressure. Stimulants, such as cocaine, amphetamines, and even caffeine, increase blood pressure and heart rate. If blood pressure remains high for any length of time, it can damage the blood vessels, causing them to thicken and deteriorate so that the heart has to work harder to pump blood. The heart may start to beat irregularly, which is called arrhythmia. Ultimately, high blood pressure may lead to heart attack, stroke, angina, kidney failure, or circulatory problems. Cocaine users also risk a fatal rupture of the aorta or sudden death from heart failure.

Drinking alcohol and smoking tobacco can result in the buildup of fatty deposits that narrow the arteries, a condition called atherosclerosis or coronary artery disease. Chronic alcohol users often show abnormally high internal pressures in the heart that weaken it so that it cannot push blood around efficiently. Symptoms include weakness and fatigue, swelling of the neck veins, and buildup of fluid in the legs and feet. This condition is called alcoholic cardiomyopathy and results in heart failure.

Smokers are prone to peripheral vascular disease, a condition that causes arteries in the extremities, usually the legs or feet, to narrow. If these vessels become blocked by a clot, oxygen and nutrients are unable to reach the surrounding tissue, which may start to die. The tissue becomes gangrenous and may have to be removed or the limb amputated. Smokers are also vulnerable to a wide range of coronary diseases including heart attack, stroke, and aneurysm (a ballooning and thinning of an artery wall that makes it prone to rupture).

Drugs that have a slowing effect on the heart rate and blood pressure include opiates and sedatives. Because these drugs depress the respiratory centers in the brain, they can bring about respiratory failure and heart attack. In the long term, lowered blood pressure and heart rate can lead to pulmonary edema, in which fluid builds up in the lungs. High doses of barbiturates can alter heart rhythm and weaken heart muscle contraction.

Liver diseases

The liver is the site where all substances that enter the body are metabolized into a form that activates them or are turned into compounds that can be eliminated by excretion. Alcohol and drugs can cause major harm to the liver and impair its function. When alcohol is present, liver cells burn alcohol rather than fatty acids for energy. This leads to a buildup of fat globules in the liver cells. As fat accumulates, the liver swells and becomes tender and may show impaired enzyme activity. This condition can be reversed with abstinence, but it is a signal that damage is being done to the liver.

Prolonged excessive alcohol consumption develops into cirrhosis, which means "scarring of the liver." Acetaldehyde, a metabolite of alcohol, is toxic to liver cells, which become inflamed and die, and are replaced by scar tissue. The liver attempts to repair itself by making new liver cells, but because the new cells are surrounded by scar tissue, they cannot grow. Blood vessels that service the cells become squeezed by the scar tissue and can rupture and hemorrhage. Not all alcoholics show symptoms of cirrhosis, and they are only detected by medical examination. Others may show signs of fluid building up in feet and hands (edema) or in the abdomen (ascites). Ascites is an uncomfortable condition, but it does not cause problems unless it becomes infected. Sometimes people with cirrhosis show signs of jaundice as bile leaks out of the liver into the blood. The spleen may enlarge because of the increased pressure the squeezed liver vessels exert on hepatic blood. The blood may show a decrease in clotting factors, which can be dangerous if the patient hemorrhages, and anemia is common. Cirrhosis is not always fatal if the alcoholic stops drinking, but unless a transplant is available the long-term prognosis is death.

Hepatitis is a viral infection of the liver. It has five different forms, described by the appendage A, B, C, D, or E. Hepatitis A is caused by ingesting food or water contaminated with the feces of an infected person. Its symptoms are similar to the flu, but it is rarely life threatening. Hepatitis B is more severe and results in a lifelong infection that can lead to liver cancer, cirrhosis, and liver failure. It is spread by sharing needles or contact with infected blood or bodily fluids. Hepatitis C is also spread in the same manner. The majority of hepatitis C carriers have no obvious symptoms but their liver-enzyme levels may fluctuate or stabilize for periods of time. Around 70 percent have chronic liver disease, but few deaths result. Hepatitis D and E are rare forms of the disease and are not often seen in the United States.

The other main danger to the liver comes in the form of accidental overdoses. While most drugs are not directly toxic to the liver, some undergo changes that are harmful. Acetaminophen, a common ingredient of painkillers, can cause acute liver failure and death if dosages are not observed. Alcoholics are at even greater risk because their liver is already compromised. People who take sedatives may find that their effect is exaggerated because a damaged liver takes longer to eliminate them. Barbiturates, on the other hand, can speed up the elimination of other therapeutic drugs, which may be dangerous in anyone taking drugs for heart disease or a stroke.

Mental disorders

The contribution of drug abuse to the development of mental illness and vice versa is often difficult to determine. Many drugs are known to cause symptoms such as anxiety, panic attacks, depression, paranoia, antisocial behavior, or hallucinations with prolonged use. Long-term use of amphetamines is known to provoke psychotic episodes similar to those of paranoid schizophrenia. These are typified by violent mood swings, delusions, paranoia, and aggressive behavior. Continued use can eventually cause damage to the dopamine and serotonin neurotransmitter systems in the brain, resulting in permanent psychological problems.

Alcohol has well-documented effects on the brain. Abrupt abstinence from prolonged use can bring on alcoholic hallucinosis, in which patients have terrifying visual and auditory hallucinations and frightening dreams. Delirium tremens is a more aggressive form of withdrawal with mental symptoms that may include disorientation, insomnia, hallucinations, anxiety attacks, confusion, and irritability. Specific brain disorders associated with alcoholism are: Wernicke-

Korsakoff's syndrome, characterized by confusion, lack of coordination, and a loss of short-term memory; Marchiafava-Bignami disease, in which patients show signs of progressive dementia; and pathological intoxication, in which episodes of uncontrolled irrational behavior are followed by prolonged sleep and amnesia of the event.

Marijuana has long been known for its long-term effects of lethargy, apathy, and loss of motivational drive. Increasingly, evidence is showing that it can trigger schizophrenia in teenagers predisposed to the condition and paranoia among smokers of stronger strains of marijuana, such as skunk.

The other side of the drug abuse and mental illness debate is the link between an existing mental condition and substance use as a means of relieving its symptoms. Anxiety disorders, depression, bipolar disorder, and attention deficit disorder are all conditions that may tempt sufferers to self-medicate with substances that relieve some aspect of their illness. Behavioral disorders such as antisocial personality disorder (APD), conduct disorder, and oppositional defiant disorder feature risk taking, lack of self-control, and impulsive behaviors among their symptoms, which may lead to drug use as a stimulatory experience. Many of the risk factors for these disorders are the same as those for substance abuse. Studies have shown that between half and three-quarters of people with antisocial personality disorder abuse alcohol, and half abuse other substances. People with APD also tend to become severely alcoholic and abuse drugs at an early age, while teenage drug abuse increases the risk of developing APD later in life.

Overview

Substance abuse is a profoundly unhealthy lifestyle. As well as the major conditions outlined here, drug abuse takes its toll on the hormonal and immune systems and has negative social and emotional effects on the lives of the abuser and the people with whom he or she comes into contact. Drugs are valuable when they are used to treat people under the supervision of a physician. Used for nonmedical reasons, they can have a detrimental impact on a person's mental and physical well-being.

Wendy A. Horan

Sunburn and sunstroke

Sunburn is the skin's reaction to too much exposure to the ultraviolet radiation of the sun. A person's skin type may determine how quickly the burn occurs. Extreme exposure to sun may cause sunstroke, a life-threatening condition in which the body's heat-regulating mechanism shuts down.

From the time of the ancient Egyptians, who worshipped the sun god Ra, the sun has been recognized as an essential for life. But the sun can also be a source of great agony if precautions are not taken. In addition to heat and light, the sun gives off invisible ultraviolet radiation in three types: UVA, which penetrates into deeper skin layers and damages the production of new skin cells and causes tanning and wrinkling; UVB, which is even more damaging because it affects the surface of the skin by releasing chemicals that dilate the blood vessels; and UVC rays, which are absorbed by Earth's atmosphere before they strike earth. Sunburn results from too much sun on the skin; sunstroke occurs when the body's mechanisms are overwhelmed by a very hot and humid environment or by strenuous physical activity.

Causes, risk factors, and symptoms

Unlike a thermal burn, sunburn is not immediately apparent. Once the skin appears painful and red, the damage has been done. The skin turns red about 2 to 6 hours after exposure, and peak effects are noted at 12 to 24 hours.

Melanocytes in skin produce melanin for protection from UV rays. However, if the UV rays exceed the blocking power of melanin, sunburn occurs. Because their level of melanin (skin pigment) is sparse, certain light-skinned and fair-haired people are at greater risk for sunburn.

Symptoms of severe sunburn include chills, fever, nausea, vomiting, flulike symptoms, and blisters, which may vary from very fine to large water-filled blisters that have red, raw skin underneath. Medical care should be sought if pain is severe.

Sunstroke is a type of heatstroke that occurs when the body's thermostat cannot keep it cool. When temperature rises, evaporation of perspiration cools the body. In humid air, sweat does not evaporate, causing the body temperature to rise rapidly. If not treated, heatstroke can cause organ shutdowns, brain damage, and death. Treatment includes cooling the body core and giving intravenous injections to restore lost fluid.

Prevention

The best prevention is to avoid the sun. Other strategies include covering up with wide-brimmed hats, long-sleeved shirts, and long pants; wearing a sunscreen with a sun protection factor (SPF) of at least 15; and drinking plenty of water but avoiding alcohol and caffeine. Chronic sun exposure may lead to premature aging, severe wrinkling, and various cancerous skin tumors. Premature cataract formation may also occur.

Evelyn B. Kelly

KEY FACTS

Description
Sunburn is the skin's reaction to the sun; sunstroke occurs when the body's heat-regulating system shuts down.

Risk factors
Sunlight and humid temperatures.

Symptoms
Red, tender, blistered, and swollen skin; sunstroke includes elevated body temperature, hot dry skin, and often unconsciousness.

Diagnosis
Severe burn and blisters; hot dry skin, fainting, confusion, and dizziness are all indications.

Treatments
Home treatments for mild sunburn include medication for pain, cool compresses, or cool baths; for severe cases or stroke, IV fluids may be given upon admission to a hospital.

Pathogenesis
Untreated severe sunburn can lead to complications; repeated sunburns precede premature wrinkling, sunspots, and skin cancer.

Prevention
Sunscreen, wide brim hats, covering, and avoiding sun in the hottest part of the day.

Epidemiology
Sunstroke kills 10 percent of its victims.

See also
- Burns • Cancer, skin • Cataract
- Melanoma • Skin disorders

Syphilis

Syphilis is a sexually transmitted disease (STD) that can cause chronic infection and irreversible health problems if left untreated. It can be transmitted during pregnancy from mother to infant, causing a serious and sometimes fatal condition called congenital syphilis. In other parts of the world where there are crowded and poor hygienic conditions, syphilis may also be transmitted though close nonsexual contact.

Syphilis has been known as a disease for thousands of years and is still a prominent STD. Syphilis is caused by *Treponema pallidum*, a motile corkscrew-shaped bacterium known for its undulating behavior, which belongs to the order Spirochaeta, commonly called spirochetes. *T. pallidum* enters the body through a break in the skin or mucous membranes of the reproductive tract or mouth after sexual contact (oral, anal, or vaginal) with an infected person.

Syphilis goes through four stages of infection that sometimes overlap. In the first stage, primary syphilis, a small, round, painless sore called a chancre (pronounced "shanker") generally develops 10 to 90 days after exposure at the entry point of *T. pallidum*, usually on the penis, vulva, or cervix, or in the vagina or rectum, on the mouth, tongue or lips after oral sex, or other parts of the body. The sore contains *T. pallidum*, so it is highly contagious. Since the sore is painless, if it is on the cervix, inside the vagina, or inside the rectum, a woman may not even know she has been infected. Because the sore heals on its own, men and women may not seek treatment, and the disease progresses. The open sore increases the risk of HIV transmission.

The secondary stage begins about two to ten weeks after the sore appears, as *T. pallidum* spreads through the bloodstream. The result is a non-itchy rash, usually on the palms of the hands and soles of the feet, but also in the mouth, other areas, or the entire body. Symptoms can include fever, swollen glands, fatigue, headache, muscle aches, or hair loss. Because many of these symptoms can be found in many other diseases, syphilis is called "the great imitator." The rash contains the bacterium *T. pallidum*, so the secondary stage is also highly contagious. Despite being able to provoke an immune response in the body, untreated *T. pallidum* can last in the body for decades.

The third stage is called latent (hidden) syphilis. There can be few or no symptoms, and this stage can last for years. The early part of this stage is still infectious, the later part much less so, and risk of transmission is low. If not treated, some people progress to tertiary, or late syphilis. During this stage *T. pallidum* can damage the heart, blood vessels, brain, nervous system, bones, liver, and joints. Some of the results are blindness, mental illness, memory loss, heart disease, stroke or even death.

KEY FACTS

Description
Sexually transmitted disease; untreated can lead to serious health problems; can be passed from mothers to babies at any stage of pregnancy.

Causes
The bacterium *Treponema pallidum*.

Risk factors
Sexual activity; multiple sex partners; living in area with high rates; inconsistent use of condoms.

Symptoms and signs
Painless sore, then may have skin rash, general flulike symptoms, mouth sores, swollen glands, headache, muscle aches, weight loss, hair loss. Symptoms may cease. Final stage: neurological, cardiovascular, and musculoskeletal damage.

Diagnosis
Detecting *T. pallidum* from sore using darkfield microscopic exam; blood tests.

Treatments
Antibiotics, usually penicillin; in later stage damage cannot be reversed. Partner notification.

Pathogenesis
T. pallidum penetrates broken skin or mucous membranes and progresses in stages. First stage: sore at site of infection. Second stage: spreads through blood, damaging organs. Increases likelihood of HIV transmission.

Prevention
Sexual abstinence. Avoiding contact with infected people; monogamous relationship with uninfected person; consistent and correct use of condoms.

Epidemiology
Lowest rate of highly infectious forms, primary and secondary syphilis, in 2000 (less than 6,000 reported cases) since reporting began in 1941 (600,000 cases). Rates from 2000 to 2004 have increased (almost 8,000) mostly due to infection of men who have sex with men.

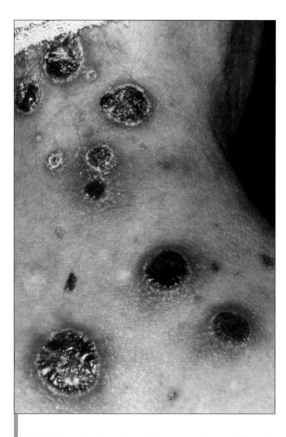

This inflamed rash on the neck is a secondary syphilis rash, which occurs about 6 to 12 weeks after infection with Treponema pallidum. *The rash is accompanied by headache, fatigue, and fever. Treatment is with antibiotics.*

Pregnant women with untreated syphilis can pass the infection to their unborn babies, resulting in miscarriages, premature births, or stillbirths. Newborns can have deformities, seizures, liver problems, anemia, and developmental delays, and as many as 40 percent of babies will die. Blood tests for syphilis are recommended routinely in pregnant women.

Diagnosis

Darkfield examination of a sample from the sore or skin rash uses a special lighting technique that makes *T. pallidum* easier to see than with standard microscope lighting. The VDRL (Venereal Disease Research Laboratory) blood test measures antibodies to the bacterium. This test may be positive when syphilis is really not present, so a more specific blood test, the FTA-ABS (fluorescent treponemal antibody absorption), can confirm the infection. If advanced syphilis involving the brain, called neurosyphilis, is suspected, a spinal tap is done to test the cerebrospinal fluid.

Because many people who have the infection may have no symptoms, many states still require a blood test for syphilis before marriage. Syphilis remains an important public health problem in poor and urban areas. The Centers for Disease Control has launched a program to eliminate syphilis in the United States, focusing on high risk populations.

Treatments

In the early stages, syphilis is easily curable with antibiotics, usually penicillin. *T. pallidum* divides slowly, so the long-acting forms of penicillin are used. During the later stages, *T. pallidum* divides even more slowly, and this requires a longer course of antibiotics. Damage from late syphilis cannot be reversed. Neurosyphilis is treated with daily intravenous (in the vein) penicillin.

Partner notification identifies sex partners of those people with HIV and other STDs so that they can be tested, evaluated, and treated for STDs.

Prevention

Prevention includes abstaining from sexual contact. Condoms used consistently and correctly and a monogamous sexual relationship with an uninfected person can reduce risk. Infection does not make a person immune; reinfection can occur.

Epidemiology

In the United States, rates of reported cases of the early infectious forms of syphilis, called primary and secondary syphilis, decreased during the 1990s, to an all-time low in 2000 of less than 6,000 since reporting began in 1941, when there were almost 600,000 cases. Reported cases increased in 2004 to almost 8,000, with rates higher in African Americans and Hispanics than in whites.

Rates in women remained stable but increased in men who have sex with men. The increase is thought to be due to an increase in high-risk sexual behavior (multiple sex partners, not using condoms consistently). Syphilis is known as a genital ulcer disease because during the early stage of infection an ulcer, or deep sore, appears at the site of infection.

Ramona Jenkin

See also
• AIDS • Cancer, cervical • Chlamydial infections • Gonorrhea • Hepatitis infections • HPV infection • Pelvic inflammatory disease • Sexually transmitted diseases

Tapeworm infestation

Tapeworms are long, segmented worms of the class Cestoda (cestodes). Infestation occurs either as fully developed (mature) tapeworms in the intestinal lumen or as fluid-filled masses (cysts) in the liver, lung, muscle, brain, eye, or other organs.

Cestodes that can infest humans include the intestinal tapeworms *Diphyllobothrium latum* (fish tapeworm), *Hymenolepis nana* (dwarf tapeworm), *Taenia saginata* (beef tapeworm), and *T. solium* (pork tapeworm) and the invasive tapeworms *Echinococcus spp.* and pork tapeworm. Tapeworms divide their life cycle between two animal hosts (intermediate and definitive), vary in size from several millimeters to 82 feet (25 m), lack an intestine, and absorb nutrients through their external surface.

The mature worm consists of a head (scolex) that attaches to the lining of the intestine, a neck, and a segmented body that contains both male and female sex organs (proglottids) and produces the parasite's eggs. Proglottids become gravid (full of eggs), break free from the tapeworm, degenerate in the stool, and release thousands of eggs per day into the feces.

Life cycle of tapeworms

The eggs of *Echinococcus spp.*, and pork and dwarf tapeworms infest an intermediate host (such as cattle and pigs) through ingestion of contaminated food. Once ingested, the egg hatches in the intestine and releases a larval form (oncosphere). The oncosphere penetrates the intestinal wall, reaches the circulation, and migrates to different organs to form a cyst. When a definitive host (such as a human) eats the cyst-containing tissues of the intermediate host, the cyst develops into a mature tapeworm in the intestinal lumen. Fish tapeworm eggs hatch in the water, and if the larval form is eaten by a small crustacean called a copepod, the larvae develops in the copepod's tissues. After the copepod is eaten by a fish (intermediate host), the larva migrates to its muscles and encysts. When an uncooked cyst is eaten by a human (definitive host), it develops into a mature tapeworm in the intestine.

Humans are solely definitive hosts for fish tapeworm and beef tapeworm and are solely intermediate hosts for *Echinococcus spp.*, which are located as mature tapeworms in the intestine of canines such as dogs and foxes. However, humans serve both as intermediate and definitive hosts for pork and dwarf tapeworms.

The immune response to intestinal infestations leads to an increase in eosinophil white blood cells and immunoglobulin E (IgE) levels in the blood, but it is not known whether this alters the course of the infestation. The immune response to a cyst often does not lead to its eradication but to its encapsulation with fibrous tissue, thus limiting damage to nearby organs.

KEY FACTS

Description

Parasitic infestation leading to the development of mature tapeworms in the intestine or to the development of cysts in different organs.

Causes

Long segmented worms of the class Cestoda.

Risk factors

Ingestion of cyst-containing tissues (meat) or of food contaminated with tapeworm eggs.

Symptoms

Intestinal infestation is often symptomless but can lead to nutrient malabsorption. Invasive infestation in the brain can cause seizures.

Diagnosis

Examination of stool samples for eggs or proglottids for intestine worms. Imaging techniques and antibody tests for invasive infestation.

Treatments

Antiparasitic drugs for intestinal infestations. Drugs and surgery for invasive infestations.

Pathogenesis

Intestinal tapeworms compete for nutrients with the host, and may lead to nutrient deficiencies in infested people. *Echinococcus* cysts may compress other organs, develop into abscesses, and rupture, causing seeding of new cysts and an allergic reaction. When pork tapeworm cysts die, they release parts of the parasite in the surrounding tissues, causing local inflammation and damage.

Prevention

Intestinal tapeworm infestations can be prevented by careful disposal of human sewage; using uncontaminated food for animals that serve as intermediate hosts; inspecting meat before marketing; and freezing or cooking meat.

Epidemiology

There is great geographic variability in the incidence and prevalence of tapeworm infestations, depending on the types of intermediate and definitive hosts involved in the tapeworm's life cycle.

Risk factors and epidemiology

Fish tapeworm infestation is acquired by eating uncooked freshwater fish that contain cysts. It is common in Siberia, northern Europe, Canada, Japan, Chile, and now also in the United States partly because of the increasing popularity of ceviche, sushi, and sashimi. Mature tapeworms reach up to 82 feet (25 m) long.

Dwarf tapeworm is acquired by ingestion of the eggs on fecally contaminated food and is the only tapeworm with direct human-to-human transmission. The mature tapeworm releases eggs that infest directly the mucosal lining and increase the number of mature tapeworms in the intestine of the infested host in the absence of further ingestion of eggs from the environment. It is very common in Asia, southern and eastern Europe, Central and South America, and Africa, whereas in North America it is found principally in people who are institutionalized, malnourished, or have a poorly functioning immune system. Mature tapeworms are small 0.6 to 2 inches (15–50 mm) long.

Beef tapeworm is acquired by eating uncooked beef containing the cysts. It is common in cattle-breeding areas of the world such as central Asia, the Near East, and Central and East Africa, and South America. Mature tapeworms reach up to 33 feet (10 m) long.

Pork tapeworm is acquired either by ingestion of eggs on fecally contaminated food, leading to the development of cysts in organs (cysticercosis) or by ingestion of uncooked pork containing the cysts, leading to the development of a mature tapeworm living the intestine. In 25 percent of cases, both forms are present simultaneously. It is common in Mexico, Central America, South America, Africa, Southeast Asia, India, the Philippines, and southern Europe. Mature tapeworms reach up to 6.5 to 26 feet (2–8 m) long.

In people with cysticercosis, the cysts are located in different organs, and involvement of the brain (neurocysticercosis) or of the heart can be life threatening. Echinococcosis results from the ingestion of eggs on food contaminated by canine feces. There are two forms of echinococcosis: hydatid disease, caused by *E. granulosus* or *E. vogeli*, and alveolar cyst disease, caused by *E. multilocularis*. *E. granulosus* is transmitted by domestic dogs and is common worldwide, whereas *E. multilocularis* and *E. vogeli* are transmitted by wild canines and are common in the northern regions of Europe, Asia, and North America, and in the Arctic regions of South America, respectively. Hydatid cysts of *E. granulosus* most commonly form in the liver or lungs and reach up to 2 to 4 inches (5–10 cm) in size. Cysts of *E. multilocularis*, which infest the lungs, tend to be smaller but invade surrounding tissues very aggressively and can spread to distant organs via the bloodstream.

Symptoms and diagnosis

Mature tapeworms in the intestine cause few symptoms, although nutrient malabsorption and a change in intestinal motility may occur. Fish tapeworm infestation may result in vitamin B_{12} deficiency and megaloblastic anemia. Patients with neurocysticercosis have few symptoms while the cysts are alive but can develop epilepsy and other neurological symptoms when the cysts die, swell, and release parts of the dead parasite in the surrounding tissues, causing local inflammation and brain damage. Symptoms of echinococcosis occur as a result of compression of other organs by an enlarging cyst, bacterial superinfection of a cyst, and rupture, causing release of offspring cysts or an allergic reaction to the dead parasite.

Diagnosis of intestinal infestation is made by examination under a microscope of stool samples for eggs or proglottids, but multiple stool samples are often needed because of the irregular rate of proglottid detachment. Invasive infestation is suspected on the basis of imaging techniques such as computed tomography (CT) or magnetic resonance imaging (MRI) and is confirmed by tests for specific antibodies in the blood or cerebrospinal fluid (in neurocysticercosis).

Treatment and prevention

Intestinal tapeworm infestation should be treated with the drugs praziquantel or niclosamide. Pork tapeworm cysts outside the brain can be surgically removed. For neurocysticercosis, surgery is often too dangerous, although treatment with drugs such as praziquantel and albendazole together with corticosteroid drugs may be beneficial. For *Echinococcus spp.* cysts, treatment is surgical removal after killing of cysts with ethanol injections or drugs such as albendazole and melbendazole.

Intestinal infestation can be prevented by careful disposal of human sewage; using uncontaminated food for animals that can be intermediate hosts; inspecting the meat before marketing to rule out cyst infestation; and freezing or cooking meat to kill cysts. Invasive infestations are more difficult to prevent because infectious eggs are widespread in the environment.

Corrado Cancedda

See also
- Anemia • Infections, parasitic • Liver fluke
- Vitamin deficiency

Tay-Sachs disease

First described in the late 1800s by physicians Warren Tay and Bernard Sachs, Tay-Sachs disease is an inherited and lethal disorder that affects the central nervous system. Though found predominantly in Jewish families of eastern European origin, Tay-Sachs disease also affects other ethnic groups. A mutation in the gene that makes the enzyme hexoaminidase A is responsible for causing central nervous system deterioration. Although it is not currently possible to treat Tay-Sachs disease, public education, genetic counseling, and genetic testing help reduce the incidence of this devastating metabolic disorder.

Tay-Sachs disease is named after the two clinicians who separately described this inherited condition. In 1881 the British ophthalmologist Warren Tay (1843–1927) linked the presence of a cherry-red spot located in the retina to symptoms of physical and mental decline—symptoms later observed in children. Several years later, Bernard Sachs (1858–1944), a New York neurologist, described this condition at the cellular level. He also discovered its genetic causes by noticing that most families who had babies with what he called "amaurotic familial idiocy" were Jews of eastern European origin.

Causes

Tay-Sachs is caused by an autosomal recessive disorder in which a faulty gene is inherited from both parents. People who have this inherited metabolic disorder either lack the enzyme hexosaminidase A (Hex A) or make Hex A enzyme molecules that do not work properly. Normally this enzyme breaks down the fatty substance GM2 ganglioside into materials needed to make nerve cell membranes. Without Hex A, GM2 ganglioside accumulates in nerve cells thus causing them to swell and die.

Symptoms and signs

Tay-Sachs babies appear normal at birth. By about three to six months, because of the effects of enzyme deficiency and nerve-cell damage, parents notice their baby startles easily in response to any noise, appears unaware of his or her surroundings, and has poor vision and muscle weakness, with floppy arms and legs. The baby will also show other developmental and behavioral abnormalities. By two years, most Tay-Sachs children experience uncontrollable seizures, diminishing mental capacity, and loss of physical skills, such as sitting and crawling. Eventually, the child becomes blind, paralyzed and nonresponsive. Most Tay-Sachs children die before their fifth birthday.

Risk factors

Medical researchers have known for more than 40 years that Hex A is absent in Tay-Sachs patients. Inherited in an autosomal recessive manner, people who have one Tay-Sachs gene make enough Hex A enzyme molecules to prevent damage. However, those who inherit two Tay-Sachs genes are completely deficient in this vital enzyme and do not survive.

The Hex A gene that causes Tay-Sachs disease is located on chromosome 15. Recent advances in DNA sequencing technology reveals nearly one hundred Hex A mutations that cause Tay-Sachs disease. Some

---

KEY FACTS

Description
A fatal genetic disorder in children that destroys the central nervous system.

Causes and risk factors
Absence of the enzyme hexoaminidase A causes Tay-Sachs disease. Inheriting two copies of the Tay-Sachs gene is the risk factor.

Symptoms
Vision loss, an abnormal startle response, developmental regression, seizures, diminishing mental function.

Diagnosis
DNA testing for the presence of Tay-Sachs mutations and the absence of hexoaminidase A in blood.

Treatments
Supportive care. There is no cure for Tay-Sachs disease.

Pathogenesis
The absence of hexoaminidase A causes accumulations of a lipid, GM2 ganglioside, in the brain.

Epidemiology
Primarily affects Jews of eastern European origin.

mutations prevent Hex A synthesis and others produce Hex A molecules that do not efficiently break down GM2 ganglioside. Infantile Tay-Sachs, the condition marked by Hex A enzyme deficiency, is the most severe and rapidly progressing form.

People who have late-onset Tay-Sachs disease (LOTS) make Hex A molecules that do not work properly. In this situation, the disease progresses slowly, and people usually experience poor coordinations, tremor, and slurred speech—symptoms of neurological degeneration—by the time they reach adolescence. Over time, LOTS patients develop other neurologic symptoms that may include unsteady gait, muscle weakness, and mental and behavioral changes.

Genetic testing and prevention

At the present time, there is no cure for Tay-Sachs disease, although the disease is lessening as a result of more available information. Public education, carrier screening, and prenatal diagnosis are effective preventive measures. Testing blood and DNA identifies people who carry Tay-Sachs mutations.

Blood testing identifies carriers because their single Hex-A gene produces smaller amounts of enzyme than people who have two functional genes. DNA testing identifies many Hex-A mutations, including those which cause LOTS.

Preimplantation genetic diagnosis (PGD) may be considered for couples when there is a known mutation. The technique identifies defects in embryos created through in vitro fertilization before transferring them to the uterus.

Genetic counseling and treatment

If the woman is already pregnant, genetic counselors can offer referrals for diagnostic tests to determine if the baby is unaffected, is a carrier, or has Tay-Sachs disease. Amniocentesis involves testing the fetal cells contained in the surrounding amniotic fluid for Hex A. Doctors perform this test between the fifteenth and eighteenth week of pregnancy.

Testing placental tissue, or chorionic villus sampling, provides similar diagnostic information. Doctors perform this test between the tenth and twelfth week of pregnancy. Overall, the incidence of Tay-Sachs disease in Ashkenazi Jews was 1 in every 3,600 births; as a result of extensive genetic counseling of carriers the incidence has been reduced by more than 90 percent. In Sephardic Jews and non-Jews, the incidence of Tay-Sachs disease is 1 in 250,000 people.

Genetic counselors, professionals who receive extensive education and training in genetics and psychology, believe that it is better if the family receives some genetic counseling information before testing. During the initial session, the genetic counselor explains the purpose of testing, how to prepare for the test procedure, and how to understand the range of possible test results. Often families see the counselor after having already received a positive Tay-Sachs report. In either situation, the genetic counselor helps the couple understand and interpret their test results and explains the range of available options.

The baby does not have Tay-Sachs disease if neither family member carries the Tay-Sachs gene. If either the mother or the father is a Tay-Sachs carrier, the baby has a 50 percent chance of also receiving a single copy of the Tay-Sachs gene. There are several possible outcomes if both parents are Tay-Sachs carriers. For each pregnancy, there is a 1 in 4 chance that the baby will not inherit the Tay-Sachs gene. There is also a 50 percent chance that the baby will be a carrier and a 25 percent chance that the baby will have Tay-Sachs disease. The genetic counselor, rather than telling the family what they should do, helps them make decisions that are compatible with their personal beliefs.

Options range from giving birth to having a therapeutic abortion. It is very important that counselors present information in a way that supports family discussion and does not stigmatize individuals.

There is currently no treatment for Tay-Sachs disease. All that is possible is to treat any symptoms when they occur, and to keep the child as comfortable as possible.

Pathogenesis and epidemiology

Tay-Sachs is a fatal disease for children who have inherited two Tay-Sachs genes. They rarely live beyond the age of five.

Medical geneticists estimate that everybody carries six to eight disease-causing genes. According to the Chicago Center for Jewish Genetic Disorders, nearly 1 in 30 Jewish people of eastern European or Ashkenazi descent carry a Tay-Sachs gene. By comparison, in the general population that also includes Mediterranean or Sephardic Jews, about 1 in 250 people have this mutation.

Janet Yagoda Shagam

See also
• Childhood disorders • Diagnosis • Genetic disorders • Mental disorders • Metabolic disorders • Muscle system disorders • Pregnancy and childbirth

Tetanus

Tetanus is a disorder of the nervous system caused by the bacterium *Clostridium tetani*. It typically occurs when traumatic injuries and wounds are contaminated by this toxin-producing organism. The disease is characterized by intense muscle spasms and is often fatal. With the advent of vaccination, the incidence of tetanus has decreased among the developed world. However, it is still very prevalent in developing nations.

The bacterium *Clostridium tetani* commonly exists in the environment, especially in soil. The organism produces spores that can gain access to the host through penetrating trauma or wounds. Once inside host tissue, the organism germinates into the bacterium and produces harmful toxins. Injury and wounds, including those seen in postsurgical patients, are the main predisposing factors for the development of tetanus.

Symptoms and signs

In its most classic form, symptoms include painful, involuntary muscular contractions that can involve the entire body. Muscles of the jaw may be affected, referred to as "trismus" or "lockjaw." In addition to muscle spasms, patients may experience fever, sweating, irritability, and restlessness. As spasms progress, airway obstruction and respiratory failure may ensue necessitating the use of a mechanical ventilator.

Diagnosis and treatments

The diagnosis is typically made based on the presentation of the patient, especially if any history of an injury or wound is reported. The bacteria do not grow well in the laboratory; therefore culture and other blood tests are rarely helpful in the diagnosis.

Several different treatment modalities should be implemented to treat tetanus. Antibiotics are universally recommended, and acceptable agents include penicillins or metronidazole. Antibodies to the toxin, also known as tetanus immune globulin (TIG), should be administered with the hope of neutralizing its effects. The vaccination series should also be started to confer long-term immunity. Surgical removal of devitalized tissue or wounds may be necessary. Finally, measures to decrease muscle spasms and support the respiratory system, possibly with a mechanical ventilator, are often required.

Once in host tissue, the organism produces its primary toxin, called tetanospasmin, which travels through neurons to the spinal cord and brain stem. The toxin then interferes with normal neuronal activity to induce muscular rigidity and other symptoms.

Vaccination with tetanus toxoid is recommended. In the United States, it is given as a series of five shots. Booster injections should be given every ten years to ensure lifelong immunity.

The annual incidence of tetanus in the United States is 0.16 cases per million people, or 35 to 70 cases per year. Worldwide incidence is higher, with roughly 18 cases per 100,000 people, about 1 million cases per year.

Joseph M. Fritz and Bernard C. Camins

KEY FACTS

Description
A disease of the nervous system caused by toxin-producing bacteria.

Causes
Clostridium tetani.

Risk factors
Deep injuries or wounds, postsurgical patients, drug users, neonates.

Symptoms and signs
Muscular rigidity and pain, often of the jaw; fever, sweating, and mental changes. Spasms lead to airway obstruction and respiratory compromise.

Diagnosis
Based on clinical presentation of the patient.

Treatments
Antibiotics, tetanus immune globulin to neutralize the toxin, and vaccination to confer immunity after treatment. Surgical debridement, muscle relaxants, and respiratory support.

Pathogenesis
Bacteria produce tetanospasmin toxin. Affects spinal cord and brain stem, causing muscle spasms.

Prevention
Vaccination series through childhood, followed by booster injections every ten years.

Epidemiology
35 to 70 cases per year in United States and about 1 million cases per year worldwide.

See also
• Infections, bacterial • Muscle system disorders • Prevention

Thalassemia

Thalassemias are a group of inherited diseases of the blood, in which one of the two hemoglobin proteins, alpha globin or beta globin, is reduced or absent. Anemia results from inefficient hematopoiesis (making stem cells) and shortened red blood cell lifespan.

Most thalassemias are inherited in an autosomal-recessive mode (a faulty gene inherited from both parents). Normal hemoglobin has four globin chains, two alpha and two beta. If someone has one to three faulty genes, she may only have mild symptoms, but four faulty genes usually results in the baby dying before birth. Insufficient quantitities of one of the globins prevents formation of normal hemoglobin. Abnormal hemoglobins cannot carry sufficient oxygen, and their precipitation damages the red cell membrane, leading to hemolysis (destruction of red cells).

Risk factors and symptoms

Thalassemias are observed in all ethnic groups. They occur mainly in the Mediterranean (beta-thalassemias) and in Southeast Asia (alpha-thalassemias). A nonspecific finding in all thalassemias is microcytic anemia.

Diagnosis and treatments

The diagnosis is made by hemoglobin electrophoresis, in which abnormal hemoglobins or increased quantities of normally rare hemoglobin species can be detected. Prenatal diagnosis is possible.

Thalassemia major and many cases of thalassemia intermedia are treated with transfusions to suppress stem cell production, and hence suppress the formation of blood cells. Excess iron as a result of repeated transfusions is removed by chelation therapy. Severe alpha-thalassemia may also require chronic transfusion and chelation, or transfusions during intermittent hemolytic or aplastic episodes. Bone marrow transplantation is curative and may be considered if a matched donor is available.

Pathogenesis

Children with lesser forms of thalassemia may have mild or no symptoms, while those who inherit a faulty gene from both parents will have severe anemia and enlarged bones as a result of bone marrow expansion.

Prevention and epidemiology

Genetic counseling is imperative for couples if both partners carry pathological hemoglobin genes. The thalassemias are the most common single-gene defects in the world. The highest prevalence of carriers is in the Mediterranean (mostly beta-thalassemias) and in Southeast Asia (more commonly alpha-thalassemias). Thalassemia trait is believed to confer relative resistance against lethal forms of malaria. In the United States thalassemias are comparatively infrequent, with around 1,000 severely affected patients.

Halvard Boenig

KEY FACTS

Description
Chronic anemia due to abnormal hemoglobin.

Causes
Mostly autosomal-recessive inheritance.

Risk factors
The thalassemias are common in regions where malaria is endemic.

Symptoms
Chronic anemia, bone marrow hyperplasia, iron overload with sequelae of hemosiderosis. Hemolysis (breakdown of red blood cells) in some types of thalassemias.

Diagnosis
Blood count or smear, hemoglobin electrophoresis.

Treatments
Chronic transfusion and chelation therapy, bone marrow transplantation.

Pathogenesis
Decreased lifespan of erythrocytes leads to chronic anemia. Increased red cell production and excessive iron reabsorption from the gut may ensue.

Prevention
Genetic counseling for carriers, prenatal diagnosis. Consistent iron removal (chelation) prevents complications of siderosis.

Epidemiology
While frequent in many parts of the world, in the U.S. the number of individuals afflicted with severe forms of thalassemia is around 1,000.

See also
- Anemia • Blood disorders • Malaria
- Sickle-cell anemia

Throat infections

A painful infection of the throat caused by viruses, bacteria, or fungi. Usually these infections are limited and cause no lasting effects. The incidence of throat infections is unknown but presumed to be very high.

Throat infections are usually caused by bacteria, viruses, or fungi. They produce a painful swelling of the throat, and the throat becomes red and sore. Sometimes, when the infection is isolated to a specific portion of the throat, it takes on the name of that part. For example, tonsillitis is an infection in the tonsils only. It is possible to have some of the symptoms of a throat infection without really having an infection. We call these conditions sore throats. They are often caused by irritants and pollutants in the air, such as cigarette smoke and chemicals.

Nearly 90 percent of all throat infections are caused by viruses. The remainder are due to bacteria and fungi. Although any virus can cause a throat infection, the most common causes are rhinoviruses, which are the same viruses that cause the common cold. Many other well-known infections are caused by viruses, including mononucleosis, influenza, measles, and herpes.

A strep throat infection is caused by bacteria. Other types of bacteria, such as *Corynebacterium diphtheriae*, which at one time caused plaguelike illnesses, have been largely eradicated by vaccination programs around the world. However, they still exist in some developing nations and in parts of eastern Europe.

A third type of throat infection, called thrush, is caused by fungi and is usually only seen in people with weakened immune systems due to diabetes, AIDS, medications, or chronic illness.

Risk factors

In a generally healthy population, people are not at a high risk for getting a throat infection. They become sick only when they are exposed to the virus, bacteria, or fungi that causes the illness. However, throat infections seem to be more common among certain groups. For instance, children in day care or school pass the illness to each other and to their teachers easily. Additionally, hospital workers who are exposed to infected people frequently also become sick.

Some people seem to be more prone to throat infections because they have pockets in their tonsils (called crypts), which store bacteria. The bacteria make thick impenetrable films inside these crypts, making it difficult to eliminate them. Since they are always present, they often cause throat infections.

Unlike healthy people, those with weak immune systems do not have the ability to fight off infections. Therefore, this group is at greater risk than all others because there are viruses and bacteria all around us.

Symptoms and signs

Throat infections usually begin almost unnoticed, but the common symptoms that develop quickly are unmistakable. The throat pain becomes sharp and more intense over a few days. The infected person cannot eat or drink comfortably because it hurts too much when he or she swallows. Sometimes, when the pain is very severe, the person becomes dehydrated and requires emergency intravenous fluids. Also, if the pain

KEY FACTS

Description
A painful infection of the throat.

Causes
Viruses, bacteria, and occasionally fungi create inflammation in the throat.

Risk factors
People with weakened immune systems are at increased risk. In healthy people the highest risk is among children and young adults.

Symptoms
Painful swallowing and sore throat. Drooling and difficulty breathing are occasional danger signs. Associated fever and muscle and joint aches.

Diagnosis
Patient history and findings of inflamed throat. Bacterial cultures and X-rays may be helpful.

Treatments
Generally, symptomatic treatment and hydration are adequate. If bacterial infection is present, antibiotics are used.

Pathogenesis
Develops from local throat infection by viruses, bacteria, or fungi.

Prevention
Hand washing is the best. Maintaining a healthy immune system is also important.

Epidemiology
Unknown, but believed to be very high.

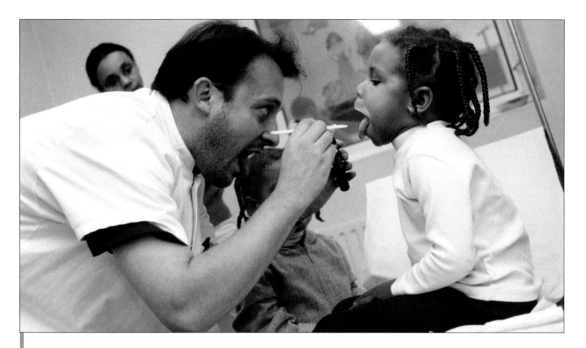

A doctor examines a child's throat. One of the most common bacteria that affects throats is Streptococcus faecalis, *hence the term* strep throat. *Left untreated, it can result in kidney problems or rheumatic fever.*

is very severe, the person may start to drool because it is too painful to swallow his or her own saliva. Lastly, a throat infection almost always causes a sore throat that changes the sound of a person's voice.

The most dangerous symptom of a throat infection is severe swelling that narrows a person's airway and results in difficulty breathing. Other significant symptoms and signs of throat infections include high fevers, rashes, headaches, aching muscles and joints, eye irritation, and general exhaustion.

Diagnosis and treatments

Doctors can diagnose a throat infection by listening to the patient's symptoms and by a routine physical examination. Sometimes it is not so obvious and the doctor has to order tests, blood sample analyses, and X-rays.

Most of the time, throat infections can be cured without long-term problems or complications. The treatment for a throat infection will depend upon the cause. The body cures most viral infections with its own disease-fighting mechanisms. Throat infections caused by bacteria are treated with antibiotics. Since strep bacteria can also cause complications such as kidney failure and heart disease, the infection must be treated aggressively and the patient must be monitored

carefully. Gargling with salty water is a popular home remedy, but there is little scientific evidence to show its effectiveness. In those people who have repeated throat infections from bacteria hiding in tonsillar crypts, the surgical removal of the tonsils may be recommended.

Prevention

The best cure for a throat infection is to prevent it before it happens. Hand washing is the most effective way of avoiding an infection. Some people recommend taking extra doses of vitamin C, vitamin E, and beta carotene. Most scientific studies have shown that these are not effective. A sufficient supply of these substances is found in a well-balanced diet, and the human body cannot use or store these extra vitamins taken as supplements.

About 15,000 cases of invasive strep infections occur each year in the United States. It is not known how many people have throat infections every year because most people do not visit the doctor with every sore throat. However, the number of missed days of work and the economic impact from throat infections is very significant, costing society millions of dollars annually.

Y. Etan Weinstock and Kevin D. Pereira

See also
• Cold, common • Croup • Infections, bacterial • Infections, viral • Kidney disorders • Rheumatic fever

Thrombosis and embolism

Thrombosis and embolism are disorders of blood clotting and circulation. Thrombosis means the development of a clot in a blood vessel; embolism means the obstruction of a blood vessel by a mass (usually a clot) that has traveled through the circulation. The most common forms are deep vein thrombosis and pulmonary embolism.

The body's ability to control the flow of blood through the arteries, veins, and capillaries is critical to survival. In normal conditions, when blood vessels remain intact (non-injured), blood flows smoothly through the vessels but quickly forms a clot at the site of any vascular injury (coagulation). Once the injury has been repaired, there is a reversible process of repair, in which the clot dissolves (fibrinolysis). The mechanisms that control the delicate balance between coagulation and fibrinolysis are known as hemostasis (arrest of bleeding).

Thrombosis and embolism are disorders in which hemostasis is unbalanced, leading to clots in arteries that obstruct blood flow to different parts of the body. Without adequate blood supply, the affected tissue or organ is damaged and ultimately loses its ability to function normally.

Depending on the location of the blood clot, thrombosis and embolism may be termed *arterial* (occurring in the arteries) or *venous* (occurring in the veins).

The most common forms are deep vein thrombosis (DVT), in which a clot forms within a vein (usually in the leg), and pulmonary embolism (PE), in which there is a blockage in the artery supplying the lungs, usually caused by a clot that developed in the leg veins and traveled to the lungs.

Causes and risk factors

Three risk factors influence the blood's tendency to clot (Virchow's Triad): the constituents of the blood itself; the vessel wall; and the flow of blood. Problems in any of these areas can lead to an increased tendency to clotting, also known as a prothrombotic or hypercoagulable state.

KEY FACTS: DVT

Description

DVT is the formation of a blood clot within a deep vein, usually in the leg. The clot may obstruct the flow of blood, causing swelling, pain, and damage to the tissues; or the clot may break free and travel to the lungs, causing pulmonary embolism, a potentially fatal complication.

Causes

Derangement in the blood's ability to flow smoothly through the vessels. Three main factors encourage the formation of blood clots: constituents in blood promoting coagulation, damage to the vessel wall, and stagnant flow through the vessels (stasis).

Risk factors

Prolonged immobility, surgery (particularly orthopedic surgery), older age, cancer, varicose veins, smoking, obesity, pregnancy, estrogen therapy, and thrombophilia (excessive clotting).

Symptoms

Many cases of DVT are asymptomatic. Common symptoms include swelling, pain, cramp, redness, and changes in the temperature and appearance of the skin of the affected limb.

Diagnosis

By ultrasound, venography, and other imaging tests to visualize blood vessels and locate the clot.

Treatments

Anticoagulant drugs to thin the blood. Less often, thrombolytic drugs are used to dissolve the clot. Compression stockings may be worn to help reduce swelling in the legs. In rare cases, a filtering device is placed in the vein to catch clots before they reach the lungs.

Pathogenesis

Without treatment, DVT can cause pain, difficulty with walking, and damage to the valves in the blood vessels, leading to venous hypertension and pulmonary embolism.

Prevention

Avoiding risk factors and prophylactic measures. For example, people who need orthopedic surgery often take anticoagulant drugs, wear compression stockings, and are mobilized one day after surgery.

Epidemiology

DVT affects around 1 person in 1,000 and is fatal in around 5 percent of cases.

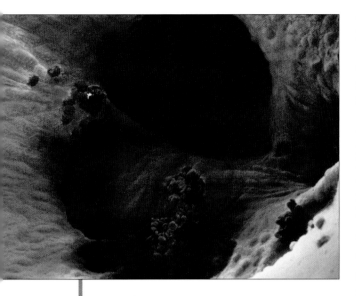

This false-color scanning electron micrograph shows a thrombus (blood clot) protruding from an arterial entrance in a chamber of the heart. This type of thrombus is called a coronary thrombosis.

Common causes of thrombosis include prolonged immobility, for example, during air travel; cancer; pregnancy; surgery, especially orthopedic surgery; oral contraceptives and hormone replacement therapy; and central venous catheters (medical devices used to deliver drugs and fluids to the body over a long period of time).

Other risk factors for thrombosis are older age, obesity, smoking, a family history of thrombosis, varicose veins, and thrombophilias (conditions in which there is an increased tendency for excessive blood clotting). The risk of thrombosis increases with the number of risk factors present.

Common thrombophilias are factor V Leiden (activated protein C resistance); deficiency of protein C, protein S, or antithrombin III; prothrombin mutation (G20210A); antiphospholipid syndrome (due to lupus anticoagulant or anticardiolipin antibodies); and high homocysteine levels (due to a genetic mutation or vitamin deficiency). Thrombophilias may be inherited (caused by genetic mutations) or acquired (caused by other medical conditions).

Symptoms, signs, and diagnosis

The symptoms of thrombosis and embolism depend on the location of the blood clot. DVT typically affects the legs (usually the thigh and calf) and may cause swelling, pain, tenderness, cramp, or changes in the color or temperature of the affected limb. DVT in the upper body may cause swelling of the arm or neck. However, many cases of DVT are asymptomatic.

The symptoms of PE are often vague or resemble other diseases. The most common symptoms of PE are sudden shortness of breath, chest pain, cough, rapid heart rate, and dizziness or fainting.

Both DVT and PE are diagnosed using tests such as ultrasound, venography (X-ray of the veins), and computed tomography to visualize the blood flow and locate the clot. A blood test may be performed to rule out thrombophilias, and other investigations may be needed to explore the underlying causes and to see how much damage the clot has caused.

Treatments and prevention

Thrombosis and embolism are serious disorders that are usually treated in a hospital. Urgent treatment is needed to reduce the risk of serious complications and death. The goals of treating thrombosis and embolism are to stop the blood clot from growing, prevent the clot from breaking off and traveling elsewhere, and to reduce the likelihood of another clot forming.

Treatment usually involves drugs to thin the blood (anticoagulants) or dissolve the clot (thrombolytics, thrombin inhibitors). Patients who cannot take these drugs may have a filtering device implanted in the large vein below the heart to stop blood clots from reaching the lungs. Patients with DVT often wear compression stockings to help reduce swelling in their legs.

Many cases of thrombosis and embolism can be prevented. Some risk factors, such as obesity and cigarette smoking, can be avoided through lifestyle changes. Other risk factors, such as being immobilized following surgery, can be modified with blood-thinning drugs, compression devices, and early rehabilitation. Preventive measures are particularly important in people with thrombophilias, who may take blood-thinning drugs on a routine basis.

DVT becomes more common with increasing age. DVT is believed to affect up to 25 percent of all hospitalized patients, although many will not have any symptoms. There is no obvious cause in 25 to 50 percent of people with DVT. Around 7 percent of people with DVT suffer a recurrence within six months.

Joanna Lyford

See also

- Aging, disorders of • Blood disorders
- Cancer • Obesity • Pregnancy and childbirth • Smoking-related disorders
- Veins, disorders of

Thyroid disorders

The thyroid gland is an endocrine gland that makes and releases thyroid hormones T3 and T4 into the blood. These hormones are responsible for regulating the body's metabolism and the way that the body uses fats and carbohydrates, affecting the tissues of every organ.

About 15 million people in the United States have been diagnosed with some form of thyroid disease. Because many people have mild forms of thyroid disease, there may be an equal number undiagnosed. The two main types of thyroid disease are hypothyroidism, an underactive thyroid gland; and hyperthyroidism, an overactive thyroid gland. More than 75 percent of people with thyroid disease are women. Symptoms of thyroid disease can be nonspecific, sometimes making diagnosis difficult. There are about 20,000 new cases of thyroid cancer each year; it is more common in men.

The thyroid gland is a two-lobed butterfly-shaped gland sitting in the front of the neck just below the Adam's apple. It produces and secretes the iodine-containing thyroid hormones T4 (thyroxine) and T3 (triiodothyronine). As part of a feedback loop to keep the body's metabolism in check, the thyroid gland works with the hypothalamus and pituitary gland, located at the base of the brain. Circulating thyroid hormones in the blood signal the hypothalamus to release TRH (thyroid-releasing hormone). TRH signals the pituitary gland to secrete TSH (thyroid stimulating hormone), and TSH signals the thyroid to produce T3 and T4. A shift in any of these hormones can cause an alteration in the feedback loop.

Causes

In hypothyroidism too little circulating thyroid hormone is present. If the hypothalamus and pituitary glands are normal, TRH and TSH levels are elevated because of lack of negative feedback by thyroid hormones. In hyperthyroidism, too much thyroid hormone signals the hypothalamus to reduce the amount of TRH secreted; this decreases the amount of TSH secreted. Because of this feedback loop, blood tests for T3, T4, and TSH are used routinely to diagnose thyroid disease. Since iodine plays a key role in thyroid hormone production and is pulled from the blood to manufacture T3 and T4, special scans of the thyroid can be made after small amounts of the harmless radioactive iodine (I-123) are swallowed or injected in a vein; the concentration in the thyroid gland indicates how much hormone the thyroid is making. Another isotope, I-131, is used to destroy normal and cancerous thyroid tissue.

Hypothyroidism

As people age, the thyroid gland may produce less thyroid hormone, more commonly in women over age 50. But the most common cause of hypothyroidism in the United States is Hashimoto's thyroiditis, an autoimmune disorder that attacks and destroys the thyroid gland. Other causes include: pituitary failure; surgical removal of the thyroid gland, or radioactive iodine or anti-thyroid medication for treatment for thyroid cancer or hyperthyroidism; previous head and neck exposure to radiation as cancer treatment; and medications, like lithium, used to treat psychiatric dis-

---

KEY FACTS

Description
Too or much or too little thyroid hormone.

Causes and risk factors
Increasing age, female gender, iodine deficiency, family history, autoimmune disorder, radiation treatment of head or neck cancers.

Symptoms
Many people have mild or no symptoms. Hypothyroidism: sluggish, weight gain, pale dry skin, fatigue. Hyperthyroidism: nervousness, sweating, tremors, weight loss, hair loss, increased heart rate.

Diagnosis
Thyroid function blood tests T3, T4, and TSH; thyroid scans; ultrasound; biopsy.

Treatments
Hypothyroidism: replacement medication for life; Hyperthyroidism: destroy thyroid tissue, thyroid replacement medication.

Prevention
Adequate iodine in the diet.

Epidemiology
About 15 million people in United States with thyroid disease; many more undiagnosed. Iodine deficiency throughout the world causes 100 million cases of hypothyroidism.

orders. Hypothyroidism due to iodine deficiency is uncommon in the United States, where iodine is added to some table salt. In other parts of the world where dietary iodine is insufficient, 100 million people suffer from iodine-deficiency hypothyroidism.

Symptoms include sensitivity to cold, slow speech, constipation, coarse hair, hoarse voice, heavy menstrual periods, pale dry skin, cold skin, weight gain, puffy face, and depression. In some cases there may be heart problems, goiter, birth defects, and myxedema, a life threatening condition due to long-standing undiagnosed hypothyroidism that can result in coma. Hypothyroidism is particularly dangerous in newborn infants (congenital hypothyroidism). Diagnosis is made by blood tests T3 and T4 (low), TSH (high), and TSAb, thyroid stimulating antibodies (high).

Hyperthyroidism

Hyperthyroidism occurs in about 1 percent of people in the United States and is at least five times more common in women, especially between the age of 20 and 60. Excess thyroid hormone causes nervousness, sweating, tremors, change in appetite, weight loss, sleep disturbances, increased heart rate, and vision changes. About 85 percent of cases are caused by Graves' disease, an autoimmune disorder that increases the size and activity of the thyroid. Graves' disease can cause inflammation of the tissues around the eyes, so they appear to bulge. Thyroid nodules can produce too much thyroid hormone and are another cause of hyperthyroidism. In thyroiditis, a general inflammation of the gland, sometimes caused by infection or unknown mechanisms, excess thyroid hormones leak into the blood. Diagnosis is made by T3 and T4 (usually high), TSH (low), and TSAb, and increased uptake on thyroid scan. Biopsy can be done for nodules. Graves' disease can be treated with radioactive iodine to destroy thyroid tissue, surgery, or both. Drugs that block production of thyroid hormone may be used. Beta blockers can treat blood pressure and heart rate. After treatment, many people become hypothyroid and need thyroid replacement medication for life.

Goiters

A goiter is a general enlargement of the thyroid gland. Causes include inadequate iodine or autoimmune disorder, such as Hashimoto's thyroiditis, and can take months or years to develop. Goiters are treated if there is trouble swallowing or breathing, from compression of the esophagus or windpipe behind the thyroid gland. Blood tests include TSH, and T3 and T4

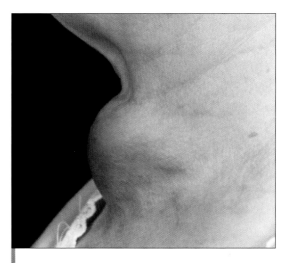

The swelling in this woman's neck is caused by carcinoma of the thyroid. Cancer of the thyroid is fairly rare and the causes are generally unknown.

(low or normal), thyroid scans, and ultrasound. Once treated, the thyroid gland shrinks back to a normal size.

Pregnancy

About 2 percent of pregnant women in the United States are diagnosed with hypothyroidism, which can lead to miscarriages, preeclampsia, bleeding after birth, and low birth-weight babies. The most common cause is Hashimoto's thyroiditis. Iodine deficiency can cause hypothyroidism during pregnancy. The most common cause of hyperthyroidism during pregnancy in the United States is Graves' disease, which occurs in 1 in 1,500 pregnancies.

Congenital hypothyroidism

Also called cretinism, hypothyroidism in a newborn occurs in about 1 in 3,000 births, twice as often in girls. It can be due to abnormal development of the thyroid or pituitary gland, or abnormal formation of thyroid hormones. The child requires rapid treatment with thyroid replacement hormone to prevent developmental problems; untreated, an infant can become mentally and physically retarded. Lifelong treatment is needed to avoid chronic symptoms. Most states require newborns to be screened for hypothyroidism.

Ramona Jenkin

See also
• Cancer, thyroid • Environmental disorders
• Genetic disorders • Immune system
disorders • Metabolic disorders

Tic disorders

Tic disorders are characterized by the presence of patterned, repetitive involuntary movements and sounds. Tic disorders can be transient, lasting between 4 weeks to less than a year, but symptoms can last at least one year, for example in Tourette's disorder. Symptoms worsen during times of stress and can be treated with various therapies or medications, or both.

Individuals with tic disorders exhibit sudden, painless uncontrolled behaviors that are either motor or vocal. The three different types of disorders (transient, chronic motor, or vocal and Tourette's) are differentiated by the severity and durations of the tics.

Causes and risk factors

Abnormal neurotransmitters are believed to contribute to tic disorders. Differences in the area of the brain concerned with movement (the basal ganglia) as well as in the anterior cingulated cortex are often present. Genetic factors are present in 75 percent of cases. Tic disorders are thought to be worsened by the use of psychomotor stimulants, either used recreationally or medicinally.

Tics may be simple: using few muscles (neck jerking), simple sounds (grunting); or complex, using many muscles (jumping) or full words and sentences, or repetition of inappropriate words.

Diagnosis and treatments

Symptoms must occur before the age of 18. Transient tic disorder consists of multiple tics which last at least four weeks, but less than 12 months. Chronic tic disorder is either single or multiple motor or vocal tics, but not both, present for more than one year. Tourette's disorder consists of both motor and vocal tics present for more than one year.

Behavioral techniques, such as habit reversal treatments, have been effective in controlling the symptoms of tic disorders. In more severe cases, most commonly Tourette's syndrome, medications such as haloperidol are effective in reducing symptoms.

Pathogenesis and prevention

Symptoms are usually present in early childhood. Transient tic disorders rarely progress to more severe cases. For chronic tics, children whose tics start between the ages of 6 to 8 seem to have the best outcomes. Tourette's disorder is usually a chronic, lifelong disease.

Very few, if any, preventive measures exist for tic disorders other than attempting to reduce stress before birth and throughout life.

From 5 to 24 percent of all school-aged children have a history of tics. Chronic tic disorders are estimated to affect 1 to 2 percent of the population, affecting boys more often than girls. The lifetime prevalence of Tourette's disorder is about 4 to 5 per 10,000 individuals.

Lori M. Lieving and Oleg V. Tcheremissine

KEY FACTS

Description

Disorders that involve the presence of tics of different severity and duration.

Causes and risk factors

Thought to involve anomalies in brain structure and function. May be also genetically linked.

Symptoms

The presence of tics, which are repetitive, patterned, and purposeless movements or vocalizations.

Diagnosis

Diagnosed when tics are observed, despite normal results on physical and neurological examinations.

Treatments

The most effective treatment has been behavioral or cognitive-behavioral therapy. Medications may also be used.

Pathogenesis

Symptoms of tic disorders may be present between 2 and 15 years of age. Symptoms appear to worsen during adolescence.

Prevention

Minimizing stress, before birth and through life, may serve limited preventive functions.

Epidemiology

Between 5 to 24% of children have some history of tic disorders. More severe cases are rare. Boys are affected up to four times more often than girls.

See also
- Brain disorders • Muscle system disorders
- Nervous system disorders

Tooth decay

Tooth decay, also known as caries, is a disorder in which a hole or defect forms in the outer mineral layer of a tooth. The normal tooth is made of a hard mineral layer, which surrounds a softer layer. The outer layer or enamel is above the gum line; underneath is dentin, which is a softer mineral layer in which the nerves and pulp of a tooth lie. When a cavity forms, the outer enamel layer has a hole, which, if deep enough, exposes the layer containing the pulp. This can lead to nerve damage, tooth loss, and even death from infection spreading past the tooth to the jaw.

Each person has numerous bacteria naturally living in the mouth, which can form plaques. When a person eats, the food meets the bacteria in the mouth, and sugars and starches are digested, leaving behind acid. This acid can then demineralize and erode the protective enamel of the teeth.

Risk factors

One of the risks for developing tooth decay is poor oral hygiene. Not brushing or flossing properly or often enough can allow plaques to develop. Not seeing a dentist can also allow early signs of decay to progress. Because the other component leading to cavities is food, a diet high in sugar and refined starch is a risk factor for decay. This includes foods such as candy, honey, sweetened snacks, and even juice. For tooth decay, how often these foods are eaten determines the risk of developing decay—that is, if a person eats these foods three separate times a day, he or she would have more risk than someone who eats them just once a day. Other risk factors include not having access to fluoride, either in the water or in items such as toothpaste or mouthwash.

Babies are at risk of developing "baby bottle caries" when they are allowed to fall asleep with sweetened liquids in their bottles or if they receive multiple feedings of sweetened liquids.

Symptoms and signs

Early tooth decay has no signs or symptoms. If the cavity enlarges, there can be increased sensitivity to cold and cold drinks or pain after having sweet drinks or food. There can also be softening of the teeth around the decay. There have also been associations with foul odors or bad breath in progressed decay.

Diagnosis and treatments

Most cavities are diagnosed by X-ray on a routine dental visit, before symptoms and signs have developed. In a dental X-ray, tooth caries can show up as darkened areas. Dentists can also find larger cavities by looking or probing with dental instruments.

There is a wide range of treatments that dentists can offer for cavities. The most important thing to re-

KEY FACTS

Description
A defect or hole in the enamel of a tooth. Also known as "cavities" or "caries."

Causes
Bacteria on teeth digest sugars from eaten food, leaving behind acid, which dissolves the outer layer of teeth.

Risk factors
Inadequate brushing, flossing, and dental care. A diet high in refined starches and sugar. Lack of preventive measures such as fluoride.

Symptoms
There are often no signs or symptoms of early decay. If the decay progresses, there can be tooth pain worsened by heat, cold, or sweet food and drinks.

Diagnosis
Dentists can find cavities on dental X-rays.

Treatments
Range from fluoride treatments, dental fillings, or root canal, depending on the extent of decay.

Pathogenesis
Can lead to tooth loss. If severe, can lead to infection of the surrounding tissues of the face and neck, and even death.

Prevention
Good oral care, diet low in refined sugars, fluoride in water, and toothpaste. Dental sealants are an option in some cases.

Epidemiology
The most common chronic disease of children. About 90 percent of schoolchildren and most adults have been affected.

member is that the earlier the cavity is found, the easier the treatment. One of the simplest treatments is topical fluoride. This treatment can be used if the cavity is very small and dental hygiene is good. Fluoride affects the enamel part of the tooth. It binds to the minerals in the enamel area, making it harder for the bacteria to stick there, and therefore harder for cavities to form. Fluoride is also used as a preventive measure in water and toothpaste.

If the decay has progressed enough into the enamel layer of the tooth, the treatment includes removing the decayed enamel by drilling it out and then replacing it with a dental filling. Many materials can be used for filling a cavity, such as gold, amalgam, resin, and porcelain. The material chosen for the filling depends on where the tooth is, what role it plays in chewing food, and how noticeable the filling will be. For example, resin and porcelain can be colored to match the color of teeth and would be used in areas where the filling would be noticeable. However, these materials are not as strong as amalgam and gold, and so may not be used in teeth that are used for chewing food.

Pathogenesis

If a cavity is not treated, it can reach the pulp of a tooth and cause the nerve to die from infection or from being exposed. For these cases, root canal treatment is necessary. In this procedure, the nerve and blood supply of a tooth are removed in addition to the decayed enamel. The tooth is filled with a rubberlike filling, and a crown is then placed over the tooth. If tooth decay progresses, the entire tooth may need to be removed, which is called dental extraction. An extraction can be necessary if the tooth is destroyed beyond an ability to repair it, or if the cost to fix it is too high. There are also severe cases of tooth decay in which an infection can spread past the tooth to include the jaw and the tissues in the mouth and neck, a condition known as Ludwig's angina. Very rarely, this condition can progress to death.

Prevention

One key way to prevent cavities is to routinely and properly brush and floss. This action prevents plaque, a pale yellow-to-white coating of bacteria on the teeth. Routine visits to the dentist to look for early signs of decay, as well as for dental cleanings, are also important. Dentists use X-rays to detect early signs of cavities.

A diet low in refined sugars and starches is key to minimizing bacteria's ability to produce decay-causing

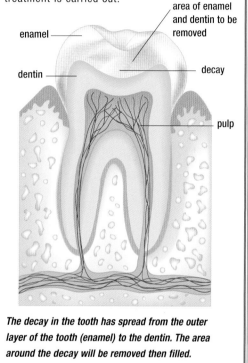

TOOTH DECAY

Decay can penetrate the enamel and dentin of a tooth and the affected tooth will have to be filled. If decay reaches the pulp, which contains the nerves and blood vessels, root canal treatment is carried out.

enamel

dentin

area of enamel and dentin to be removed

decay

pulp

The decay in the tooth has spread from the outer layer of the tooth (enamel) to the dentin. The area around the decay will be removed then filled.

acids. In fact, tooth decay only became a worldwide problem after sugar cane plantations were developed in the 1700s, which made sugar easily available worldwide. Before sugar was commonly available, cavities were less frequently encountered. Fluoridation of both water supply and toothpaste has reduced the incidence of tooth decay. Dentists may also use dental sealant on developing teeth in children to prevent cavities.

Epidemiology

By World Health Organization (WHO) estimates, nearly 90 percent of all schoolchildren and young adults have tooth decay. It is the most common chronic disease of children and is at least five times more common than asthma.

Nisha Bhatt

See also
• Dental and oral cavity disorders • Gum disease • Infections, bacterial

Toxic shock syndrome

Toxic shock syndrome is a bacterial disease caused by *Staphylococcus aureus* and *Streptococcus pyogenes*.

Toxic shock syndrome (TSS) is caused by *Staphylococcus aureus* and *Streptococcus pyogenes*. *S. aureus* is present in the nose of about 50 percent of humans; and it can affect other people. Many types of *S. aureus* exist; only some have the ability to cause TSS. *S. pyogenes*, the other cause of TSS, more commonly causes strep throat (pharyngitis). Streptococci are contracted from other humans, usually by coughing. Only certain types of streptococci can cause TSS, via breaks in the skin. TSS, whether staphylococcal or streptococcal, is caused by toxins called superantigens that are produced and released by both bacteria.

Risk factors include infections as a result of surgery, trauma, drug use, and infection with the influenza or chickenpox virus. The viruses damage both skin and mucous membranes, allowing subsequent infection by streptococci and staphylococci. Tampon usage during menstruation can create conditions favorable for staphylococcal toxin production; thus menstruating women are at greater risk of developing menstrual TSS.

The signs of TSS include flulike symptoms, vomiting and diarrhea, then a drop in blood pressure and multiple organ involvement. Other signs may include a sunburn-like rash. Streptococcal TSS is often complicated by a deep soft-tissue infection known as necrotizing fasciitis (flesh-eating disease), which causes severe pain, usually around bruised areas. Diagnosis requires drop in blood pressure or dizziness on standing, multiple organ involvement (such as vomiting, diarrhea, and confusion or combativeness), and fever. Diagnosis of TSS should include the isolation of *S. aureus* or *S. pyogenes* from mucosal surfaces or from normally sterile sites on the body. Septicemia is far more common in streptococcal TSS than in staphylococcal TSS.

The risk of menstrual staphylococcal TSS can be reduced by not using tampons or alternating with pads, and using tampons of the lowest absorbency. Nonsteroidal anti-inflammatory drugs may mask the pain of streptococcal TSS, so use of these drugs may be risk factors. Treatment options for both types of TSS are available. *S. pyogenes* responds to antibiotics such as penicillin and clindamycin; however, the selection of antibiotics can be challenging for *S. aureus*, because of

prevalent antibiotic resistance. Treatment of TSS also should include intravenous immunoglobulin (IVIG), a mixture of antibodies that neutralizes the superantigens. TSS treatment can include drainage of wounds, removal of the tampon, and surgery to remove gangrenous limbs. In the case of streptococcal TSS with necrotizing fasciitis, surgical removal of dead tissue is often required, or possible amputation of the limb.

Kristi L. Strandberg, Amanda J. Brosnahan, and Patrick M. Schlievert

KEY FACTS

Description
Uncommon illness caused by bacterial toxins.

Causes
Staphylococcus aureus (tampon disease) or *Streptococcus pyogenes* (flesh-eating disease).

Risk factors
Tampon use and vaginal barrier contraception, viruses, surgery, burns, skin trauma, and use of nonsteroidal anti-inflammatory agents.

Symptoms
Flulike symptoms, then dizziness upon standing. Symptoms of streptococcal TSS may include pain in areas of bruising that have become infected.

Diagnosis
Based on signs, changes in liver and kidney function, high fever, rash, and isolation of the organism from infection site.

Treatments
In the case of antibiotic resistance, the antibiotic vancomycin is used. Intravenous immunoglobulin to neutralize toxins, removal of tampons, and surgery.

Pathogenesis
Without treatment, multiple organ failure and death.

Prevention
Not using tampons. No preventive measures exist for streptococcal TSS.

Epidemiology
The annual incidence of staphylococcal TSS is about 3 in 100,000, affecting males and females equally. Worldwide, 5 in 100,000 are affected by streptococcal TSS; males and females and all ages affected about equally.

See also
- Infections, animal-to-human • Infections, bacterial • Throat infections

Toxoplasmosis

Toxoplasmosis is an infection caused by *Toxoplasma gondii*, a parasite that infects birds and mammals, including humans. Very few infected people show symptoms, since a healthy person's immune system usually keeps the parasite from causing illness. However, toxoplasmosis in pregnant women and people with weak immune systems can cause serious health problems.

Toxoplasmosis is an infection caused by *Toxoplasma gondii*, a parasite found in most warm-blooded animals and birds. Domestic cats can contract the parasite by eating infected birds or rodents. They shed the parasites in their feces, and infection can spread to people through direct contact with the cat's feces or with soil that has been in contact with it. People can also get toxoplasmosis from eating undercooked infected meat. Less commonly, a pregnant woman may pass the infection to her unborn baby. Though toxoplasmosis is generally asymptomatic, infection in unborn children and individuals with a weak immune system can cause serious health problems.

Causes and risk factors

Humans may contract toxoplasmosis by touching the mouth after gardening or cleaning a cat's litter box; by eating or handling undercooked infected meat; by drinking contaminated water; or, in rare cases, by receiving an infected organ transplant or blood transfusion. If a pregnant woman contracts toxoplasmosis, there is a 40 percent chance that her unborn child will also become infected. Toxoplasmosis is most dangerous for babies born to mothers who became infected during or just before pregnancy, and for people with severely weakened immune systems, such as those with HIV/AIDS, or chemotherapy or transplant patients.

Signs and symptoms

A minority of healthy individuals may develop mild, flulike symptoms that typically resolve within a few months. However, toxoplasmosis in those with weakened immune systems may damage the brain, eyes, or other organs. Unborn children infected in early pregnancy may later suffer blindness, deafness, seizures, and mental retardation, though only about 1 in 10 infected babies show signs of infection at birth.

Diagnosis and treatments

Blood testing is the routine method of diagnosis. In a pregnant woman with an active infection, amniocentesis or ultrasound may help determine if the fetus is also infected. Medical treatment is generally needed only for pregnant women and people with weak immune systems, who are given pyrimethamine (an antimalarial), sulfadiazine (an antibiotic), and folic acid. The antibiotic spiramycin can halve the chance of an infected woman passing the infection to her unborn child.

Jonathon Cross

KEY FACTS

Description
An infection caused by *Toxoplasma gondii*, a common parasite.

Causes
Contact with infected cat feces or soil; infection of fetus by pregnant mother; eating infected meat.

Risk factors
Infected soil, cat litter, and blood transfusion.

Symptoms
Usually none, though may cause flulike symptoms. Severe toxoplasmosis may damage the brain, eyes, or other organs.

Diagnosis
Blood testing. Amniocentesis and ultrasound may determine infection in a fetus.

Treatments
Generally not needed, though pregnant women and immunodeficient individuals may be treated with antibiotics and other drugs.

Pathogenesis
Symptoms in healthy people usually resolve in a few months. Severe health problems in babies infected in early pregnancy may be apparent at birth but usually appear months or years later.

Prevention
Avoiding contact with cat feces, soil, or raw meat.

Epidemiology
It is estimated that more than 60 million people in the United States have toxoplasmosis. One to two in 1,000 infected babies are born each year.

See also
- Immune system disorders
- Infections, parasitic • Pregnancy and childbirth

Trachoma

Trachoma is one of the most common infectious diseases worldwide and currently the world's most common cause of preventable blindness. Caused by the bacterium *Chlamydia trachomitis*, it is a disease that strikes underdeveloped areas with poor sanitation. The worldwide burden of this disease is huge, and international efforts are underway to eradicate it.

Trachoma is caused by repeated eye infections with *C. trachomitis*. This bacterium exists as many different serotypes and also causes infection involving the urogenital system. The strongest risk factor for this disease is residence in impoverished areas where trachoma is endemic. Typically there is poor access to water and sanitation. Most transmissions occur among household contacts.

Once the bacterium gains access to the eye, it replicates and causes inflammation of the conjunctiva, the thin membrane that lines the inner eyelid and the exposed surface of the eyeball. This is commonly referred to as "conjunctivitis." Patients develop irritated, red eyes with mucopurulent drainage. Signs of inflammation can often be seen on the underside of the eyelid. Pain and photophobia may also occur. Repeated episodes can result in significant scarring that can eventually progress to blindness if untreated, typically over the course of several years.

Diagnosis and treatments

The diagnosis is usually made based on the history and clinical exam. Tests to identify the bacteria are time-consuming, expensive, and usually not available in areas in which trachoma is endemic. Initial episodes can be treated with either topical antibiotics (tetracycline) or oral antibiotics (azithromycin or tetracycline). Patients usually become reinfected quickly because of environmental factors. If blindness occurs, there is no treatment that can restore the sight.

Pathogenesis

Infected children act as the main reservoirs in endemic areas. The bacteria can live on skin surfaces, such as the hands, and are spread through physical contact. The initial episode usually heals spontaneously, although patients often become reinfected. Repeated infections result in ongoing inflammation, lid deformities, and scarring. If untreated, corneal damage and blindness may develop.

Prevention and epidemiology

The best method of prevention is appropriate sanitation and hygiene practices; otherwise the bacteria will continue to cause worldwide disease. There is no vaccine available. About 6 million people are now living with blindness caused by trachoma, while 150 million people are living with active disease. It is most prevalent in Africa, the Middle East, and the Indian subcontinent. It is rare in developed nations. The World Health Organization has launched a mass treatment campaign to eradicate trachoma by the year 2020.

Joseph M. Fritz and Nigar Kirmani

KEY FACTS

Description
Bacterial infection of the eye.

Causes
The bacterium *Chlamydia trachomitis*.

Risk factors
Poverty and poor sanitation enhance spread.

Symptoms
A red, irritated eye with pain and drainage. The initial infection often resolves spontaneously.

Diagnosis
Based on history and physical exam.

Treatments
Topical and systemic antibiotics.

Pathogenesis
Spreads through intimate contact. Untreated, it may progress to blindness.

Prevention
Good sanitation and hygiene measures and treatment of those already infected.

Epidemiology
Occurs in underdeveloped countries. There are 150 million people worldwide with the active disease and about 6 million people living with blindness caused by repeated infections.

See also
• Blindness • Chlamydial infections
• Conjunctivitis • Eye disorders • Infections, bacterial

Trauma, accident, and injury

Trauma is a term that is frequently used to mean injury; it is a disruption or damage of living tissue caused by an external agent and can be organic or psychological, and frequently both (for example, a gunshot can cause trauma to the body but can also produce psychological trauma as a result of the circumstances associated with the event). An accident is defined as an unfortunate event resulting from an unexpected happening that causes injury. Often, unexpected events are preventable and therefore are considered more a result of ignorance or lack of proper care (for example, many deaths in car accidents happen as a result of not using the seatbelt). Injury is regarded as any damage or harm done to a person; the characteristics of injury depend on the mechanism, the affected organ, and the severity or extension of the damage (for example, a bone fracture is not as dangerous in a toe as it could be in the skull).

In general, the calculated amount of injuries in the United States is 60 million a year, with 50 percent requiring medical attention and 12 percent requiring admission to a hospital. Trauma remains the leading cause of death in the first four decades of life (in all ages up to 44 years), surpassed only by cancer and diseases related to atherosclerosis (such as heart attacks and strokes) as the major causes of death in all age groups.

In the United States approximately 150,000 people die every year as a consequence of trauma, and as many as 9 million people more are not fatally injured but become disabled (approximately 300,000 permanently and 8.7 million temporarily). Most common causes of unintentional injury deaths are as follows: motor vehicle accidents, falls, poisoning, fires and burns, drowning, airway obstruction (as a result of food or nonfood items), firearm accidents, machinery, aircraft, and suffocation. The increased number of terrorist attacks are now placing explosions in the category of common causes of injury and death in all countries of the world.

Risk factors

Using the term *accident* implies a random circumstance resulting in harm, when in fact injuries occur in patterns that are predictable and preventable. The reasons for accidents are a combination of high-risk individuals with high-risk environments, which together provide the chain of events that results in trauma.

RELATED ARTICLES

Motor vehicle accidents. The most common age group population involved is young males, and the highest mortality is related to motorcycle collisions. Around 40 percent of adult automobile victims are legally classified as intoxicated by alcohol. These statistics suggest that young people, and especially males, have a higher probability of motor vehicle accidents, apparently due to behavior that includes driving at a higher speed, as well as a sense of invincibility.

In the same respect, alcohol and recreational drugs decrease driving abilities and encourage aggressive behavior. The nonuse of safety devices (that is, seatbelt, helmets, or car seats for children), as well as improper vehicle maintenance, may increase the frequency of motor vehicles accidents and the severity of the injuries.

Falls. Falls are the most common accidental injury in people more than 75 years of age, and they are the second most common accidental injury in people between 65 and 74 years. Remarkably, most individuals who fall will do so on a level surface and will suffer an isolated orthopedic injury. No doubt aging has added problems of decreased visual capacity, motor strength, balance, memory, and difficulty in recognizing a hazardous environment.

Extreme sports and occupational exposure have a higher probability of fatal falls, but prevention is accomplished by the proper protective equipment and precautions.

Poisoning. More than half of reported poisoning events are accidental and occur in children between the ages of one and five, with 5 percent fatalities. A child's normal curiosity commonly leads to toxic exposure in an unsupervised environment.

On the other hand, adults may be accidentally poisoned at the workplace, but more frequently are poisoned after intentional exposure as the result of a recreational drug overdose or suicide attempt.

Fires and burns. Household and industrial settings provide a great variety of hazards that lead to fires or burns, including inhalation, ingestion, flames and spilling of hot fluids or caustics on the skin.

Inadequate storage of caustic substances frequently found in cleaners and detergents is a source of hazard that can lead to fire accidents and burns. Unattended hot liquids, flammables, as well as manipulation of

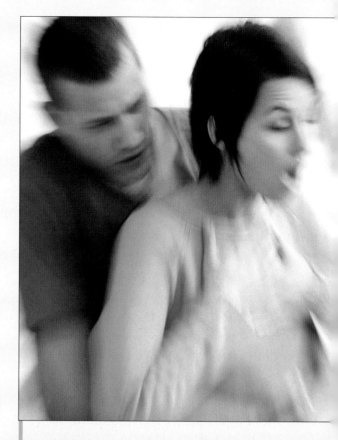

If a person is choking and does not dislodge the object by coughing vigorously, or when a slap is given on the back, the Heimlich maneuver must be attempted. This involves standing behind the person and doing abdominal thrusts.

chemicals, gas pipelines, or flames indoors make the kitchen, garage, storage units, and pantries the perfect places for burning catastrophes. Many fires occur when personnel have not been given appropriate training or instructed about what precautions to take.

Drowning. About 4,500 people die of drowning every year in the United States; the most common occurrence is among children under age four, followed by teenagers. Unattended children make up the greatest number of casualties in swimming pools, but a significant percentage of drownings happen in bathtubs, not only of small children, but also of elderly individuals. Medical conditions such as seizures, as well as alcohol consumption and drug use by victims or supervising adults, often play a role in drowning accidents.

Airway obstruction. Different mechanisms can

cause airway obstruction. Choking accounts for approximately 3,000 deaths annually. In adults, this usually occurs during eating, and meat is the most common cause. In children, choking is frequently related to foreign bodies like food products (particularly meat), toy parts, coins, and small objects. Other causes of airway obstruction are secondary to inflammation or edema in response to allergic reactions to food or medications (angioedema). In the event of choking, a lifesaving tactic such as the Heimlich maneuver may be the only effective resource if used in time.

Firearms. Given that most firearm injuries are intentional, a great number are still considered accidental, and many of them have deadly outcomes. Easy access to firearms and their presence in households significantly increases the possibility of intentional and unintentional injuries; improper storage, presence of children, hostile family dynamics, and use of alcohol and drugs make conditions more favorable for the occurrence of firearm accidents.

Machinery. Accidental injuries related to machinery are frequently associated with permanent disabilities and fatal outcomes. Some risk factors include the operators' inexperience, lack of safety protocols, distraction, alcohol use, and exhaustion.

Aircraft. Because the prevention of injuries related to aircraft accidents is the responsibility of the makers and operators of the aviation industry rather than the users, little can be done by passengers except to follow the safety recommendations.

Suffocation. Incidents of suffocation occur with infants by accidental hanging from curtain cords, or even in a friendly environment, for example, restricted breathing in a crib as a result of bulky pillows. The lack of motor and developmental skills to react to a threatening situation, such as obstruction of the respiration with a pillow or a plastic bag, and the lack of an appropriate preventive child-proof environment are the usual factors in these types of incidents.

Mechanisms of trauma

Trauma is a dynamic process, and multiple factors play a role in the severity and extension of the injuries. The type of accident is relevant (whether it is a car collision, fall, or fist blow); the acceleration applied (that is, falling from a chair presents far less acceleration than falling 15 feet (4.5 m) from a ladder); and the internal resistance of each tissue, (for example, muscles can tolerate more trauma than the brain). The velocity, as opposed to acceleration, is important. Velocity is the magnitude of energy transmitted to an object (a bullet has much higher velocity than a thrown rock; therefore it can cause more damage). Other factors are: heat conduction or temperature of the bodies in contact (for example, the hotter the object the more harmful); the time of exposure (crucial in burns and poisoning); and finally, age, preinjury condition, and any other diseases make an individual more susceptible to harm by trauma.

Blunt injury. This is a direct blow with a nonsharp object without disruption of the skin but with potential for internal injuries, depending on the severity of the force. The damage is usually more pronounced in the area of the impact, but the force transmission can involve other organs in the pathway of the trauma. Externally blunt trauma can be seen as bruising, swelling, hematoma, malfunctioning of the organ, or pain but can cause bone fractures and destruction of internal organs. Blunt mechanism is the most common type of injury and is present in almost every trauma (for example, falls, assault with fist or baseball bat, car collision, and falling objects).

Penetrating injury. This type of injury usually presents with evidence of disruption of the skin or scalp. It can be classified as high speed, for example bullets or projectiles from explosions, and low speed, such as stab wounds with sharp objects. Injuries range from small skin lacerations or cuts to severe hemorrhage and perforation of fatal organs, such as the heart or the lungs.

Crush injury. The effect of this injury is to compromise the normal blood circulation and macerate the tissues. This can result from prolonged or forceful compression, creating a toxic environment that causes the death of the involved parts and eventually the release of those toxins to the circulation in a process called rhabdomyolysis. This type of trauma is most commonly observed in events like earthquakes and presents high probability of death and loss of limbs (amputations).

Blast injury. Explosions are the result of an extremely fast transformation of the explosive into gaseous material that occupies a much larger space and creates a powerful pressure wave.

When the body is exposed to a blast, the most frequently damaged organs are those containing air. These are the ears, bowels, lungs, and eyes, and an explosion can cause rupture, contusion, edema, and hemorrhaging. In the case of explosions, injuries are not only secondary to the blast mechanism but are also associated with flying objects and the possibility that the body will be thrown as a missile.

Burn injury. A severe rise or decrease in the temperature of the body tissues can cause alteration of the normal biological functioning, severe inflammation, and denaturalization or melting of the affected areas. The skin is the most directly exposed structure, but deeper organs can also be affected. In burn trauma, the length of time of exposure, extremes of temperatures, and rapidness of treatment will determine the severity of injury.

Radiation injuries. The magnitude of the radiation injuries depends on the dose of the radioactive material; the duration of the exposure; and the route of contamination, which may be inhalation, ingestion, or absorption from contaminated mucous membranes or skin wounds.

Radiation damage occurs at cellular level; it can induce mutation and alter the ability of cells to reproduce (mitosis). Organs such as the skin, gastrointestinal, hematological, and reproductive systems can be affected, and there is likely to be damage to the immune system. Organ failure can occur years after exposure to the radiation, and there may be long-term complications of radiation, such as cancer.

Poisoning. Even innocuous substances such as oxygen and water are toxic when they are taken in excessive amounts. Poisons and toxins produce injury mostly at the chemical level of cell functioning by altering vital functions or overwhelming the body's metabolism. The effects of some poisons can be counteracted with antidotes; others will be cleared from the body over time.

It is important to note that in most severe trauma cases more than one type of injury is present, and a vigilant mind, trained personnel, and teamwork are required to increase the chances of a better outcome.

Diagnosis

The most important diagnostic tool in trauma, if it is available, is detailed information about the events and circumstances surrounding the accident. The time of onset of trauma, ingestion of poison, or exposure to radiation or other damaging substances may be indicative of the severity of the injuries and the need for treatment. For example, lacerations need suturing within the first six to eight hours after occurrence; after that time frame, lacerations may be left open in order to prevent infection. Also, some toxic ingestions require no treatment if no symptoms are present after a reasonable period of time.

The dynamics of the trauma of a motor accident, such as the person's position in the car, ejection, speed, severity of the car damage, and use of protective equipment, like a helmet, help anticipate the sort of injuries present and inform the treatment plan to follow.

Initial findings and intervention by a rescuer, such as the induction of vomiting immediately after poison ingestion, decreases the chance of toxicity. Observed transient loss of consciousness after trauma may be an indication of brain injury. Ideally, the information about the event is obtained from the victim, as well as a complete medical history, including past medical conditions, allergies to medications, related symptoms like shortness of breath and dizziness, and location and intensity of the pain. However, in many cases, abnormal mental conditions, intoxication, young age of the victim, unconsciousness, language barrier, or placement of artificial respiration devices makes the interrogation of the victim an unrealistic task.

Once in the presence of a physician, minor injuries rarely need diagnostic tests after a physical exam, but in more severe trauma, extensive tests may be indicated in order to rule out other injuries that are not immediately obvious. The armamentarium of blood tests and imaging diagnostic techniques may be necessary in the trauma setting; it includes X-rays, computed tomography (CT) scans, ultrasonography, magnetic resonance imaging (MRI), and electrocardiography (ECG) (see DIAGNOSIS).

Some diagnostic procedures may be indicated, and for severe trauma victims, these procedures may prove to be lifesaving. They include pericardiocentesis, peritoneal lavage, and endotracheal intubation.

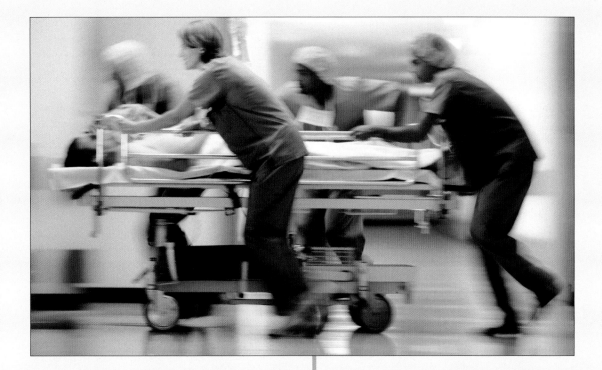

In many cases when the victim presents in critical condition due to suspected intraabdominal or intrathoracic injuries, there is no chance to perform diagnostic tests in the emergency room, and the patient should then be transferred immediately to the operating room.

A patient is given oxygen, which is considered a necessity in emergency medicine, while being rushed by a team of doctors and nurses from the emergency room to an operating theater for urgent lifesaving treatment.

Treatments

There are written protocols such as ATLS (advance trauma life support) used for the care of trauma victims; they are implemented by the American College of Surgeons to standardize initial care of severe trauma cases. In this protocol a sequential "ABC" or "ABCD" intervention is focused on preserving life and preventing disability.

"A" represents "airway." The first lifesaving intervention is to guarantee air passage to the lungs. The multiplicity of trauma scenarios can be associated with inability to transport air into the lungs. Sometimes this is because of altered mentation, which impairs the voluntary respiration. This may be a result of intoxication, drug overdose, or head trauma. It can also be because of physical obstruction of the airway by vomiting, bleeding, foreign bodies, disruption of the anatomy, and most commonly due to relaxation of soft tissues, including the soft palate, uvula, and tongue

into the posterior part of the pharynx. In all cases the consequences of inadequate transportation of oxygen to the lungs and subsequently to the rest of the body reduces the normal functioning of vital organs such as the brain, the heart, and the kidneys. A reduction in oxygen increases the damage of organs, and often this is the direct cause of death. Therefore "securing the airway" can be the single most important lifesaving intervention in trauma. It can be achieved by simple head positioning, or suctioning and removing obstructing material from the mouth, or advanced interventions, such as orotracheal intubation or cricothyroidotomy (tube inserted in the anterior aspect of the trachea through a surgically opened wound).

"B" represents "breathing." If the victim is not breathing properly, the next intervention is to assist respiration. In chest trauma, blood or air and sometimes both can accumulate between the lungs and the thoracic wall (hemothorax and pneumothorax, respectively). This event is usually secondary to rib fracture or direct laceration of intercostal or intrapulmonary vessels; such mechanical compression of the lungs, combined with pain, impairs expansion of the lungs, and the proper respiration process. This can have fatal consequences if not properly treated.

In the case of a pneumothorax, a temporary lifesaving procedure is the insertion of a large gauge needle through an upper intercostal space to decompress the thorax and facilitate lung expansion, but a definitive treatment must follow. The procedure is similar to that for hemothorax; it consists of a plastic tube insertion in an intercostal space (thoracostomy) to connect the space containing air or blood to a negative pressure trap and drain the compressing elements.

"C" represents circulation. These measures include stopping bleeding and replacing lost blood. Bleeding decreases the capacity to oxygenate, collect cellular waste, and supply nutrients to vital organs; some compensation mechanisms are activated but have limited efficiency. External bleeding can be controlled with external compression, elevation of limbs, and ligation of bleeding vessels. A, B, and C can be accomplished in the field or in the emergency room. On many occasions the bleeding is internal and needs repair in the operating room. When there is obvious bleeding, blood replacement can be achieved temporarily with intravenous fluids designed to increase the circulating volume and help the perfusion of the vital organs, but if the blood loss is not sufficiently replaced by the intravenous fluids, blood transfusions are indicated.

"D" represents "disabilities"; the following initial interventions are focused on preventing further injury and on early repair of non–life-threatening injuries. Once most lifesaving interventions have been performed, the next strategy in trauma management is the correction of limb-threatening injuries and less serious injuries such as fractures, luxations, and lacerations, and to prevent further damage from the present injuries. This part of the treatment includes pain management, oxygen supplementation, and sedation as needed. The aim is to ensure a proper recovery by preventing infections with antibiotics, regulating electrolytes and sugar abnormalities, and doing more detailed diagnostic studies, such as CT scans, special view X-rays, and angiographies.

Overall, the treatment of any injury is summarized in the following basic concepts. Preservation of life, regardless of the severity of the injuries, and despite the possibility of major secondary disabilities, is a doctor's main concern. Cerebral death, amputations, severe deformities, or coma are not sufficient reasons to stop efforts to keep a victim alive.

Prevention of further damage is essential once life-threatening interventions are not needed. The following are preventive measures: decontamination of radioactive material, giving an antidote for a specific poison, controlling bleeding by direct compression, establishing venous access for blood transfusions, or realigning a fracture that is blocking blood circulation.

Some injuries need no specific treatment or therapy except time to heal and supportive therapy. For example, pain control and swelling management with elevation, ice packs, and immobilization are indicated for sprains, contusions, hematomas, abrasions, and even small fractures. Other injuries need a more specific approach, such as suturing, debris removal, hematoma drainage, fracture reduction, grafting of lost tissue, reconstruction of distorted parts, or amputation of nonsalvable organs. Prevention of complications for a faster recovery include antibiotics to combat infection, pain management, wound care, tetanus vaccine, and education of patients. Rehabilitation depends on the extent of the injury; most injuries are mild to moderate and are followed by a complete recovery; however, severe trauma can be associated with residual psychological or physical suffering that becomes part of a new lifestyle in which physical therapy and rehabilitation play a major role.

Prevention

Since trauma can reach epidemic magnitude, government agencies, private organizations, and proactive citizens spend resources and funds to educate the public, push for new legislation, and enforce safety at all levels. Educational institutions, the media, and nonprofit organizations usually manage to reach the general population, but the most effective level of education starts at home with parents and older relatives acting as role models in regular daily living. Everyone would benefit by bearing in mind that, after all, prevention is always better than treatment.

Carlos J. Roldan

Treatment

It is a principle in medicine that, except in acute emergencies, treatment should not be started until the doctor is reasonably confident that he or she knows what is wrong with the patient. Diagnosis should always, if possible, precede treatment. Treatment without diagnosis is bad medicine. Many doctors are concerned about alternative therapies and the availability of powerful drugs on the Internet.

Treatment is commonly classified into medical (in which drugs are used), surgical (which involves operative intervention), and psychiatric disciplines (in which both drugs and counseling are used). The professionals involved in these are known, respectively, as physicians, surgeons, and psychiatrists. Effective treatment in all three disciplines must, however, always include a fourth and equally important element in the interaction between doctor and patient: that of sympathetic concern involving discussion, reassurance, advice, and the conveying of medical information. This element should be present in all medical consultations of whatever kind, and it is a serious deficiency in the quality of medical care if this element is neglected. Clinical medicine, although based on science, is actually an art requiring communication, awareness, and empathy. Good

doctors must be both knowledgeable and humane. In addition to these four broad categories, treatment commonly involves the activities of a range of people who work in other fields. These include general, specialized, and community nurses, dentists, optometrists, physical therapists, counselors, dietitians, orthopedists, occupational therapists, speech therapists, and podiatrists.

Medical treatment

With the development and rapid expansion of medical knowledge, specialization has become inevitable. No single person can possibly hope to master the whole range of the knowledge and skills needed to provide even an adequate level of care.

Although primary care physicians trained in general family practice, pediatrics, and internal medicine still handle many of the new cases, an increasing proportion of physicians in the United States now specialize. In 1998 half of internal medicine residents elected to enter primary care, but by 2006 more than 80 percent became specialists or hospital doctors.

The specialities for physicians include cardiology, dermatology, urology, gynecology, geriatrics, oncology, hematology, neurology, pediatrics, psychiatry, and radiotherapy. In all of these cases the principal treatment measure available to practitioners is

RELATED ARTICLES

pharmacology, which is the science of the characteristics and uses of drugs.

The whole face of medicine was changed in the late 1930s when the antibacterial drug sulfanilamide began to become available to doctors. This was quickly followed in the 1940s by penicillin and, after that, by a long succession of other antibiotic drugs. The idea of producing new and effective drugs by research and clinical trials led to a revolution in medicine, and today there are thousands of valuable drugs capable of curing or relieving important illnesses. Now almost all medical, as distinct from surgical, treatment involves the use of drugs, so any account of treatment must necessarily deal with them.

Medical drugs are now organized into classes, according to the effects they have or to the diseases they are designed to treat. There are many of these classes of drugs, but only the most widely used will be discussed here.

Treatment of infections

The most important measure in the treatment of infections is the use of antibiotic drugs. This is a very extensive range of drugs that have the ability to kill bacteria in the body without harming the patient. All the early antibiotics were obtained from cultures of living organisms, such as fungi or bacteria, but many are now chemically synthesized. Although antibiotics have greatly advanced the effectiveness of treatment of bacterial infections, they have not yet succeeded in eliminating any bacterial diseases.

The main disadvantage of antibiotics is the inevitable development of the ability of bacteria to resist the drug. This occurs because bacterial genetic variation allows natural selection of resistant bacteria to survive and reproduce, while susceptible bacteria are destroyed. Evolutionary changes in bacteria occur very rapidly because the interval between generations is only a matter of a few hours. The inappropriate use of antibiotics and inadequate dosage encourages the development of resistance. Biochemists thus have to produce ever new and more effective antibiotics.

This general class of drugs also includes antifungal drugs that kill or remove from the body other living organisms capable of causing disease. These drugs kill small single-celled parasites such as malarial parasites, and amoebae that cause amebic dysentery,

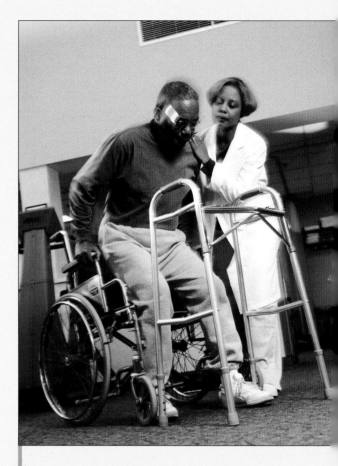

An occupational therapist helps a patient who is wheelchair-bound to attempt to stand. The aim of the treatment is to help people to be as independent as possible and to reach the best level of functioning for their particular disability.

and the large class of drugs (anthelmintics), which are used to kill or dislodge parasitic worms.

Treatment of viral infections

The development of effective antiviral drugs is a comparatively recent development, and many of the advances have come about as a result of strong pressure to develop a treatment for AIDS. Currently, the way to treat this condition is to use a combination of drugs, each of which can attack the human immunodeficiency virus (HIV) in a different way. HIV is called a retrovirus because its genome consists of a single strand of RNA from which normal double-stranded DNA is synthesized under the influence of an enzyme called reverse transcriptase. Prior to the discovery of retroviruses, it had been assumed that all

RNA derived only from the splitting of DNA. In this case, the reverse occurs. Drugs used to treat AIDS, or to prevent the development of AIDS in HIV-positive people, include those that inhibit the action of reverse transcriptase, those that bind directly to reverse transcriptase, those that block the action of another enzyme, HIV protease, so that it is incapable of forming new HIV, and those that prevent the fusion of viruses with helper T cells.

Other antiviral drugs used to treat other viral infections include acyclovir (Zovirax), which inhibits the enzyme DNA polymerase, and is used to treat herpes virus infections of the lips, mouth, skin, and genitals; amantadine and rimantadine, which inhibit replication of some of the viruses that cause influenza; and the reverse transcriptase blocking drug adefovir, which is too toxic for general use but which is effective, in safely low doses, in treating hepatitis B.

Treatment of pain

Pain provides warning that something is wrong in the body and should never be ignored unless the cause is known. There is always a mental component to pain, and this may be harder to bear than the pain itself. When a new pain occurs, it is essential to discover the cause. It is not a good idea simply to seek relief of pain without proper investigation of its significance. When the cause of a new pain is obvious, or has been discovered, it should be treated effectively. Reassurance, when appropriate, and explanations are important. Painkillers (analgesics) should not be withheld until pain is severe but should be given repeatedly in expectation of pain. Acute, self-limiting pain is easily dealt with by the prescription of analgesic drugs appropriate to the severity. Long-term pain is more difficult to manage successfully and should ideally be treated by a multidisciplinary team in a pain clinic. In addition to analgesics, pain may be relieved by electrical stimulation of the skin by acupuncture, skilled massage, cold sprays, injections of local anesthetic drugs, or, in extreme cases and very rarely, by permanent destruction of sensory nerves by cutting or by alcohol injection.

Treatment of heart disorders

Depending on the type of disorder, heart problems may be treated surgically or medically. On the medical side, many different drugs may be used. Various drugs are effective in regularizing the rate and regularity of the heartbeat. Those that correct beat irregularity are called anti-arrhythmic drugs. The large class of beta-blocker drugs are valuable for their selective blockade of the action of adrenaline, a hormone that speeds the heart and increases its tendency to contract prematurely. Beta-blockers are used to treat weakness of the heart (heart failure), angina pectoris, heart irregularities, and its associated anxiety. Drugs in the inotropic class can increase the power of the heartbeat. Among the most valuable drugs for treating heart failure are the ACE inhibitors. These block an enzyme called angiotensin-converting enzyme (ACE). This enzyme converts an inert substance in the blood into angiotensin II, which tightens arteries and raises the blood pressure. When this enzyme is blocked by ACE inhibitor drugs, the arteries relax, the blood pressure drops, and the load on the heart is much reduced. ACE inhibitors can reduce the symptoms of heart failure, improve the quality of life of patients with heart failure, and substantially prolong their lives.

Reducing blood cholesterol levels

Anticholesterol drugs work in various ways to achieve the same effect; they lower the level of cholesterol in the blood. Currently the most effective and widely used anticholesterol drugs are the statins. Cholesterol is synthesized in the liver, and statin drugs reduce the liver's production of cholesterol by interfering with the action of an essential enzyme. Many large trials have shown their benefits in preventing heart attacks and the effects of atherosclerosis, in which cholesterol is deposited in arterial walls.

Other drugs that lower cholesterol include fibrates that also interfere with cholesterol synthesis, bile acid sequestrants that bind and remove bile acids from the intestine, and others that interfere with the release of fats from body fat stores and increase the activity of fat-splitting enzymes.

Many critics are now challenging the prevailing belief that high blood cholesterol, which can be caused by eating saturated fats is, in itself, an important cause of diseases such as heart attacks. They point out that when different populations are compared, the association of high blood cholesterol values with high mortality from coronary heart disease is not consistently found. Further research is necessary in this important field.

Prevention of blood clotting

Drugs that can prevent blood from clotting within the bloodstream are called anticoagulants; they are used in conditions in which dangerous blood clots can form in veins and arteries. Such clots can be carried in the bloodstream to sites where they can block the circulation with dangerous or even fatal results. Anticoagulant treatment must be carried out cautiously because overdosage carries the danger of internal bleeding within and around the brain, which results in stroke. Elderly people with high blood pressure are most at danger of stroke, and those on anticoagulants must have regular checks of their blood clotting time. It is also important for people on anticoagulants to avoid head injury.

Treating high blood pressure

High blood pressure is a principal cause of heart damage and stroke. It can usually be helped by losing weight and getting more exercise, but if these measures are not effective, drugs must be used. These are called antihypertensive drugs, and they fall into several classes. Prescription of diuretic drugs, which increase the outflow of urine and reduce the blood volume, is usually the first stage in treating high blood pressure. The thiazide group of diuretic drugs have the additional effect of relaxing and widening arteries. In many cases these effects will suffice. If a more powerful action is required, the most commonly used drugs are the ACE inhibitors and the beta-blockers. A newer class of antihypertensive drugs is that of the calcium antagonists. These act by blocking microscopic channels on the membranes of the muscle cells in the walls of arteries. Calcium is necessary for muscle cell contraction so, by limiting inward movement of calcium ions, this drug causes muscle fibers to relax. Because these muscle cells are circularly arranged in arteries, their tightening narrows the arteries. The action of calcium channel blockers allows the arteries to relax and widen so that the resistance to blood flow is less and the blood pressure is reduced. Another class of antihypertensive drugs, the alpha-1 antagonists, work by blocking

receptors for adrenaline, a hormone that tightens the muscle fibers in the walls of blood vessels.

Medical treatment of cancer

Many cases of cancer are, of course, treated by surgery, and if all of the cancer can be removed in this way, no further treatment is needed. However, many cancers have already spread at the time of diagnosis, and it then becomes necessary to use radiation or drugs. If the cancer is widespread, radiation therapy may be inappropriate, and not all cancers are sensitive to radiation. All anticancer drugs are damaging to healthy body cells, especially those that are most actively reproducing. Enormous effort has been expended by pharmacologist researchers to increase what is called the therapeutic index. This is the ratio of the effectiveness of the drug in performing its desired function (in this case, killing cancer cells) to its toxic effect on normal body cells.

Cytotoxic drugs are those that act to stop the division (reproduction) of cancer cells. They act in various ways. Earlier drugs were simple poisons that had been found to be slightly more damaging to cancer cells than to healthy cells. More recent anticancer drugs are more sophisticated. Some of them work by interfering with an enzyme necessary for the topological manipulation of DNA. DNA must be unwound before it can replicate. This occurs in short segments and is achieved by an enzyme called topoisomerase, which cuts one strand so that the free end can be rotated around the unbroken strand. The topoisomerase inhibitors prevent this and interfere with the rapid replication of DNA in cancer cells.

An innovative new class of anticancer drugs acts by blocking the growth of new blood vessels on which cancers depend for their survival. Another new class of drugs prompt cancer cells to carry out the suicide process known as apoptosis, which is normal in old and worn-out body cells. Other new drugs interfere with the action of abnormal proteins within cancer cells that instruct them to grow. An important recent development is the use of monoclonal antibodies that block the receptors on certain cancer cells of a growth factor that promotes cancer growth and spread. The drug herceptin (trastuzumab), currently being used to treat women with a particular type of breast cancer, functions in this way.

Drug treatment for other conditions

Other important groups of drugs include anticonvulsants, used to prevent or reduce the severity of epileptic attacks; antidotes, to neutralize or counteract the actions or effects of poisons; antiemetics, to prevent vomiting; antiepileptic drugs, used to prevent, or reduce the liability to, epileptic seizures; anti-inflammatory drugs, such as the corticosteroids, which reduce inflammation; antimalarial drugs to prevent and treat malaria; antioxidants, which inhibit destructive oxidative changes in molecules; antiparkinsonism drugs to control the effects of Parkinson's disease; antiperspirants to inhibit perspiration or prevent excessive perspiration; antipruritic drugs to relieve itching; antipsychotic drugs used in the treatment or control of severe mental illness such as schizophrenia or bipolar emotional disorder; antispasmodic drugs, which relieve sustained muscle contraction; and antitussives, which prevent or relieve cough.

Surgical treatment

Surgery, too, has undergone major changes since the 1990s and has also become more fragmented into specialities. The general surgeon, ready to undertake almost any operation, is a thing of the past. Today there are accident and emergency surgeons; cardiovascular surgeons; ear, nose, and throat surgeons; gastrointestinal surgeons; gynecological surgeons; neurosurgeons; oncological surgeons; orthopedic surgeons; ophthalmic surgeons; plastic (including cosmetic) surgeons; thoracic surgeons; urological surgeons; and vascular surgeons. Even these classes have been further subdivided.

The other great advance in surgery is the development of minimally invasive surgery, sometimes called laparoscopic surgery or keyhole surgery. The principal reason for this development was the realization that most of the pain, discomfort and disablement that usually followed a surgical operation was not the result of what was done inside the body, but from the usually large wound, the surgical incision, that had to be made to gain access to the interior. It

During microsurgery, a closed-circuit camera is attached to a fiber-optic device at the end of an endoscope, which is inserted into the patient. Surgeons can control exactly what they are doing by looking at a high-definition monitor.

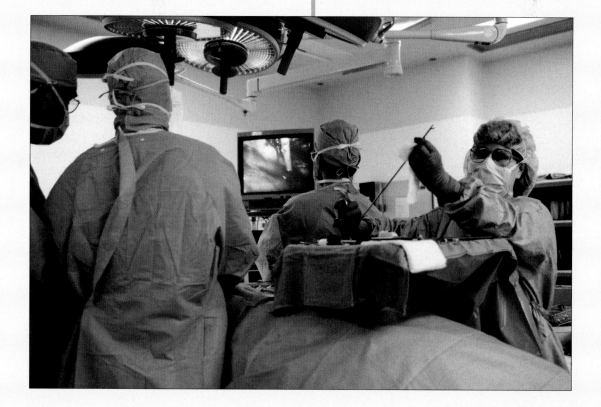

was also well known that many patients were unhappy about unsightly scars left after an operation.

Keyhole surgery began to be made possible with the development and increasing use of the examination technique known as endoscopy. The inside of the body can be examined by means of a narrow tube, either by direct vision or by fiber optics. Video technology and internal illumination allow for inspection of many body structures. The gynecologists were among the first to use this technique at an early stage in its development for operations on the fallopian tubes and the ovaries. This led to the development of specialized surgical instruments that could be passed through these narrow tubes—instruments with functioning tips for manipulating, clamping, cutting, cauterizing, stitching, and stapling that were controlled from the outside.

The next step was to improve the view of the inside of the body by linking closed-circuit television cameras to fiber-optic viewing and illuminating devices. Soon surgeons using the method were controlling their instruments by watching what they were doing on a high-definition television monitor. One of the first minimally invasive operations, outside gynecology, to become standard was removal of the gall bladder (cholecystectomy), and it is now routine for patients to have this type of keyhole surgery and be back at work, fully recovered, within a few days of having such an operation.

The last few years have seen a progressive extension of keyhole surgery to an ever-widening range of surgical procedures. Today, it is commonplace for surgeons to use minimally invasive methods to perform operations such as appendectomy, abdominal wall hernia, hiatal hernia, reflux disease treatment, esophageal, gastric, and colon cancer treatment, lymph node biopsy, splenectomy, diverticular disease treatment, rectal prolapse, internal inspection of joints, knee joint cartilage removal, carpal tunnel release, and rotator cuff damage repair. Another application is a wide range of gynecological procedures, including endometrial ablation for excessive menstruation, hysterectomy, benign ovarian cyst removal, repair of vesico-vaginal fistulas, and treatment of pelvic endometriosis.

Remote control surgery. Because the instruments used in keyhole surgery can be computer operated, it is not even necessary for the surgeon to be in the same room as the patient, or even in the same country.

Operations are being performed over the Internet with the surgeon thousands of miles distant from the patient. Robotic surgery is still in its infancy, but a beginning has been made, and the most advanced centers are currently actively exploring this important area of development.

Microsurgery. In the second half of the twentieth century, as surgery gained in refinement, it became apparent that better results could be achieved and the scope of surgery could be extended if finer manipulation of tissues was possible and if very small structures could be operated upon. The pioneers in this movement were otolaryngologists who had found that surgery on the tiny structures of the middle ear was virtually impossible without high magnification. They became the first surgeons to use microscopes in surgery. The ophthalmologists were quick to follow and, for them, the use of the operating microscope transformed ocular surgery.

About the same time, vascular surgeons discovered that by using a microscope in the operating room it was possible to join up tiny arteries and veins, making possible grafting procedures that would otherwise always have failed. Neurosurgeons were now able to join small but essential nerves that had been cut, and orthopedic surgeons could do a much better job of joining delicate severed tendons. The operating microscope has made possible the replacement of complete limbs that have been traumatically removed, and it has vastly extended the scope of donor grafting. One of the most recent examples of this is facial grafting. Now the operating microscope is an essential part of the tool kit of every surgeon whose work can be improved by its use.

The operation for cataract is a good example of how the use of the microscope has radically improved surgery. In the 1960s a cataract operation involved an incision half way around the outside of the cornea, the opening of the eye, and the insertion of a freezing probe that adhered to the lens so that the whole opaque lens could be pulled out. Many fine stitches were required to close the incision. The patient then needed heavy magnifying spectacle lenses to refocus the eye. Today, a tiny incision is made near the edge of the cornea, an opening is cut in the front of the lens

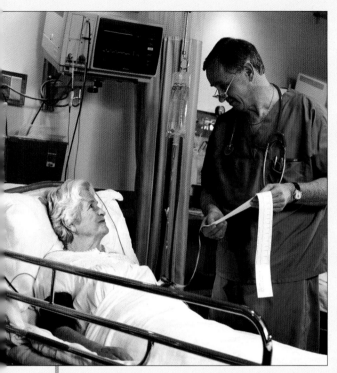

A doctor gives his patient the results of some tests taken in the hospital. From these, the doctor can prescribe a treatment plan to alleviate or control the symptoms.

capsule, and a fine ultrasonic probe is used to emulsify the opaque lens, which is washed out, leaving the capsule intact. A delicate, rolled-up plastic lens is then inserted though the incision into the capsule and allowed to unroll, and the operation is complete. No stitch is required for this procedure.

Microsurgery has greatly improved the results of corneal grafting and operations for glaucoma. It has allowed the restoration of hearing in certain types of deafness. It is widely used by gynecologists to open up blocked fallopian tubes and restore fertility in women, and by urologists to reverse vasectomies in men.

The scope of plastic surgery has been extended because microsurgery now allows successful free grafting of muscle and full-thickness skin by connecting blood vessels. Replantation of severed thumbs and large toes is now commonly performed using microsurgery to ensure an adequate blood flow. Various other parts, including the external ear, the nose, the scalp, and the penis, have been successfully replanted.

Psychiatric treatment

Psychoanalysis based on the ideas of Freud and his successors no longer has the dominant position it once enjoyed in psychiatric treatment. Various forms of psychotherapy for treating nonpsychotic mental disorders are in use at present. Currently one of the most effective treatments appears to be cognitive behavior therapy.

The purpose of cognitive behavior therapy is to adjust patients' attitudes and behavior so that both conform more closely to accepted mores. Treatment studies the beliefs and personalities of patients in relation to their emotional problems and how these determine the way they behave. The time taken for the treatment is very much shorter then earlier forms of psychotherapy and lasts for, at the most, a few months rather than years. It is conducted in weekly sessions of about an hour during which the patient and the therapist work together to develop a new strategy for dealing with the problems. Sound principles of thought, which can be applied whenever necessary, are explained so that they become lifelong habits. The method employed in cognitive behavior therapy demonstrates the importance of understanding the thinking patterns that patients have developed from childhood and how these influence behavior and can lead to problems.

Other forms of psychotherapy include family therapy, group therapy, expressive therapy (therapy through dance, drama, art, music), marriage guidance, and various kinds of counseling.

Treating schizophrenia. Today, schizophrenia is treated with antipsychotic drugs in order to control the most acute features and to prevent relapse. By means of these drugs, most people suffering from schizophrenia can be maintained within the community and do not need to be hospitalized.

Schizophrenia is not a curable condition, but effective drug treatment can prevent recurrence of psychotic episodes, and it can minimize damaging symptoms such as mood upsets and cognitive deficit. Psychiatrists are now recognizing that these benefits are essential for the quality of life of patients. A major problem in treating schizophrenia is to ensure continuity of treatment. Many patients resent the effect the drugs have on them, preferring to be left with their delusions and hallucinations. In addition, antipsychotic drugs tend to have distressing side effects, such as muscle spasms of the face, neck, and back (dystonias); restlessness, causing constant movements (akathisia); and dry mouth, nasal stuffiness, and difficulty in urination.

The earliest antipsychotic drugs, such as largactil, melleril, and stemetil, have been succeeded by the "atypical" antipsychotics such as clozapine, risperidone, and olanzapine, which may be effective in lower dosage and produce fewer distressing side effects. None of these drugs, however, is without risk, and all must be used with great care.

Treating depression. Severe depression is dangerous and should always be treated by an expert. The large number of antidepressant drugs fall into three main classes. The cyclic drugs have structures involving two (bicyclics), three (tricyclics), or four (tetracyclics) rings of atoms.

Most used are the tricyclic drugs, which act by blocking the reuptake of two neurotransmitters: serotonin and norepinephrine (noradrenaline) from synapses, thus prolonging their action. These neurotransmitters promote brain function and elevate mood.

The second class of drugs is the selective serotonin reuptake inhibitors (SSRI), which act at the clefts of synapses in the brain by blocking the reuptake of only one neurotransmitter, serotonin, and stop its removal from the synapse, thus increasing its action as a neurotransmitter. Selective serotonin reuptake inhibitors include fluoxetine, which has the brand names Oxactin or Prozac.

The third class is that of the monoamine oxidase inhibitors (MAOIs). These work by blocking the action of enzymes found in brain cells and elsewhere that break down noradrenaline, dopamine, and serotonin. By preventing the breakdown, the levels of these essential substances are raised. The MAOIs have the disadvantage that they can react dangerously with certain foods such as cheese, yeast extracts, protein extracts, wines, beers, banana skins, and fava bean pods. The list must be known and such foods avoided while the drugs are being taken.

A feature of many antidepressant drugs is that they must be taken for a period of up to three weeks before they act fully to relieve depression. It is important for patients to be aware of this, as disappointment in apparent lack of improvement may lead to suicide. In the case of the bipolar form of depression, the mainstay of the treatment is the drug lithium.

Complementary medical treatment
Complementary medicine is used in conjunction with conventional medicine and includes acupuncture, chiropractic, homeopathy, and osteopathy. Alternative medicine, which is often confused with complementary medicine, is used in place of conventional medicine. This class of treatments includes a wide range of interactions, none of which have been reliably proved to be effective according to the criteria required by the medical establishment. Proof of such efficacy requires trials uninfluenced by any form of bias. In drug trials the most widely used form is the double blind trial, in which the effect of the drug is compared with the effect of a placebo. During the trial, neither the patients nor the researchers know which drugs the patients are taking. Many alternative remedies, as a result of being tested in this way, have failed to demonstrate medically useful results. Alternative treatments include reflexology, radionics, iridology, faith healing, naturopathy, aromatherapy, Alexander technique, Feng Shui, sound therapy, Bates method, anthroposophical medicine, and orthomolecular therapy.

Complementary medicine flourishes for several reasons, including: general public ignorance of the rational basis of, and of the sciences underlying, conventional medical treatments; public dislike of medical authoritarianism; reports of dangerous side effects of some medical treatments; and the relative ease with which people are able to set up as complementary medical practitioners.

Another, and perhaps more important, reason why complementary medical practices flourish has to do with the fact that practitioners often have the time to take a genuinely holistic view of their patient's problems and are able to concern themselves more fully with many relevant aspects of their patient's lives, physically and psychologically, rather than simply with the presenting complaint.

Good medicine should, ideally, be holistic, but orthodox practitioners are often so driven by the pressure of work that they are unable to fulfill this aspiration.

Robert Youngson

Trichomoniasis

Trichomoniasis is one of the most common sexually transmitted diseases worldwide. Over 8 million new cases are reported yearly in North America. It is the third leading cause of vaginitis (inflammation of the vagina) in American women.

Trichomoniasis is caused by a microscopic parasite, *Trichomonas vaginalis*. The disease is transmitted by sexual contact, so risk is increased among people with multiple sexual partners. The use of condoms may reduce the risk of transmission. The infection can be a risk factor for infertility in women, cervical dysplasia, premature labor, and enhanced HIV transmission.

Symptoms, signs, and diagnosis

Women may be asymptomatic carriers of the disease but will more often have a malodorous, thin green-yellow discharge from the vagina. Associated symptoms may include vaginal itching, burning, painful sexual intercourse, or urgency and pain on urination. Men are usually asymptomatic, or they may have urgency and burning on urination, or the presence of a thin, malodorous discharge from the penis. Trichomoniasis is most often diagnosed by visualization of the parasite under a microscope from a vaginal (women) or urethral (men) swab sample. An increase of inflammatory cells in the specimen and an elevated vaginal pH may also accompany infection. Microscopic examination alone may result in some false negative diagnoses (up to 30 to 50 percent). Culture of the vaginal or urethral specimen is more accurate but takes longer (3 to 7 days) for diagnosis. Because trichomoniasis is a sexually transmitted disease, people who are diagnosed should ideally be tested for other sexually transmitted diseases.

Treatments and prevention

The treatment of choice is metronidazole, an oral antibiotic that can be given at a low dose for seven days or as a single high dose. Tinidazole is a suitable alternative or is often used in cases resistant to metronidazole. All sexual partners should be treated, otherwise reinfection is highly likely. The need to treat asymptomatic pregnant women is not established and remains controversial. For patients with persistent symptoms, a trial of repeated treatment is warranted, along with testing for other sexually transmitted diseases. Special testing for suspected antibiotic-resistant trichomonas is available through the U.S. Centers for Disease Control and Prevention.

Abstinence from sexual intercourse, the proper use of condoms, and limiting the number of sexual partners will all lower the risk of disease transmission. People with the infection should abstain from sexual intercourse until they have completed antibiotic therapy for themselves and their sexual partners.

Kristin Mondy

KEY FACTS

Description

Trichomoniasis is a sexually transmitted infection of the vaginal and urethral tissues.

Causes

Trichomonas vaginalis, a flagellated parasite.

Risk factors

Multiple sexual partners or coinfection with other sexually transmitted diseases.

Symptoms

Can vary from none (particularly in men) to the presence of a green-yellow malodorous discharge with vaginal or urethral itching, redness, burning, painful sexual intercourse, or painful urination.

Diagnosis

Microscopic examination of the parasite taken from a vaginal or urethral swab. Specialized culture of the parasite is also available.

Treatments

Antibiotics (metronidazole or tinidazole), which are given to the affected person and his or her sexual partner(s).

Pathogenesis

Trichomonas vaginalis causes local invasion of surrounding urethral and vaginal tissues, leading to inflammation of these tissues.

Prevention

Abstinence from sexual intercourse. Use of condoms.

Epidemiology

Highly prevalent worldwide. Symptomatic disease primarily affects sexually active women. More than 8 million cases yearly in North America.

See also

- Female reproductive system disorders
- Infertility • Sexually transmitted diseases

Tuberculosis

Tuberculosis (TB) is a life threatening infection that worldwide kills nearly 2 million people per year. The World Health Organization has predicted that this number will increase. Presently, one new TB infection occurs every second. The bacterium *Mycobacterium tuberculosis* causes most cases of tuberculosis infections. It usually affects the lungs but can result in a localized lesion or lesions throughout the body.

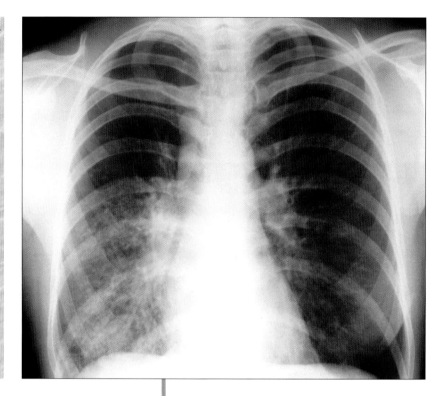

This colored chest X-ray of a woman with pulmonary tuberculosis shows black areas, which are the lungs; the areas affected by tuberculosis are red.

Tuberculosis has been known to cause disease from ancient times to the present. Egyptian mummies have been found with tubercles, which are tuberculous lesions. The most common form of TB is tuberculosis of the lungs. The bacteria are spread in the air and enter the body through the respiratory tract. General symptoms include fever and weight loss. The symptoms of tuberculosis depend upon the area of infiltration of the microorganisms. For example, Pott's disease is a presentation of TB that affects the spine. Tuberculosis is the most common major communicable disease today, infecting 2 billion people, equating to one-third of the world's population. Some famous people who had or are believed to have had TB include Jane Austen, Robert Burns, Edgar Allan Poe, Fredric Chopin, and Stephen Foster.

Causes and risk factors

Tuberculosis is a bacterial infection which may or may not cause disease. *Mycobacterium tuberculosis* is the bacterium responsible for most cases of tuberculosis as a respiratory disease. This disease, also known as consumption, has occurred in all eras and worldwide climates. In 1882 Robert Koch discovered a stain that he used to microscopically identify *Mycobacterium tuberculosis*. His accomplishment provided a new approach to fighting this deadly disease. *Mycobacterium bovis*, *Mycobacterium bovis BCG*, and *Mycobacterium africanum* are other species that cause tuberculosis. *Mycobacterium tuberculosis* and *Mycobacterium bovis* cause infections worldwide. The organism *Mycobacterium africanum* causes human infections mainly in East and West Africa. *Mycobacterium bovis* can cause respiratory or intestinal tuberculosis and is contracted by drinking contaminated milk or through airborne transmission. Humans and a wide host range of animals, including cattle, goats, cats, dogs, and pigs, can be infected with *Mycobacterium bovis*. This species of mycobacterium is mainly seen in countries that have tuberculous dairy cows and unpasteurized milk.

After human immunodeficiency virus (HIV), tuberculosis is the leading infectious cause of death in the world. Individuals with HIV are highly susceptible to rapidly active tuberculosis because their bodies are being immunosuppressed by the virus. Studies have shown there is a connection between the rise in HIV infections and the increasing rate of TB infections. Mycobacterial organisms can live for a considerable period of time in dust or air. Tuberculosis is most commonly acquired by person-to-person transmission of airborne droplets of mycobacterial organisms from a person with active disease to a susceptible person, the host. When a person with infectious (active) tuberculosis coughs or sneezes without covering the mouth, the tubercle droplets are expelled into the air. Other people may inhale the air containing these airborne droplets of mycobacteria and become infected.

Some populations are at higher risk for the active (infectious) TB disease because they are more likely to be exposed or infected. Tuberculosis thrives wherever there is poverty, crowded living conditions, and chronic illness (for example, HIV, diabetes mellitus, and alcoholism). In jails and homeless shelters, the crowded conditions and inadequate testing and treatment also lead to extremely high TB infection rates. Also, people born in regions of the world where tuberculosis is highly prevalent, elderly people, people who inject illegal drugs, and health care workers are all at a much higher risk of becoming infected with TB.

In 1993 the World Health Organization (WHO) declared TB a global health emergency since one-third of the world's population is infected. Regions and countries afflicted by wars, poverty, and natural disasters are seriously affected. The highest incidences are seen in countries with the lowest gross national products, in Africa, Asia, and Latin America. As the HIV and AIDS epidemic spreads in Africa, TB rates are increasing, not only in those afflicted with AIDS, but also in the general population.

Symptoms and signs

The tuberculosis infection begins when the bacterial organisms enter the lungs and multiply in the small air sacs of the lungs. Some of these tubercle microorganisms enter the bloodstream and spread throughout the body, but the body's immune system usually keeps the bacterial organisms under control. The primary infection is contained and, in many cases, the infection is permanently stopped. Thus, the infection does not cause any symptoms. This controlled disease is referred to as latent TB infection (LTBI). If the body's immune defenses decrease, the tuberculosis disease may break out again and become active. It is highly probable for a person infected with HIV to have LTBI progress to active TB disease. Most people who have

latent TB infection never develop the active TB disease, and they cannot spread the infection to others. Latent TB infection is detected through a positive reaction to the tuberculin skin test or the QuantiFERON TB Gold blood test, used to diagnose both latent and active TB infections.

Patients with a tuberculosis infection may or may not have symptoms. Common presenting symptoms include fever, cough, loss of appetite, night sweats, weight loss, weakness, or chills, or all the symptoms. Also, the person may cough a small amount of yellow, green, or bloody sputum (saliva, pus, blood, and other matter discharged from diseased lungs). These symptoms are seen in those people with mainly tuberculosis of the lungs. Other regions of the body that can become infected with the mycobacterial organisms include the bones, lymph nodes, joints, abdominal cavity, pericardium (membrane around the heart), kidneys, reproductive organs, and central nervous system.

KEY FACTS

Description

A life-threatening infection that usually affects the lungs. Commonly called TB.

Cause

Bacteria in the genus *Mycobacterium*, particulary *M. tuberculosis*.

Risk factors

Contact with infected people or animals or contaminated food; chronic illness such as HIV infection; poor and unsanitary living conditions.

Symptoms

In latent TB, no symptoms; in active TB of the lungs, there may be fever, cough, loss of appetite, night sweats, weight loss, and chills; coughing up yellow, green, or bloody sputum.

Diagnosis

Tuberculin skin test; QuantiFERON TB Gold blood test; chest X-ray; sputum smear and culture.

Treatments

Antibiotics such as isoniazid, rifampicin, pyrazinamide, and pyridoxine.

Pathogenesis

Mycobacterium causes lesions called tubercles in the lungs. Without treatment the infection can spread to other body organs.

Prevention

Vaccination; isolation of infected people.

Epidemiology

Affects one-third of the world's population. Most common in Africa, Asia, and Central America.

Many people with untreated TB develop shortness of breath as the infection spreads in the lungs. The kidneys and lymph nodes are the most common sites of the body affected by TB outside the lungs (extrapulmonary tuberculosis). Tuberculosis that infects the central nervous system tissues covering the brain is called tubercular meningitis.

Diagnosis

When a person has symptoms that suggest tuberculosis, a tuberculin skin test (PPD-purified protein derivative test) or QuantiFERON TB blood test, a chest X-ray, a sputum smear, and a culture are normally ordered by the physician. A person who has contracted the type of tuberculosis that affects the lungs will have tubercules (lesions) that will appear on a chest X-ray. The tuberculin skin test is performed by injecting a small amount of protein derived from TB bacteria between the layers of skin on the forearm of the patient. Two days later, the injection site is checked and measured. A positive test result is indicated by swelling that feels firm to the touch and is larger than the specified normal size. The tuberculin skin test may show false-positive results due to a recent vaccination against tuberculosis. The QuantiFERON TB blood test requires that a sample of blood be taken from the patient and tested in a clinical laboratory with special chemical reagents that identify if a person has a TB infection.

The patient's sputum is examined in the clinical laboratory by smearing some of the sputum on a glass slide, staining the smear, and looking at this stained smear using a microscope. When the stained smear is viewed microscopically, the tuberculosis bacteria will appear as red rods. Also, some of the sputum is placed on culture media and in an incubator to see which microorganisms grow. Cultures do not provide results for several days because mycobacteria organisms grow slowly. A positive culture for *Mycobacterium tuberculosis* confirms that the patient has TB disease. After the culture has identified the TB bacteria, a drug susceptibility test is performed, which will help the physician choose the correct medication for use in the patient's treatment.

It is extremely important that TB disease be diagnosed as early as possible since pulmonary tuberculosis can cause permanent lung damage if not treated early.

Prevention and treatments

The infectiousness of a patient with TB disease is directly related to the number of tubercle bacteria that he or she expels into the air from the lungs. Patients who expel many mycobacteria are more infectious than patients who expel few bacteria. Patients who have signs and symptoms of tuberculosis must be placed in an area separated from other people, promptly evaluated, then given treatment to avoid spreading the disease. Infectiousness decreases very rapidly after treatment is started. Patients who have been receiving appropriate medication for TB for two to three weeks, whose symptoms have improved, and who have three consecutive negative sputum smears collected on different days can usually be considered noninfectious.

Latent tuberculosis infection in a patient must be treated with antibiotics so that the patient does not contract active TB disease. The usual medication for latent tuberculosis infection, isoniazid, abbreviated as INH, is given daily for nine months to the patient. The patient must be checked by a physician monthly since this TB medication and others may cause side effects such as skin rashes, upset stomach, or liver damage. Taking the medication rifampin for four months is an alternative treatment for latent tuberculosis infection. The patient must not miss taking the daily medication and must take all of it to avoid the possibility of TB disease.

TB disease in the lungs must be treated much more rigorously than latent TB infection. The disease is usually treated with daily doses of rifampin, isoniazid, pyrazinamide, and pyridoxine over a six-month period. All of the medications are given since resistance to one or more of these drugs occurs in many patients. Because it is so important to take all of these medications on a daily basis, the patient may be required to see a nurse who will administer the medications every day.

Treatment of tuberculosis in other parts of the body, such as the bones or central nervous system, must occur over nine months to one year for full effective recovery from the disease.

Prevention of TB infection and disease has occurred through vaccination with BCG (bacilli Calmette–Guerin). It is given to school children in some countries to decrease the risk of developing tuberculosis.

Kathleen Becan-McBride

See also
- AIDS • Antibiotic-resistant infections
- Diagnosis • Infections • Infections, bacterial • Prevention • Respiratory system disorders • Treatment

Turner's syndrome

Turner's syndrome is a genetic condition named after one of the physicians who first described patients with this condition. Turner's syndrome affects only females. About 99 percent of affected pregnancies do not survive to birth. The life expectancy of those who do survive to birth is generally lower than that of the general population, primarily as a result of the frequency of heart disease in this syndrome.

The hallmark features associated with Turner syndrome include short stature (an average adult height of 4 feet 8 inches, or 1.4 m), loose skin around the neck in infancy, a low hairline at the back of the neck, and infertility. Affected individuals are at an increased risk for birth defects, including heart defects and kidney abnormalities. Although mental retardation is not associated with classic Turner's syndrome, deficiencies in certain areas of learning are common, including visual-spatial perception and mathematical skills. For example, an affected individual may find it difficult to follow a map because they are unable to mentally visualize their location based on the map's information. Other subtle variations in physical development include underdeveloped nails, a broad chest with widely spaced nipples, and an inability to fully extend the arms at the elbow. Prenatal symptoms identified by ultrasound include the presence of a fluid-filled cyst at the back of the neck, called a cystic hygroma, and edema (an excess of fluid) found throughout the body.

Causes

Turner's syndrome is caused either because one X chromosome is missing, one of the chromosomes is normal and one is faulty, or a mixture of problems in which some cells have a missing chromosome and others have an extra chromosome.

Diagnosis and treatments

When a diagnosis of Turner's syndrome is suspected given the presence of associated clinical features, chromosome analysis by karyotype is typically used to confirm the diagnosis. A karyotype is a laboratory test used to evaluate the overall number and structure of the chromosomes; it can be carried out both before and after birth. A female without Turner's syndrome has two normal X chromosomes. Karyotyping identifies the presence of cells with only one normal X chromosome in all females with classic Turner's syndrome. Treatments such as growth hormone are given at an early age to manage clinical symptoms. This can help affected girls reach near-normal stature.

Cheryl B. Thomas and Brian C. Brost

KEY FACTS

Description

A genetic syndrome due to a sex chromosomal abnormality that affects females.

Causes

A sporadic error in the division of the chromosomes during development of the egg or sperm, resulting in an abnormal number of sex chromosomes in a fetus.

Risk factors

No known risk factors contribute to an increased risk for Turner's syndrome.

Symptoms

Short stature, gonadal dysgenesis (defective development of the ovaries) birth defects, extra skin and a low hairline at the back of the neck, infertility, specific learning problems, and a characteristic physical appearance.

Diagnosis

Physical examination and laboratory analysis by karyotyping.

Treatments

Treatments are aimed at managing clinical symptoms; for example, growth hormone treatment is given for short stature.

Pathogenesis

There are numerous genes on the X chromosome; it is the absence of one set of these genes that causes the associated symptoms. These symptoms can vary greatly, from death before birth to short stature and infertility in adults.

Prevention

There is no prevention.

Epidemiology

Turner's syndrome occurs in about 1 in 2,000 to 1 in 5,000 live births.

See also
- Birth defects • Genetic disorders
- Heart disorders • Kidney disorders

Typhoid and paratyphoid

Typhoid is a life-threatening, feverish disease caused by the bacterium *Salmonella typhi*, which seriously affects the digestive system. Paratyphoid is a less severe disease caused by *Salmonella paratyphi*. Most cases of both diseases are reported in developing countries where hygiene is poor.

Salmonella typhi is a bacterium that is exclusive to humans. While other animals, such as birds, cows, and turtles, may pass other types of *Salmonella*, this hardy bacterium has a protective coat that helps it hide from the human immune system. The bacterium is transmitted with water and foods and can withstand drying and freezing. Also, certain humans may carry the disease without being ill themselves. *Salmonella paratyphi* causes paratyphoid fever, a condition that is similar in the way it is spread but that has milder symptoms than typhoid.

Signs and symptoms

Typhoid fever makes its victims feel very ill. Classic typhoid goes through two phases. In the first phase, the bacterium gets into the intestine from water or food that has been contaminated by the feces or urine of people who have the disease or are carriers of the disease. The bacterium penetrates the intestinal lining, or mucosa, to the underlying tissue. If the immune system does not stop the infection there, the bacteria multiply and spread to the bloodstream, causing the first observable symptoms of fever and sweating. The patient will have loss of appetite and may have a fever pattern of as high as 105°F (40.6°C), which may gradually rise and fall and last for weeks at a time. Then the bacteria penetrate the bone marrow, liver, and bile ducts, and are excreted into the bowel contents. Rose spots on the trunk appear in about 25 percent of Caucasians.

The second phase of the disease occurs when the bacteria penetrate the immune tissue of the small intestine, causing violent and prolonged diarrhea, interspersed with constipation. Usually this happens in the second or third week. Severe abdominal pain and blinding headache with a continued cough and slow heart rate begin within one to two weeks after exposure, but this period can be from three days to three months. In the third week, severe diarrhea resembling pea soup may also contain blood. In severe cases, the person may lie motionless, appearing as dead, with eyes half open, a state referred to as "typhoid state."

Around the fifth week, the fever may drop and the condition may slowly improve.

Left untreated, complications such as potentially fatal intestinal bleeding can occur. Other complications include pneumonia, psychosis, meningitis, bladder and kidney infection, a condition known as typhoid spine, and coma.

Diagnosis

It took several years for people to connect unsanitary conditions with disease, especially with typhoid. During the early decades of the nineteenth century, physicians proposed the "filth" theory of disease. As the industrial revolution brought people into crowded cities, diseases like typhoid and typhus, a disease carried by lice, became endemic. Some speculated that conditions spontaneously generated from the bad air and open sewage.

In 1839 Englishman William Budd argued that typhoid did not arise from filth but that it was a contagious disease. After investigating several epidemics, he found that some students became ill from using a common well and concluded that the well water was poisoned. By the 1870s it was accepted that the poison of typhoid was from sewage-contaminated water. With the advance of microbiology, the organism was finally grown in culture, and by 1896 physicians had tools for diagnosing the bacteria.

Because early symptoms resemble other conditions, such as malaria, the doctor's clinical picture must include information on travel and which countries have been visited. The final diagnosis should include analysis of stool, blood, and tissue samples. Stool samples are teeming with *S. typhi*. Food and water contaminated by feces and urine transmit typhoid fever. In some countries, shellfish taken from sewage-contaminated beds, particularly oyster beds, may transmit the organism. Fruit and vegetables that are fertilized by "night soil" (human feces) can be sources of typhoid infection. Other sources include contaminated milk and milk products. Flies may infect foods in which the organism can multiply to an infective dose.

Epidemiology

Typhoid fever is common in certain parts of Asia, Africa, and Latin America. With the development of sanitary facilities, the disease has been eliminated in many areas, with most cases occurring in endemic areas. Six countries—India, Pakistan, Mexico, Bangladesh, the Philippines, and Haiti—accounted for 76 percent of the cases. Strains resistant to chloramphenicol and other antibiotics have been recently reported.

Treatments

Treatment requires admission to a hospital, where antibiotics and in some cases steroid medicines are administered. In addition, treatment for dehydration (loss of fluids and electrolytes) demands a high-calorie, nonbulky diet and possibly intravenous feeding. In the hospital, infected people are isolated, and the staff must be vigilant to avoid unprotected contact with contaminated clothing or bedding.

If the appropriate antibiotics are administered, the prospects of cure are very good, and the person may be discharged when the condition is stable. Choice of antibiotic depends upon the strain of *S. typhi*.

At present 107 types of typhoid can be distinguished by a technique called phage typing; three types of *S. paratyphi* are recognized. However, care must be taken because the bacteria may be excreted for several more weeks.

Paratyphoid fever is caused by a different bacterium called *Salmonella paratyphi*. The incubation is shorter, and although there may be carriers, they are not as likely to transmit the disease in the way that typhoid carriers do.

Paratyphoid has a similar clinical picture to typhoid but is much milder, and the fatality rate is much lower. No generalized symptoms occur; rather, the patient suffers an acute bout of gastroenteritis. The ratio of disease caused by *S. typhi* to *S. paratyphi* is about 10 to 1. Some experts believe paratyphoid occurs more frequently than reports suggest and may be infrequently identified in Canada and the United States.

If a traveler is in a developing country and becomes very ill, there is reason to suspect typhoid fever. The U.S. consulate is the source for a list of recommended doctors. Immediately, the physician will start the patient on the most common antibiotics to treat the disease: ampicillin, ciprofloxacin, and trimethoprim-sulfamethoxazole. As soon as the antibiotics are in the system, the person begins to feel better in a few days, and deaths rarely occur.

Although the symptoms go away, a person may be carrying *S. typhi*, so the illness could return or be passed on to other people. If the person works in food service, he or she may be legally barred from going back to work until it is proven that he or she no longer harbors the bacteria.

A person being treated for typhoid should take the prescribed antibiotics until the whole course is finished. Good hygiene practices should be observed, such as washing hands carefully with soap and water after each bathroom use. Someone with typhoid should not prepare or serve food to other people, and the doctor should arrange for a series of stool cultures to be performed until it can be demonstrated that no *S. typhi* remain in the body.

KEY FACTS

Description

Bacterial diseases that affect the digestive system; typhoid is the most serious, paratyphoid has milder symptoms.

Causes

The bacteria *Salmonella typhi* causes typhoid; *Salmonella paratyphi* causes paratyphoid.

Risk factors

Unsanitary food and drinking water.

Symptoms

Typhoid: fever, headache, weakness, sore throat, cough, diarrhea. Paratyphoid: acute gastroenteritis, but without the general malaise.

Diagnosis

A physician takes a blood or stool sample to identify the bacteria.

Treatments

Antibiotics.

Pathogenesis

Without treatment for typhoid, mortality is high; as many as 20 percent die from complications of the infection. Only rarely is paratyphoid fatal.

Prevention

Vaccination, care in eating food and drinking water. Rigorous hygiene such as washing hands after bathroom use, peeling fruit and vegetables, and drinking bottled water.

Epidemiology

Worldwide the annual incidence of typhoid is estimated at about 17 million cases with about 600,000 deaths. Only about 400 cases occur in the United States each year, and these are related to travel to developing countries. The global annual incidence of paratyphoid fever is estimated to be 5.4 million people.

TYPHOID MARY

Mary Mellon, an Irish immigrant, was the first person to be identified as a carrier of typhoid in the United States. She was the picture of health when the New York health inspector knocked on her door in 1907. She was informed that although healthy and immune to the disease, she spread disease while working as a cook in the New York City area. Charles Henry Warren, a wealthy banker, hired Mary to be the cook at their summer home in 1906. Soon, 6 out of 11 people in the household came down with typhoid. George Soper, a sanitary engineer, found that Mary had worked at several jobs where 22 people had become ill. When he asked Mary for stool samples to test for typhoid, she refused and ran away. Soper found her and obtained a court order incarcerating her for examination, but she was freed after three years on the condition that she would never take a job as a cook. Mary disappeared, but five years later, Soper found her working as a cook in a hospital under another name. In 1914 she was confined in a former isolation hospital, Riverside Hospital, on North Brother Island (an island in the East River), where she was institutionalized for more than two decades until she died in 1938. Mary, who became known as "Typhoid Mary," had unwittingly caused three typhoid deaths and 47 cases of typhoid. She died showing complete unwillingness to admit there was a problem or to comply with restrictions.

Typhoid is a very serious disease when untreated. Even when treated, a small number of people may not survive. Elderly people or those with disabilities may be vulnerable; however, in children the disease is usually milder. Typhoid can adversely affect many organs of the body, and when complications develop, the outlook is poor.

This light micrograph shows gram negative, rod-shaped bacteria called Salmonella typhi. *They are magnified 500 times.* Salmonella typhi *are the causative agent of typhoid fever in humans, and they are transmitted through contaminated food or drinking water.*

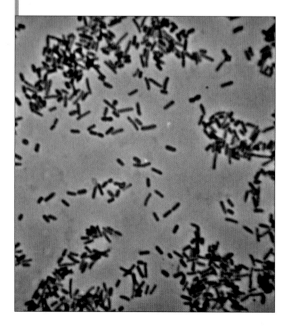

Prevention

Travelers to areas where the disease is common are recommended to visit a doctor or a travel clinic to get vaccinated. TY21a is an oral vaccine; four doses are necessary and last about six years. A booster is needed every five years. VICPS is an injectable vaccine in which one dose is given; a booster is needed every two years. Vaccines are not completely effective, so it is wise to continue to take food and drink precautions. There is no effective immunization for paratyphoid.

Other preventive measures include carefully selecting food and drink while visiting a developing country. This measure will also protect from cholera, dysentery, and hepatitis A. Drinking water should be bottled or boiled. Bottled carbonated water is safer than noncarbonated drinks. Drinks should be taken without ice; when brushing teeth, bottled water should be used rather than tap water. Foods should have been thoroughly cooked, and hands washed with soap and water after bathroom use. When eating raw fruits or vegetables that can be peeled, a good procedure is "boil it, cook it, peel it, or forget it." It is best to avoid foods and beverages from street vendors, which are a common source of illness for travelers.

Pathogenesis

With prompt treatment, typhoid usually clears up, but if not treated, the consequences can be fatal.

Evelyn B. Kelly

See also
• Infections • Infections, bacterial
• Meningitis • Pneumonia • Prevention

Typhus

Typhus is a group of infectious diseases transmitted to humans by lice or fleas. It is characterized by high fever, a transient rash, and intractable headache.

Typhus is prevalent worldwide and is transmitted to humans in the feces of body lice, which contaminate wounds on human skin. There are three kinds of typhus: murine, epidemic, and scrub typhus. They are caused by different rickettsial bacteria.

Murine typhus occurs in the southeastern region of the United States, mainly southern Texas and southern California. It is primarily transmitted by the rat flea *Xeonpsylla cheopis*. Murine typhus is mild and is seldom fatal; less than 100 cases are reported annually. This disease is often seen in the summer and fall and lasts for two to three weeks.

Epidemic typhus may have caused more deaths in the twentieth century than any other infectious disease. Epidemic typhus occurs in conditions of war, poverty, famine, crowding, and poor hygiene (called "jail fever") when the temperature is cold. The disease spreads by lice, although it is rare in the United States. Outbreaks of the disease occur in Ethiopia, Uganda, Rwanda, and Peru. Brill-Zinsser disease is a reoccurrance of epidemic typhus, years after the initial attack. This is more common in the elderly when the host defense mechanism falters. Acute sporadic infections occur during the winter months in the eastern and southern United States. It appears to be associated with contact with the parasites of flying squirrels.

Symptoms

Murine (endemic) typhus is an uncommon flea-borne infectious disease caused by *Rickettsia typhi*. After an incubation period of 7 to 14 days, headaches, fever, backache, and arthralgia (joint pain) occurs. Temperatures of 105°F–106°F (40.5°C–41°C) may last two weeks with slight remission in the morning. A rash begins on the trunk and spreads to the periphery, sparing the face, palms, and soles. Nausea, vomiting, dry cough, and abdominal pain are common symptoms.

In contrast, epidemic typhus is characterized by shaking chills, headaches, and fever lasting 12 days, then returning to normal. Rash and other symptoms are similar to murine typhus but are not as severe.

Hypotension and stupor or delirium, or both, occurs in the more seriously ill patients. Without treatment, death occurs in 10 to 60 percent of patients with epidemic typhus. Less than 2 percent of untreated patients with murine typhus may die; however, appropriate antibiotics will cure virtually all patients.

Diagnosis and treatments

Blood tests may show anemia and low platelets; liver function enzymes are mildly elevated. Antibody test to typhus should be elevated. Definitive diagnosis is best made by analysis of typhus group antigens. Because these tests take time, many physicians begin treatment based solely on a patient's symptoms.

Symptoms and signs are alleviated if an effective antibiotic, such as tetracycline, is given when the rash first begins. Intravenous fluids and oxygen may be required to stabilize patients with epidemic typhus.

Immunization and lice control are highly effective. Dusting infected persons with DDT, malathion, or lindane may eliminate lice. However, no effective vaccine exists. Keeping out rats and rat fleas from food depots and granaries is a preventive measure.

KEY FACTS

Description
Infectious diseases transmitted by fleas or lice.

Causes
Typhus is a rickettsial disease caused by *R. prowazekii* and *R. typhi*.

Risk factors
War, poverty, overcrowding, poor hygiene, cold temperature, rat fleas, rat feces, or fleas.

Symptoms
Headache, myalgias, arthralgia, backache, high fevers, a rash, nausea, vomiting, dry cough, gut pain. Other symptoms include low blood pressure, delirium or stupor, and photophobia.

Diagnosis
By analysis of acute and convalescent phase sera for typhus antibodies.

Treatments
Antibiotics.

See also
• Infections, bacterial • Lassa fever • Lice infestation • Lyme disease • Malaria

Urinary tract disorders

The urinary tract is a vital system in the body. It is made up of two kidneys, the bladder, and the urethra. The kidneys act like filters for the blood, removing waste and toxins and creating urine in the renal pelvis. Urine passes down the ureters to be stored in the bladder until there is a signal to void, when urine leaves the body through the urethra. Disorders of the urinary system can be classified as developmental or congenital, functional, infectious, or cancerous.

The kidney is a complex organ with many structures that are specifically designed to filter blood. A congenital abnormality can occur when parts of the kidneys do not develop properly. If an infant is born without working kidneys, he or she will die shortly after birth. If only one kidney is abnormal, the other kidney can do the filtering work necessary for life. Multicystic disease occurs when the kidney tissue of one or both kidneys does not develop correctly and is replaced by fluid-filled structures that do not function.

All the structures of the urinary tract begin their development in the pelvis. As the fetus grows and the body becomes longer, the kidneys migrate toward the head into their final position at the lower edge of the ribs, near the spine. As they grow, one or both kidneys may not rise and will remain in the pelvis. Both kidneys can also end up together on one side of the body or can even fuse into one larger kidney. An example of this is a horseshoe kidney, which looks like a horseshoe in the abdomen. Some people have an extra kidney, double ureter, or double bladder; for

example, a double ureter would have two tubes connecting one kidney with the bladder. These duplicate systems often have abnormal positions in the body. Some ureters do not develop properly, and a person can have urinary reflux. Normally, the ureter has a one-way valve, so urine cannot go backward from the bladder up to the kidney. If it is abnormal, urine can go backward and cause complications, such as infections or poor kidney function. Urine exits the bladder when a muscle called the urethral sphincter relaxes to let urine pass through the urethra. In about 1 in 5,000 male births, a boy will be born with urethral valves. In this condition, a piece of tissue blocks the urethra channel. If this happens, it causes obstruction, and urine is unable to exit the bladder; this can be corrected by a simple procedure.

Functional

Even if all of the parts of the urinary system are present and in their correct locations, they may not function properly for various reasons. If the kidneys' filtering capacity does not work, this condition is termed renal failure. This can develop acutely or over a long period of time. Acute renal failure may be reversible; it can be caused by infections, toxic reactions, trauma, or urinary tract obstruction. Chronic renal failure occurs over a long period of time and is often related to high blood pressure and diabetes. If renal failure causes the kidneys to shut down, a person may require a substitute filter system called dialysis, a procedure in which a person's blood is pumped through a machine, filtered, then returned to the body.

RELATED ARTICLES

Obstruction occurs when one or both kidneys become blocked; this can be due to a kidney stone, tumor, or anatomical abnormality. The blockage can be in the kidney, the ureter, or the urethra. When the drainage of the kidney is blocked, urine backs up and causes very high pressure in the kidney, which causes damage that may or may not be reversible. Often surgery is required to reverse the obstruction. A functional problem can also prevent urine from exiting the bladder properly. Injury to the nerves to and from the bladder can result in loss of ability to expel urine. This condition, called a neurogenic bladder, can occur because of disease or trauma, such as a spinal cord injury. The reverse problem occurs if the bladder cannot store urine. Incontinence is uncontrolled loss of urine from the bladder and can be caused by weak muscles around the bladder or overactivity in the bladder. When a person coughs or sneezes, he or she may lose urine because of the sudden pressure change in the abdomen. This is seen in around 3 million people in the United Kingdom and 13 million in the United States.

Infections

The urinary tract is usually a sterile environment; when bacteria or other microorganisms get into the system, they can multiply and cause infections. The simplest infection is cystitis, which is inflammation of the bladder, often caused by bacterial infections. If the infection travels to the kidneys, pyelonephritis occurs. Kidney stones harbor bacteria, which can cause recurrent infections. A urinary system with obstruction is prone to infections because the urine remains static and bacteria can grow more easily. Sexually transmitted diseases can also cause infection in the urethra or bladder. Treatment for urinary tract infections is with antibiotics. If an infection is severe, a patient may have to be hospitalized and given intravenous antibiotics.

Cancer

There are many types of cells in the urinary tract, and any of those cells can change into cancer cells. When cancer cells grow, they create tumors that can cause symptoms locally, and the cells can spread to other sites in the body. Cancer that starts in the kidney is known as renal cell carcinoma. A kidney tumor can grow even larger than the original kidney or cause

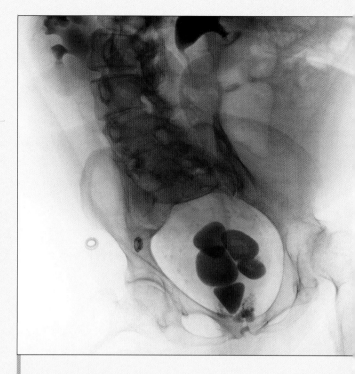

This colored urogram of the abdomen of a man shows five large stones in the bladder. Stones as large as these require removal by a surgical procedure.

problems, such as bleeding in the urine or pain. Treatment of this cancer often involves removing part of the kidney. The cells lining the renal pelvis, ureter, bladder, and urethra are similar, and the most common type of cancer in these cells is transitional cell carcinoma. Tumors can grow in the bladder and cause bleeding and pain. A doctor can cut out the cancer; if it is more invasive, the bladder must be removed. Other types of cancer can also arise in the prostate, urethra, and penis. Some of these can be treated with chemotherapy or radiation therapy. Cancer can be fatal, but many patients with cancers in the urinary tract can live for many years with treatment.

The incidence of development of urinary tract infection in the United States is approximately 6 million people each year. Urinary tract cancers are divided into kidney, bladder, and prostate cancer. Kidney cancer makes up about 3 percent of all cancers. Bladder cancer is the fourth most common cancer in men and the eighth most common cancer in women. Prostate cancer is the most commonly diagnosed cancer among men.

Jennifer M. Taylor and Run Wang

Usher syndrome

Usher syndrome is the most common cause of deafness and blindness. It is estimated that more than 50 percent of adults who are deaf and blind have Usher syndrome.

All three subtypes of Usher syndrome are inherited in an autosomal recessive manner (a pair of abnormal genes is inherited; usually, both parents are unaffected carriers). Eight different genes are associated with this disease; an individual must have two mutations in any one of these genes to exhibit features of Usher syndrome. These mutations cause degeneration of hair cells in the cochlea (inner ear), resulting in deafness. They also destroy the rod cells in the retina. Vision loss in Usher syndrome usually begins as night blindness and loss of peripheral vision ("tunnel vision") and progresses to blindness (retinitis pigmentosa).

Symptoms and diagnosis

Usher syndrome type 1 is characterized by profound hearing loss present at birth, which does not worsen over time. To date five genes and two loci are known for Usher syndrome type 1. Affected people also have balance problems resulting from changes to their inner ear (vestibular ataxia). The onset of vision loss begins in childhood.

People with Usher syndrome type 2 generally have milder hearing loss than in type 1. These people do not have the balance problems experienced in type 1, and vision loss does not usually occur until adolescence, but vision problems progress with age. The hearing loss in Usher syndrome type 3 worsens with time and generally starts after children have begun speaking (postlingual hearing loss). Balance problems of varying severity may be present. The onset of vision loss ranges from adolescence into adulthood.

Diagnosis of Usher syndrome is usually made based on combined deafness and blindness. Because vision loss occurs later in life, most individuals with Usher syndrome are first diagnosed as having nonsyndromic hearing loss (hearing loss not associated with other features). Genetic testing for Usher syndrome is mainly on a research basis, but some clinical testing is offered.

Treatments

Because hearing loss is severe in Usher syndrome type 1, cochlear implants can help these individuals hear some sounds and speech. Hearing aids can be helpful for milder hearing loss in Usher syndrome types 2 and 3. Patients with Usher syndrome should consider limitations in driving motor vehicles secondary to the loss of peripheral vision and difficulty with night vision. Vitamin A supplementation may reduce the average rate of retinal degeneration. Researchers are currently considering gene therapy to slow or halt the progression of vision loss.

Cheryl B. Thomas and Brian C. Brost

KEY FACTS

Description
There are three subtypes of Usher syndrome, all characterized by varying degrees of deafness and blindness.

Causes
Usher syndrome is an autosomal recessive genetic disease. To date, eight genes have been identified that are associated with the syndrome.

Risk factors
A family history of Usher syndrome may indicate that other individuals in the family are at risk. However, there may not be a family history due to its autosomal recessive inheritance.

Symptoms
The severity of hearing loss and age of onset at which vision loss occurs depends on the subtype of Usher syndrome. Individuals with Usher syndrome types 1 and 3 also have balance problems.

Diagnosis
Hearing loss and progressive vision loss later in life.

Treatments
Cochlear implants and hearing aids may be beneficial to individuals with Usher syndrome. There is currently no treatment for vision loss.

Pathogenesis
Degeneration of cells in the inner ear and retina result in hearing loss and progressive blindness.

Prevention
No known prevention for Usher syndrome.

Epidemiology
Usher syndrome is estimated to occur in 4.4 per 100,000 live births in the United States.

See also
- Blindness • Deafness • Ear disorders
- Genetic disorders • Retinal disorders

Uterus, prolapse of

Prolapse of the uterus is a common condition affecting women of varying ages, in which loss of pelvic support results in protrusion of the uterus into the vagina. Prolapse may be caused by multiple factors, such as genetic factors and injury to pelvic floor tissues. It is often asymptomatic, but it can cause symptoms that affect a woman's physical, social, or sexual activity.

Uterine prolapse is one of a constellation of conditions collectively referred to as pelvic organ prolapse in which loss of pelvic support results in the protrusion of pelvic organs (uterus, bladder, or bowel) into the vagina. Uterine prolapse is a common problem for women and may occur concurrently with either bladder prolapse, bowel prolapse, or both. Recent reports have estimated that as many as 40 to 76 percent of women will have some degree of prolapse during their lifetime. Although many women are affected by this condition, the exact number is not known. This is due to the fact that prolapse is often asymptomatic; therefore, women often do not seek medical care. In addition, many women may not report the problem to their physician because of the embarrassing nature of the symptoms, or the lack of sympathy or understanding by the health provider.

Support of the pelvic organs is provided by an overlapping system of ligaments, fascia, and muscles. There may be many reasons for loss of this support. A combination of genetic factors, denervation or ischemic injury to the musculature, and mechanical failure of the connective tissues can lead to pelvic organ prolapse. Vaginal childbirth appears to be among the greatest risk factors for pelvic organ prolapse; the more children a woman has, the more it is associated with advancing prolapse. Damage to pelvic support tissues during childbirth is likely due to compression and extreme pressures from the fetal head and maternal expulsive efforts. These high pressures can cause temporary or permanent stretch and tear injury (mechanical injury), as well as ischemic or neurological injury. In addition to vaginal childbirth, other risk factors include pregnancy, advancing age, low estrogen, obesity, chronic constipation, chronic cough, chronic obstructive pulmonary disease, cigarette smoking, and repetitive heavy lifting. The therapeutic options to treat uterine prolapse are variable and are determined by age, health status, severity of symptoms, and degree of prolapse. No treatment is necessary with mild prolapse, especially if asymptomatic. For more severe degrees of prolapse or if the woman is suffering from symptoms, treatment options include both nonsurgical and surgical therapy. The primary nonsurgical method involves placing a pessary in the vagina to support the pelvic organs. The traditional surgical treatment includes hysterectomy, then repair of the support mechanism, but uterine preservation with reconstruction of the support tissues is under investigation. Currently, focus is on prevention, such as elective cesarean section and aggressive treatment of chronic conditions that increase intra-abdominal pressure.

Stephanie Beall and Charles Rardin

KEY FACTS

Description
Uterus protrudes into or past the vagina.

Causes
Genetic predisposition; direct or indirect injury to pelvic muscles, connective tissue, and nerves.

Risk factors
Vaginal delivery, pregnancy, aging, chronically increased intra-abdominal pressure, menopause, hypoestrogenism, trauma, genetic factors, musculoskeletal disease, chronic disease, smoking, and prior surgery. A combination of risk factors that varies from patient to patient.

Symptoms
Urinary incontinence, fecal incontinence, sexual dysfunction, sensation of vaginal bulging or protrusion, and pelvic pain.

Diagnosis
Pelvic examination and urodynamics.

Treatments
Pessary or surgery.

Pathogenesis
Disease may be secondary to damaged pelvic muscles, connective tissue or nerves, or both.

Prevention
Treatment of underlying conditions.

Epidemiology
Around 40 to 76 percent of women are affected.

See also
- Female reproductive system disorders
- Pregnancy and childbirth

Veins, disorders of

After arteries deliver oxygen-carrying blood to the body's organs and tissues, veins return the blood to the heart to receive more oxygen. An exception is in the pulmonary (lung) circulation, in which oxygenated blood from the lungs is taken to the left part of the heart by pulmonary veins. Another exception is the portal vein that transports blood from the intestines to the liver.

Venules are minute vessels that function to collect deoxygenated blood from capillaries. Many venules unite to form a vein. Many veins, particularly those in the arms and legs, have one-way valves that aid the return of blood to the heart by preventing blood from flowing in the reverse direction. Also, the valves in the veins prevent blood from pooling in the legs and elsewhere due to gravity pull. The wall of a vein surrounds a central carrying canal, known as the lumen. The walls of veins consist of three layers of tissues that are thinner (0.5 mm thickness) and less elastic than the walls of arteries. Veins that lie near the surface of the skin are called superficial veins. The blood flow from the superficial veins is mainly directed toward the deep veins, which are veins buried in the muscles or deep tissues of the body. The muscles that surround the deep veins compress them and help force the blood upward toward the heart. The veins that connect the superficial and deep veins

are called communicating or perforating veins.

The longest vein in the body is the great saphenous vein, which extends from the groin to the ankle and is a deep vein. Other important veins in the body include the femoral vein, inferior vena cava, superior vena cava, portal vein, and pulmonary vein. Deep veins in the arm include the brachial vein, radial vein, and ulnar vein. Deep veins in the leg include the femoral vein, profunda femoris vein, popliteal vein, anterior tibial vein, and posterior tibial vein. The deep veins have a major physiological role in propelling blood upward to the heart. These deep veins also carry 90 percent or more of the blood from the legs toward the heart. The deep large veins typically parallel the large deep arteries.

Varicose veins

The main disorders that affect the veins include clotting, inflammation, and defects that lead to abnormal enlargement (distention) and varicose veins. The leg veins are especially affected because a person's standing position requires blood flow to be forced upward, against gravity, to the heart. Varicose veins result when the valves that control the blood flow in the veins fail to work properly, and the pull of gravity causes blood to pool in a vein, causing it to enlarge. Weakness in the walls of the veins may contribute to this disorder. Varicose veins usually occur in the superficial veins of the upper and lower legs, although they may sometimes occur elsewhere. The pooling of the blood results in a backflow, causing the veins to enlarge and stretch. Many people with varicose veins also have spider veins, which are enlarged blood capillaries. Primary varicose veins result because of a genetic tendency toward the development of varicose veins. Secondary varicose veins occur because of another factor, such as long periods of standing and long airplane or automobile rides. Also, pregnancy, obesity, increased pressure within the abdomen, and aging are factors that may increase the risk for the development of varicose veins or the aggravation of an already existing varicose vein disorder. It is estimated that 15 to 20 percent of the general population eventually develop varicose veins. Women are more likely than men to have varicose or spider veins. Also, women over 30 years old are most often affected by varicose veins.

Most often, varicose veins have no symptoms other than the appearance of purplish, knotted veins protruding under the surface of the skin. Varicose veins can cause leg, feet, and ankle pain, swelling, and aching. Also, these veins are unsightly in appearance, and the skin at the ankle can become discolored to a reddish brown tint. A small percentage of people with varicose veins may have complications that lead to inflammation of the veins (phlebitis), itchy rash, sores or ulcers on the skin, and bleeding.

Varicose veins can usually be seen as the purplish, knotted veins under the skin, but symptoms may develop before these veins are visibly detected. Thus, a doctor will check for them by palpating the leg as the patient is standing or is seated with the legs dangling. If the doctor detects a problem with the deep veins, such as swollen ankles, skin ulcers, or changes in the skin color, then an ultrasound exam or X-ray may be performed to assess the functioning of the deep veins and to rule out other disorders of the legs.

The patient will usually be told to avoid excess standing and to elevate the legs when resting or sleeping. Also, elastic stockings (support hose) compress the veins; when they are worn, the veins are prevented from stretching and hurting. Varicose veins can be removed (vein stripping) by surgery (phlebectomy) or injection therapy.

Surgery can remove many of the varicose veins in the leg, except the saphenous vein. This vein must be preserved because it can be used as a bypass graft if the patient requires heart bypass surgery in the future. Vein stripping is a very extensive surgery, requiring a general anesthetic. This procedure usually relieves the pain and swelling but does not eliminate the tendency to develop new varicose veins.

An alternative to surgery is injection therapy (sclerotherapy of veins). In this procedure, a solution is injected into the vein to cause scarring and closing of the vein. Injection therapy is more time-consuming than surgery, but anesthesia is not necessary, and new varicose veins can be treated as they develop.

Deep vein thrombosis

Deep vein thrombosis, also known as DVT or deep venous thrombosis, is the formation of a blood clot (thrombus) in a deep vein. The tendency of blood cells to stick together to form blood clots can develop in any vein within the body. DVT occurs when a blood clot forms, usually in the femoral vein of the legs or the deep veins of the pelvis. DVT can lead to pulmonary embolism (blockage), a potentially fatal complication in which the blood clots break away in the veins and travel in the blood to the lungs, plugging the lung arteries. Over 60,000 people die of pulmonary embolism each year. DVT is also known as thrombophlebitis (*thrombo* means "clot," and *phlebitis* means "inflammation of a vein"), venous thromboembolism, or phlebothrombosis. People who have had orthopedic surgery or abdominal, thoracic, or pelvic surgery are at high risk for DVT. Also, cancer patients, patients having congestive heart failure, and those who have suffered a heart attack are also at high risk for thrombophlebitis. Other risk factors for DVT include the use of oral contraceptive pills; long-distance flights, such as international flights; a history of miscarriage; and a genetic tendency to venous thromboembolism.

Sluggish blood flow from sitting still or lying down for a long period of time can slow the flow of blood and lead to clot formation. Many hospitalized patients will develop DVT, which is not clinically apparent unless a pulmonary embolism occurs. Veins that have had injuries or have been traumatized, or pockets in the deep veins of the calf, or all of these conditions, can lead to DVT. Substances in the blood that regulate the formation of clots, referred to as clotting factors,

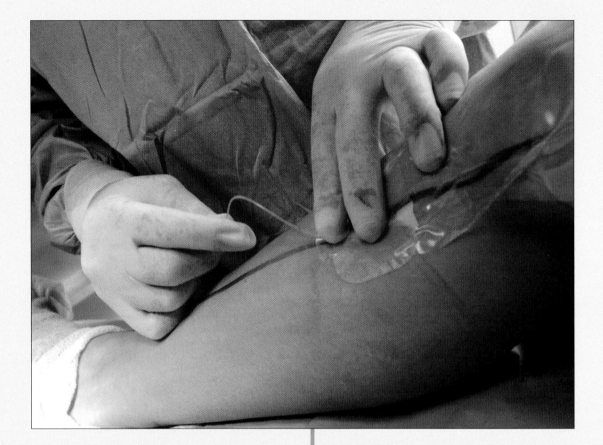

A patient undergoes a procedure to treat varicose veins. An optical fiber is introduced into the affected vein, and a continuous wave endovenous laser is used to treat the varicosities. This treatment is an alternative to stripping the veins.

may increase after an injury, surgery, or during pregnancy and can lead to DVT. A person may or may not have any symptoms. Typically, the clot occurs suddenly and without warning. The classical symptoms of DVT include pain, swelling, and redness of the affected leg.

Venography is the most accurate test to diagnose DVT. However, it is not used very often because of the radiation exposure for the patient, as well as the reactions and complications that can ensue. Compression ultrasound scanning, also known as Doppler ultrasonography, is the preferred procedure for detecting deep vein thrombosis. This diagnostic test uses sound waves to measure blood flow through leg veins and arteries. It is very accurate in detecting a clot and the location of the clot, for example, whether it is below or above the knee. Impedence plethysmography is another noninvasive procedure to detect DVT. It records changes in blood volume and vessel resistance in the legs.

Blood tests that may be performed to diagnose DVT include D-dimer levels; complete blood count (CBC);

prothrombin time (PT); activated partial thromboplastin time (APTT), fibrinogen (coagulation tests); liver enzymes; electrolytes (sodium, potassium chloride, bicarbonate); and kidney function tests.

Blood thinners (anticoagulants) are the usual treatment for DVT. An anticoagulant, such as heparin, will be injected to prevent clots from increasing in size. After the heparin therapy, the anticoagulant warfarin (Coumadin) will be given to the patient over a period of three to six months to prevent the clot from growing. Sometimes, additional medication has to be administered by the physician to dissolve the clot.

In patients who cannot tolerate anticoagulant therapy because of the possibility of hemorrhaging, a filter may be inserted into the main vein in the abdomen (inferior vena cava) to prevent loose clots in leg veins from lodging in the patient's lungs.

Taking a walk or moving the legs regularly when sitting, or both, will help in preventing a blood clot from forming. Also, drinking plenty of fluids and stretching the leg calves at least once an hour is a good preventive technique.

Superficial thrombophlebitis

Superficial thrombophlebitis (SVT, or ST) is a condition in which inflammation due to a blood clot occurs in a vein just under the skin. Superficial (on the surface) thrombophlebitis may develop in varicose veins, usually in the legs, but less frequently in the arms, pelvis, or neck. SVT occurs when a clot forms in a vein because blood flow stops or slows down.

SVT can occur due to a sudden injury, such as a bruise, or after medication or fluid is administered intravenously into a vein. Intense exercise can also lead to SVT. Superficial thrombophlebitis differs from DVT in that an inflammatory reaction occurs immediately, which causes the thrombus (clot) to adhere to the superficial vein wall and lessens the chance that it will break away and travel in the bloodstream. Also, superficial veins do not have muscles surrounding them. Thus, a thrombus is not likely to be dislodged from a superficial vein since muscle tissue does not squeeze these small veins in the way that occurs in deep veins. For these reasons, pulmonary embolism infrequently occurs with SVT.

Symptoms of superficial thrombophlebitis may include warmth and redness of the skin around the inflamed vein; tenderness of the vein that is very sensitive to pressure; a hardened area over the vein as a result of the clot in the vein; and swelling in the area around the vein.

The physician will usually detect from the physical symptoms described above that the patient has ST. However, if the doctor is concerned that the patient may also have DVT, ultrasound technology may be used as described in the DVT section above.

The physician usually will recommend an anti-inflammatory drug, such as aspirin or ibuprofen, to relieve the pain and inflammation. In addition, he or she will recommend that the patient rest and elevate the leg or arm that has the pain and swelling from the ST, typically for five to seven days. Sometimes, placing warm (not hot) moist compresses on the inflamed area can assist in relieving the pain and inflammation. Usually the inflammation will decrease gradually and disappear in a few days. However, the symptoms of tenderness and hardened feeling of the vein are usually present for several weeks before they subside completely.

Portal vein thrombosis

The portal vein provides 75 percent of the blood flow to the liver. Portal vein thrombosis is another type of vein thrombosis affecting the portal vein. This type of thrombosis can lead to a reduction in the blood flow to the liver.

Portal vein thrombosis (PVT) can be caused by any condition that causes blood to back up in the portal vein, such as heart failure. It can also be caused by pancreatitis (inflammation of the pancreas), cirrhosis (severe scarring of the liver), diverticulitis (inflammation in the intestinal walls), or by cancer of the pancreas, liver, or stomach. Also, inherited blood clotting disorders can lead to portal vein thrombosis. Many patients with this disorder are young. In newborn infants, PVT may result from an infection of the umbilical vein.

PVT frequently occurs as slowly and silently as other conditions, such as cancer and pancreatitis, which will have preexisting symptoms, shadowing the PVT. Portal vein thrombosis may not be discovered until sudden bleeding (hemorrhaging) in the upper gastrointestinal tract is evident. Patients may have abdominal pain due to the pressure in the vein caused by the blockage.

Doppler ultrasound, a CT scan, or MRI are all useful imaging techniques to diagnose portal vein thrombosis. These techniques will show the blockage. To confirm the findings from the listed imaging procedures, a liver biopsy may be performed. A small piece of liver tissue is removed with a needle and examined microscopically by a pathologist, who can detect changes in the cells if PVT has occurred in the patient. Also, blood tests for liver function will usually be abnormal for a patient with PVT.

Treatment is used to reduce the pressure in the portal vein from the blockage. Various types of surgical procedures may be performed, depending on the underlying condition that originally led to the portal vein blockage.

Kathleen Becan-McBride

Vitamin deficiency

Vitamins are small noncaloric, carbon-containing organic compounds that are essential for normal physiological functions, such as growth and development, maintenance, and reproduction. Vitamins are required in minute amounts, but they are either not synthesized by the body, or they are produced in insufficient quantities to meet the requirements for the normal functioning of the body.

Vitamins are classified as either fat- or water-soluble. The fat-soluble vitamins include Vitamin A, Vitamin D, Vitamin E, and Vitamin K. They are absorbed along with dietary fat. After being transported to the liver, they are either used immediately or stored there or in fatty tissues for future use.

The water-soluble vitamins include the vitamin B complex group comprising thiamine (vitamin B_1), riboflavin (vitamin B_2), niacin (vitamin B_3), biotin, pantothenic acid, pyridoxine (vitamin B_6), folic acid, and vitamin B_{12}. Vitamin C (ascorbic acid) is also water soluble. Water-soluble vitamins are absorbed from the intestine into the bloodstream and are transported to various cells to be used as needed. Since these vitamins are not stored in large amounts, any excess will be excreted by the kidneys in the urine, so water-soluble vitamins need to be consumed at least weekly, if not daily. If not consumed on a regular basis, deficiency symptoms or, in some cases, disease may develop fairly quickly.

Although vitamins are sometimes grouped in terms of general function, ultimately each has a specific purpose in the body and, when deficiencies develop, they are specific to the vitamin or vitamins that are lacking. Vitamin deficiencies may come about due to inadequate intake, poor absorption as a result of various medical conditions, or even the use of medication (drug-nutrient interaction). Although a deficiency of the fat-soluble vitamins or vitamin C may occur singly, deficiencies of B vitamins usually appear together. Deficiency symptoms will be addressed individually for each vitamin.

Treatment and prevention of deficiencies are similar for all vitamins. They include a diet high in foods rich in the missing nutrient, and if necessary, use of a high-dose vitamin supplement. If a medical condition causes malabsorption, it must be treated and corrected. If the deficiency is caused by a drug-nutrient interaction, physicians often consider changing the medication or utilizing large doses of a supplement to overcome the effects of the drug.

The following discussion will focus on each of the above-named vitamins, first detailing functions of the vitamin, and then concentrating on the deficiency of each, including the causes and risk factors, symptoms, and diagnosis. Treatment and prevention will not be discussed unless it differs from that stated above. Vitamin A will be discussed in the Key Facts Box.

Fat-soluble vitamins

Vitamin A (retinol) is involved in a number of functions in the human body. These functions include roles in night and color vision; cell differentiation of epithelial cells (the cells that line the body surfaces, including the skin mucous membranes, mouth, stomach and intestines, lungs, urinary tract, uterus, vagina, cornea, and sinus passageways); sperm production in men and fertilization in women; maintaining healthy bones; and contributing to a healthy immune system. Beta-carotene, a precursor (provitamin) of Vitamin A acts as an antioxidant.

Vitamin A deficiency is most common in individuals who do not consume dark-green, orange, and deep-yellow fruits and vegetables (excellent sources of beta-carotene) or animal foods such as liver, eggs, or dairy products. Disorders of the intestine can also impair absorption, and liver disorders negatively impact storage of the vitamin.

Night blindness, the inability to see in dim light, is the earliest symptom of a deficiency. If left untreated, it may progress to xerophthalmia, which is irreversible total blindness as a result of hardening of the cornea. Other deficiency symptoms include impairment of growth, immunity, and reproductive function. Vitamin A deficiency affects as many as 5 million people, mainly infants and children in developing countries. Diagnosis of vitamin A deficiency is based on symptoms and a low level of the vitamin in the blood.

Vitamin D promotes the absorption of calcium and phosphorus from the small intestine; regulates blood calcium levels; is required for bone mineralization, growth and repair; and is important in cell differentiation (maturation). Interestingly, the body can actually synthesize vitamin D when sunlight strikes the skin. Thus it is not considered an essential nutrient if individuals spend enough time in the sun.

Vitamin D deficiency is more common in people who are not exposed very often to the sun (10 or 15 minutes of exposure on hands, face, and arms on a summer day appears to be all that is needed) or have dark skin (less vitamin D is made by these individuals), in infants who are breastfed without any supplementation, and in those who do not use fortified milk or fortified margarine (major sources of vitamin D).

The classical vitamin D deficiency is known as rickets in children and osteomalacia in adults. Children develop bowed legs because the leg bones cannot support their body weight and a protruding abdomen due to weakened musculature. Rickets is still a problem in many less developed nations. Adults who develop osteomalacia exhibit softened bones of the legs and spine, causing some individuals to become bowlegged and bent. Diagnosis of rickets or osteomalacia is based on symptoms, the appearance of abnormal bones on X-rays, and a low level of vitamin D metabolites in the blood.

Vitamin E functions as an antioxidant, protecting the cells against oxidative damage by free radicals (unstable, highly reactive products of normal cellular activity). It is especially important in stabilizing cell membranes and protecting polyunsaturated fatty acids and vitamin A.

A deficiency of vitamin E from a poor intake is rare, since the vitamin is so widespread in foods. However, newborn premature infants who are not supplemented are at risk for a deficiency. They may develop a hemolytic anemia, causing red blood cells to rupture. Disorders that impair fat absorption, such as liver, gall bladder, or pancreatic disease, can also reduce vitamin E absorption and may cause a deficiency. Symptoms of deficiency include difficulty walking, loss of coordination, and muscle weakness; these symptoms are the result of nerve damage (peripheral neuropathy). Blood tests are available to detect vitamin E deficiency.

Vitamin K functions in the synthesis of proteins involved in blood clotting and bone metabolism. Besides being found in green leafy vegetables, vitamin K is synthesized in the body by bacteria in the colon.

Because people depend on bacterial synthesis for vitamin K, deficiency is unlikely except in newborns (whose intestinal tracts are not inhabited by bacteria) and individuals taking antibiotics (which destroy both harmful and helpful intestinal bacteria), anticoagulants, and anticonvulsants. The main symptom of a deficiency is impaired blood clotting and uncontrolled bleeding. Additionally, there are possible negative effects on bone health, such as weakened bones. Newborns are routinely given a vitamin K injection at birth to protect them from hemorrhagic disease. Blood tests to measure clotting function are used to assess vitamin K status.

Treatment consists of vitamin K injections or adjusting the dose of medications.

KEY FACTS: VITAMIN A DEFICIENCY

Description

A deficiency of vitamin A in the body.

Causes

Inadequate intake of preformed vitamin A or the precursor beta-carotene. Disorders involving malabsorption of fat, liver disease, or protein-energy malnutrition (vitamin A requires retinol-binding protein for transport inside the body).

Risk factors

Poor diet, impaired intestinal absorption, liver disease.

Symptoms

Night blindness, xerophthalmia with Bitot's spots (foamy deposits in the whites of the eyes), leading to irreversible blindness. Increase in infections.

Diagnosis

Based on dietary history, symptoms, and low level of vitamin A in the blood.

Treatments

Large oral doses (200,000 IU or 60,000 RE) of vitamin A supplements and correction of protein-energy malnutrition.

Pathogenesis

Low intake leads to depletion of liver stores. Night blindness, xerophthalmia progresses to keratomalacia (softening of the cornea), which leads to irreversible blindness. Accumulation of keratin, a water-insoluble protein, is responsible for the increase in infections.

Prevention

Diets adequate in vitamin A or beta-carotene, protein, and energy.

Epidemiology

Around 3 and 10 million people, mainly infants and preschool children in developing nations, suffer from vitamin A deficiency. About 275 million more children suffer from mild deficiency that impairs immunity and promotes infections. Severe vitamin A deficiency causes more than 500,000 preschool children to become blind each year.

Water-soluble vitamins

Vitamin B$_1$ (thiamine) functions as a coenzyme (thiamine pyrophosphate), a small molecule that promotes enzymatic activity in energy metabolism of the cells. Enzymes are catalysts that allow cellular reactions to take place in a timely fashion. Thiamine is most important in carbohydrate and amino acid metabolism, but it also has a role in nerve function.

A deficiency of thiamine results in beriberi, a disease involving the nervous and cardiovascular systems. Lack of thiamine in the diet is no longer a problem in most developed nations due to the enrichment of flour with B vitamins, but people whose diet consists mostly of polished rice are at risk for deficiency. Alcoholics, who often have a poor food intake, are also at risk. They may develop Wernicke-Korsakoff's syndrome, with memory loss, mental confusion, difficulty walking, and eye problems. Diagnosis of a thiamine deficiency is based on symptoms.

Vitamin B$_2$ (riboflavin), like many B vitamins, functions as a coenzyme (flavine adenine dinucleotide and flavin mononucleotide) in energy metabolism of the cells. Its function is in carbohydrate and fat metabolism, in which it carries hydrogen ions and electrons during various reactions. Riboflavin also serves as an essential component of energy production via the electron transport systems (respiratory chain).

Deficiencies of riboflavin generally occur in concert with other B vitamins. Thus symptoms are often secondary to those arising from other nutrient deficiencies. In the laboratory, an induced lack of riboflavin brings about sensitivity to light, tearing, burning, and itching of the eyes with a loss of visual sharpness, as well as soreness and burning of the lips, mouth, and tongue. Often fissures and cracks develop in the lips and corners of the mouth. Diagnosis is based on the above symptoms and evidence of general malnutrition.

Vitamin B$_3$ (niacin) also functions as a coenzyme (nicotinamide adenine dinucleotide and nicotinamide adenine dinucleotide phosphate) in the energy metabolism of the cells. It is most important in carbohydrate, fat, protein, and alcohol metabolism, DNA replication and repair, and cell differentiation, in which it carries hydrogen ions and electrons during various reactions. Niacin also has an important role in energy production via the electron transport system (respiratory chain).

A lack of niacin leads to pellagra, a deficiency disease with symptoms of diarrhea, dermatitis (a reddened rash similar to sunburn), dementia (confusion, disorientation, hallucinations, and memory loss), and

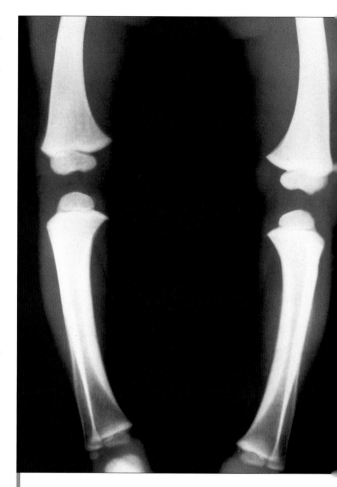

A colored X-ray of a child's legs shows that the long bones are abnormally curved. This severe deformity is a result of rickets, caused by a nutritional deficiency of vitamin D, which is needed for the absorption of calcium from food.

eventually death. In those nations where enrichment of flour with B vitamins occurs, deficiencies are rare. However, in countries where individuals consume a low-protein diet consisting of mostly corn or maize, niacin deficiency may occur. Diagnosis of a deficiency is based on a diet history and symptoms.

Pantothenic acid is part of the chemical structure of coenzyme A (coA), an essential coenzyme involved in the synthesis of fats, neurotransmitters, steroids, and hemoglobin. As coA, it is also an important metabolic intermediate, serving as an entrance point to the tricarboxylic acid (TCA) cycle.

Since pantothenic acid is widespread in foods, deficiency is quite rare. If present, symptoms include fatigue, gastrointestinal problems (nausea, vomiting, cramps), and neurological disturbances.

Pyridoxine (vitamin B_6), in common with a number of other B vitamins, functions as a coenzyme (pyridoxal phosphate) in amino acid, carbohydrate, and fat metabolism. Also, pyridoxine is involved with the synthesis of neurotransmitters and red blood cells.

Dietary deficiencies of pyridoxine are relatively rare; however, a number of drugs interfere with vitamin B_6 metabolism. These include isoniazid (an antibiotic and chemotherapeutuic agent), hydralazine (an antihypertensive), and penicillamin (used to treat arthritis and Wilson's disease). Deficiency symptoms include seizure in infants, microcytic anemia, dermatitis, numbness and prickling in the hands and feet, depression, confusion, and convulsions. Diagnosis of a deficiency is based on symptoms that respond to supplementation.

Biotin functions as a coenzyme in carbohydrate, fat, and protein metabolism. It is involved in the addition or removal of carbon dioxide to and from various compounds. Deficiencies of biotin are rare due to its widespread occurrence in foods and synthesis by intestinal bacteria. Avidin, a protein found in raw egg whites, binds with biotin, making it unavailable. Hence a diet high in raw egg whites (cooking destroys avidin) may precipitate deficiency symptoms, which include dermatitis, hair loss, pallor, nausea, vomiting, and anorexia. Diagnosis of deficiency is based on dietary history.

Folic acid (folate or folacin) functions as a coenzyme in DNA and RNA synthesis and amino acid metabolism. Specifically, it transfers one-carbon compounds in many different reactions, including those involved in formation of red and white blood cells and the metabolism of homocysteine, an amino acid that can build up and may increase the risk of heart disease.

A deficiency of folate leads to changes in DNA and RNA metabolism, leading to poor growth, megaloblastic anemia, neural tube defects in a developing fetus, elevated homocysteine levels, and gastrointestinal tract disturbances. A number of drugs, including antacids, aspirin, oral contraceptive agents, chemotherapeutic agents, and anticonvulsants, have been shown to interfere with the body's use of folate. Pregnant women and alcoholics are at high risk for deficiency. Some researchers suggest that folate deficiency may be the most common vitamin deficiency in humans.

Folate is found in many foods, although brewer's yeast, liver, leafy green vegetables, and legumes have the greatest levels. Recently, flour in the United States has been enriched with folate. Diagnosis of folate deficiency is by a blood test that detects large red blood cells (macrocytic anemia), followed by additional tests that specifically measure folic acid in the blood.

Vitamin B_{12} functions as a coenzyme in the synthesis of new cells. Specifically, it is used to transfer methyl groups in various metabolic reactions. Vitamin B_{12} is necessary for the synthesis of nucleic acids, maturation of red blood cells, normal nerve function, and activation of folic acid.

Vitamin B_{12} is found only in animal products; hence, strict vegetarians (vegans) are at increased risk of deficiency. Since the vitamin requires an acidic environment to be released from food, elderly people whose stomach acidity is low may also be at risk. Intrinsic factor, a protein made in the stomach, is necessary to protect the vitamin until it reaches the end of the small intestine, where it is absorbed. Thus, individuals with stomach injury or an autoimmune disorder that destroys intrinsic factor would also be at risk.

Deficiency symptoms include megaloblastic anemia (called pernicious anemia if it is caused by lack of stomach acid or intrinsic factor); nerve damage, in the form of tingling and numbness of the arms and legs; memory loss; disorientation; and dementia. The anemia develops slowly since the body can store enough vitamin for up to five years. Diagnosing a deficiency can be complicated, since large doses of folic acid will mask symptoms, although nerve damage will proceed unchecked. An anemia with large red blood cells is often the first sign of a deficiency. Blood tests or a Schilling test using a small amount of radioactive vitamin B_{12} can confirm the diagnosis. Treatment of a deficiency is vitamin supplementation by mouth if the deficiency is due to diet, or by injections if it is due to a lack of stomach acid or intrinsic factor.

Vitamin C (ascorbic acid) functions in the synthesis of collagen (a protein necessary for the structure of connective tissue, cartilage, bone matrix, tooth dentin, skin, and tendons) and thyroid hormone; as an antioxidant; in amino acid metabolism; and to increase the absorption of iron. It also promotes resistance to infection.

Vitamin C deficiency causes scurvy, with symptoms that include rough skin, swollen, inflamed, and bleeding gums, loose teeth, dry mouth and eyes, and hair loss. There may also be bleeding under the skin that resembles bruises, poor wound healing, frequent infection, muscle degeneration and pain, and anemia. Diagnosis is based on symptoms followed by a blood test.

Alan Levine

See also
- Anemia • Blindness • Bone and joint disorders • Eating disorders • Kwashiorkor • Nutritional disorders • Prevention

Vitiligo

Vitiligo is a common skin disorder characterized by the loss of pigment within the epidermis, leading to depigmented white patches.

Melanocytes are pigment-producing cells in the basal layer of the skin. Vitiligo is a condition in which the melanocytes have disappeared from an area of the skin so that white areas replace pigmented areas. Generally, these areas start as small white spots that enlarge with time. The patches can be localized (one body site), generalized (multiple body sites), or universal (entire skin surface). The white areas are usually asymptomatic, and affected individuals are usually most disturbed by the cosmetic appearance.

Vitiligo can affect any area of skin but appears most commonly on the backs of hands and elbows, as well as around the mouth, eyes, rectum, and genitalia. Often the hair in the area is also depigmented. Ultraviolet dark light may be used to help confirm the diagnosis of vitiligo. This light is shone on the lesion, and if the pigment contrast is accentuated, the lesion is consistent with vitiligo.

Although the cause of vitiligo is unknown, it has been associated with thyroid disease, pernicious anemia, Addison's disease, diabetes, and alopecia. Therefore, blood tests to measure thyroid function and glucose levels and a complete blood count should be ordered. It is also important to realize that depigmentation of the retina may occur. Generally, it is unnecessary to take a skin biopsy to diagnose vitiligo. However, if a sample of skin is taken, it will show absence of melanocytes; there may also be evidence of inflammation.

One theory is that the body produces antibodies against the melanocytes, leading to an immune system response. Lymphocytes may play a direct role in killing these cells. Another theory proposes that neurochemical mediators may be responsible for destroying melanocytes. Others believe that toxic compounds accumulate within the pigment-producing cells and destroy them. In addition, up to 30 percent of vitiligo patients have an affected relative; however, the disease seems to have a multifactorial genetic basis.

Treatments

Often the goal of treating this disease is to help the patient deal with the cosmetic appearance. One option is topical agents, such as corticosteroids that suppress inflammation. Another option is taking a psoralen pill to make the skin more sensitive to light and then expose it to long-wave ultraviolet A light (PUVA). These treatments are often of limited success, and some patients prefer to use cosmetic makeup to even out the skin tone. In severe vitiligo, patients may prefer to depigment the rest of their skin.

The disease is usually chronic, unpredictable, and often progressive, although there can be spontaneous repigmentation starting around the hair follicles, so the area looks as though it has been sprinkled with pepper.

Nina Pabby and Richard S. Kalish

KEY FACTS

Description

A skin disorder in which there is loss of pigment, leading to depigmented white patches.

Causes

Unknown; however, theories involve immune mechanisms, neurochemical mediators, or toxins that may destroy melanocytes.

Risk factors

No known genetic inheritance pattern, but there seems to be a multifactorial genetic basis.

Symptoms

Asymptomatic white areas replace areas of skin that were previously pigmented. Generally, these areas start as small white spots that enlarge.

Diagnosis

A clinical diagnosis. Skin biopsy may help.

Treatment

Topical corticosteroids, light treatments, topical immunomodulators, and cosmetics.

Pathogenesis

Chronic, unpredictable, and often progressive.

Prevention

No reliable method to prevent vitiligo is known.

Epidemiology

Vitiligo is reported to occur in 1 percent of the population, with the peak age group being between 10 and 30 years old. No gender-related difference in prevalence is reported.

See also

- Adrenal disorders • Alopecia • Anemia
- Diabetes • Immune system disorders
- Skin disorders • Thyroid disorders

Von Willebrand's disease

Von Willebrand's disease is the most common inherited bleeding disorder in the world. It was named for, and by, its discoverer, Erik Adolf von Willebrand, a Finnish pediatrician who first described it in 1926. It is caused by an abnormality of the von Willebrand factor (vWF), which is a large multimeric (subunits held together by weak bonds) glycoprotein that functions as the carrier protein for factor VIII, a critical blood coagulation protein; it also is required for normal platelet adhesion.

The abnormality in vWF can be either qualitative or quantitative; due to different genetic mutations, an individual may have either defective vWF or not enough vWF. In primary hemostasis (arrest of bleeding), vWF binds to a receptor on platelets, glycoprotein Ib, and acts as a bridge between the platelets and damaged subendothelium at the site of vascular injury. In secondary hemostasis, vWF protects factor VIII from degradation and delivers it to the site of injury.

vWF is composed of dimeric subunits that are linked by disulfide bonds to form complex multimers of low, intermediate, and high molecular weights. The small multimers function mainly as carriers for factor VIII, whereas the high molecular weight multimers have higher numbers of platelet-binding sites and greater adhesive properties. The high molecular weight multimers are therefore the most important for normal platelet function.

Symptoms

There are three types of von Willebrand's disease. Type 1 vWD accounts for 70 to 80 percent of cases. It is characterized by a partial quantitative decrease of qualitatively normal vWF and factor VIII. A person with type 1 vWD generally has mild clinical symptoms, and this type is usually inherited as an autosomal dominant trait. However, penetrance may vary dramatically in a single family. In addition, clinical and laboratory findings may vary in the same patient on different occasions. Typically, a proportional reduction in vWF activity, vWF antigen, and factor VIII is observed with type 1vWD.

Normal or near-normal levels of dysfunctional vWF protein characterize type 2 vWD, which accounts for 15 to 20 percent of cases. Patients with the type 2a

variant (the most common one) exhibit a deficiency in the high and medium molecular weight forms of the vWF multimer. The high molecular weight multimers have higher numbers of platelet-binding sites and greater adhesive properties, so are therefore the most important for normal platelet function. Those with the type 2b variant also lack the high molecular weight

KEY FACTS

Description

Von Willebrand's disease is the most common hereditary bleeding disorder in the world. Von Willebrand's disease is caused by a deficiency of von Willebrand factor (vWF). Von Willebrand factor helps platelets to clump together and stick to the blood vessel wall, which is necessary for normal blood clotting.

Causes

Genetic; vWD is inherited as an autosomal dominant trait.

Risk factors

Parents with the disease.

Symptoms

Bleeding, ranging from mild (only after trauma or surgery) to severe (spontaneous gastrointestinal, urogenital, or oral mucosal bleeding). Also, easy bruising and long bleeding times.

Diagnosis

A diagnostic blood test is generally the vWF antigen assay, which tells how much protein is circulating in the blood. The ristocetin cofactor assay indicates how well the vWF protein works; and a factor VIII level test is also often done. Von Willebrand factor binds to factor VIII, a clotting protein that is lacking in people with one type of hemophilia. Factor VIII levels may be low in people with von Willebrand's disease.

Treatments

Administration of cryoprecipitate—a plasma fraction enriched in vWF—or factor VIII concentrates that contain vWF; alternatively, a vasosuppressive analog called DDAVP.

Prevention

People with this disease should avoid medications that have known antiplatelet effects; these include aspirin, ibuprofen, antihistamines, caffeine, and ethanol.

Epidemiology

Von Willebrand's disease affects both men and women. Its prevalence worldwide is estimated at 0.9–1.3 percent.

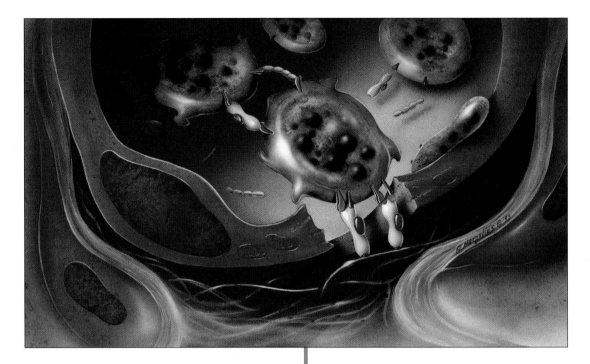

multimers, whereas in type 2a vWD these proteins are made and then destroyed; in type 2b vWD their lack is due to the inappropriate binding of these proteins to platelets. A similar disease, platelet type vWD, is due to a mutation in glycoprotein Ib, the receptor protein the platelets use to bind to vWF.

Type 3 vWD is very severe, and relatively rare; approximately one in one million individuals have type 3. Unlike the other two types, it is inherited in an autosomal recessive manner; those affected are usually the offspring of two parents with mild, even asymptomatic, type 1 vWD. These patients have no detectable vWF. They mimic mild hemophiliacs in that they can have severe mucosal bleeding.

Treatments

Two therapeutic options exist to deal with vWD. The first involves the use of cryoprecipitate, a plasma fraction enriched in vWF, or factor VIII concentrates that are highly purified, are heat treated to destroy HIV, and that retain high molecular weight vWF multimers. These are appropriate treatments for all inherited forms of vWD.

The other option is the use of DDAVP (1-desamino-8-D-arginine vasopressin). This may be preferable, as it avoids the use of plasma. Also called desmopressin, it is a synthetic analogue of antidiuretic hormone. It works by causing release of vWF from endothelial storage sites. Patients with type 1 vWD are the optimal candidates for treatment with DDAVP. DDAVP is usually given either by nasal spray or by injection.

Patients suffering from this disease can benefit from seeking out a hemophilia treatment center. These centers often have a dedicated physician, nurse, and other medical personnel who see many types of bleeding disorders. Usually, a center is federally funded to have a hematologist, nurse coordinator or practitioner, dentist, geneticist, physical therapist, or social worker who have experience in all the issues of von Willebrand's disease and other bleeding disorders.

Bleeding disorders tend to be rare in the general population. Thus it is usually in the best interest of patients, or people who suspect they might have a bleeding disorder, to go to a center that is experienced in these disorders. Hemophilia treatment centers have the resources, expertise, and experience to properly assess and diagnose the condition.

Diana Gitig

See also
- Blood disorders • Genetic disorders
- Hemophilia

Wart and verruca

Warts and verrucas are harmless, contagious viral infections of the skin that cause small unsightly growths. Over 80 types of the human papilloma virus (HPV) cause four different types of warts. Verrucas (plantar warts) are warts on the bottom of the feet.

Warts or verrucas are growths that occur on the top layer of skin; the overgrowth of cells develops into a small lump. Warts on the soles of the feet are commonly called verrucas.

Causes and risk factors

Scientists now know that the unsightly but harmless growths are caused when the human papillomavirus (HPV) enters the skin through small cuts. Most common in children and teenagers, the lesions appear on the hands, feet, and face and come in many shapes, colors, and sizes. HPV is passed by direct and indirect contact. For example, if a person touches the damp towel of someone who has warts, the person may pick up HPV. Children who bite their fingernails or pick at hangnails get warts more often than children who do not. Why some people get warts and others do not is still unknown. One theory is that certain individuals are immune to the virus. Others have recurring warts; those people may harbor the virus, which may lie dormant in underlying skin tissues.

Symptoms and signs

There are several types of warts. Common warts appear most often on tops of fingers, hands, along the cuticles, knees, and elbows. Looking like a rough cauliflower, they may have small black dots, which are tiny blood vessels. The wart may appear alone or with small satellites. Flat or juvenile warts are about the size of a pinhead and have flat tops that are pink, light brown, or yellow. Usually occurring in children, the warts can grow in clusters of as many as 100. Plantar warts or verrucas grow thick calloused areas on the ball of the foot and feel like a stone in the shoe. Filiform warts are those depicted on witches in fairy-tale books. This wart has a fingerlike shape and grows around the mouth, eyes, and nose. Genital warts are lesions that may be sexually transmitted and can extend internally into the reproductive organs. Most are painless, but some can increase the risk of cervical cancer. A vaccine has been developed to prevent these types of warts.

About 50 percent of warts go away untreated, but others need a doctor's attention. Over-the-counter preparations with salicylic acid may be helpful. Genital warts respond to podophyllin, a topical resin. Cryosurgery freezes warts with liquid nitrogen, and this may get rid of them. Laser treatment is used for stubborn warts, especially plantar warts, which may respond to this treatment. Surgery is not the best treatment because it may leave scars and residual virus. Immunotherapy is now commonly used; a variety of techniques involve painting or injecting a medication at the site of the wart to stimulate immune clearance and to prevent recurrence.

Evelyn B. Kelly

KEY FACTS

Description
Small growths; verrucas are warts on the feet.

Causes
More than 80 types of the human papillomavirus (HPV) cause warts; the virus is passed from person to person.

Risk factors
Virus enters through cracks in the skin; some types are transmitted sexually.

Symptoms
Painless, flesh-colored small cauliflower-like growth with tiny black dots or minute blood vessels.

Diagnosis
Observation.

Treatments
Ranges from no treatment to physical or chemical destruction, or immunotherapy.

Pathogenesis
Warts are generally not harmful; rarely will they become cancerous.

Prevention
Avoid contact with warts or objects that have touched the growths in other people; scratches or cuts on feet or hands may lead to verrucas.

Epidemiology
Most commonly seen in children and teenagers.

See also
- Cold, common • HPV infection
- Infections, viral • Skin disorders

West Nile encephalitis

In 1999, West Nile virus (WNV) was introduced into the Western Hemisphere, perhaps through importation of an infected bird or mosquito, and has since spread rapidly. The emergence of WNV has raised awareness about the introduction of new viruses into naive ecosystems.

West Nile virus (WNV) is a member of the virus family *Flaviviridae*. The virus was first isolated in 1937 from the West Nile district in Uganda. WNV is maintained in birds and transmitted to humans and other vertebrate animals by mosquitoes, primarily *Culex* species. Bird infection is usually benign, although some species, such as crows and jays, have shown mortality rates exceeding 90 percent. Humans and other vertebrates are incidental hosts and may contribute to viral amplification. Transmission of WNV has also occurred through blood transfusions, organ transplants, laboratory exposures, and transplacental passage from mother to child.

Signs and symptoms

Most human infections are asymptomatic or mild. The incubation period is usually around two to six days. People with symptoms experience fever, chills, headache, rash, joint and muscle pains, diarrhea, nausea, and vomiting (West Nile fever). Less than 1 percent of humans infected with WNV, primarily the elderly and immunocompromised, develop neuron-invasive disease (West Nile encephalitis), with signs of meningitis or encephalitis, including muscle weakness, disorientation, tremors, convulsions, paralysis, coma, and death in 3 to 15 percent of cases. Previous infection provides protective immunity.

The infection is diagnosed by tests to detect WNV or antibodies in blood or tissues. Treatment is supportive.

Pathogenesis and prevention

Early infection in the skin and regional lymph nodes seeds the blood, leading to widespread organ infection, including the spleen, liver, lungs, and central nervous system. Viremia normally lasts only a few days and ceases with the onset of symptoms but may be prolonged in the elderly and immunocompromised. Prevention centers on avoiding mosquito bites. Screening blood donations for WNV in the United States in 2003 has greatly reduced the risk of infection via blood products. A vaccine is in clinical trials.

Epidemiology

After WNV was first introduced to the Western Hemisphere in 1999, subsequent migrations of infected birds have resulted in spread of WNV across North America, encroaching further into the Southern Hemisphere of the Americas with each passing year. From 2002 to 2005, annual averages of almost 5,000 cases were reported in the United States.

Ian H. Mendenhall and Daniel G. Bausch

KEY FACTS

Description
Acute viral infection from an infected mosquito.

Cause
West Nile virus, in birds and transmitted to humans and other vertebrates by mosquitoes.

Risk factors
Spending time outdoors during peak mosquito-biting season. More rarely, blood transfusion or transplantation with infected tissues.

Symptoms
Most infections are asymptomatic or result in mild fever. Elderly and immunocompromised are at risk of central nervous system involvement.

Diagnosis
Test of blood or tissues for antibodies or virus

Treatments
Supportive. No specific antiviral drug available.

Pathogenesis
Combination of direct viral damage from replication in organs and pathologic effects of the immune response.

Prevention
Covering exposed skin and using insect repellants. Monitor mosquito and bird populations for infection. Eliminate mosquito breeding.

Epidemiology
Found in Africa, southern Europe, the Middle East, western Asia, Australia, and North America.

See also
- Infections, animal-to-human • Infections, viral • Lyme disease • Meningitis
- Nervous system disorders • Rickettsial infections • Rocky Mountain spotted fever

Whiplash

The term *whiplash* is commonly used to describe a soft tissue injury of the neck caused by hyperextension and hyperflexion of the neck, also called a "neck sprain" or "neck strain." The injury may involve the muscles, nerve roots, intervertebral joints, disks, or ligaments of the neck.

Motor vehicle collisions are the most common cause of whiplash, although the injury may occur with assaults, falls, or with sports activities that cause hyperextension and hyperflexion of the neck. Increasing age and preexisting neck conditions may increase the severity of the condition.

Symptoms

The patient presents with neck pain, stiffness, and tenderness of the neck musculature. The patient may also present with less common symptoms of headache, muscle spasms of the neck, decreased range of motion of the neck, paresthesias (skin sensations) of the upper extremities, pain in the shoulders or between the shoulder blades, dizziness, fatigue, sleep disturbances, or depression. Whiplash is sometimes also associated with memory loss, impaired concentration, irritability, and nervousness. The pain associated with whiplash typically resolves within days to weeks, with complete resolution for most patients within three months. Patients with six weeks or more of pain should have a reevaluation by a physician to determine possible alternate causes for the pain.

Diagnosis

The diagnosis of whiplash is by history and physical exam with a complete neurological exam. X-rays of the cervical spine are done according to the judgment of the physician; if there is pain, palpation of the neck is undertaken to exclude bony injury. In patients with negative X-ray studies who have persistent pain or neurological problems, additional imaging with computed tomography (CT) or magnetic resonance imaging (MRI) may be necessary to further delineate the underlying anatomy and injury.

Treatments and prevention

Treatment of whiplash may include ice or heat application to the affected area. Medications, such as nonsteroidal anti-inflammatory drugs (NSAIDs) or a short course of narcotics or muscle relaxants, may be administered. Additional treatment options include physical therapy, range of motion exercises, traction, massage, local injections, ultrasound, or short-term use of a soft cervical collar. Antidepressants may be prescribed if a patient has associated depression with ongoing pain.

Since motor vehicle collisions are the most common cause of whiplash, prevention has been aimed at the use of head rests on car seats, which, on impact, decrease the range of motion of a person's head.

Joanne L. Oakes

KEY FACTS

Description
Soft-tissue injury of the neck.

Causes
Motor vehicle collisions, falls, and assaults.

Risk factors
Increasing age and prior neck injury.

Symptoms
Localized pain, neck tenderness, decreased range of motion of the neck, headache, paresthesias of the upper extremities, pain in the shoulders or between the shoulder blades, dizziness, fatigue, sleep disturbances, depression, impaired concentration, irritability, and nervousness.

Diagnosis
History and physical exam with a complete neurological exam.

Treatment
Oral pain medications, muscle relaxants, local application of ice or heat, physical therapy, traction, massage, local injections, ultrasound, and temporary use of a soft cervical collar.

Pathogenesis
Hyperextension and hyperflexion of the neck.

Prevention
Use of head rests in cars.

Epidemiology
Common, although actual incidence unknown due to underreporting.

See also

- Bone and joint disorders • Depression
- Muscle system disorders • Nervous system disorders • Sleep disorders

Whooping cough

Also called pertussis, whooping cough used to be a common childhood disease in industrialized countries. Thanks to vaccination, it is now much less common in the United States, though outbreaks still occur.

Whooping cough is a sometimes severe respiratory infection caused by the bacterium *Bordetella pertussis*. Young children are particularly at risk from the disease. Today it is most common in less developed countries of the tropics.

Cause and symptoms and signs

Whooping cough results from *B. pertussis* infecting the lining of the upper respiratory system. The incubation time between infection and symptoms appearing is usually around 7 to 10 days. The first symptoms are nonspecific, such as sneezing and a runny nose. Usually it is another week or two before the characteristic coughing fits begin. These fits are often accompanied by a distinctive "whooping" sound, as the sufferer gasps for breath. Coughing fits can go on for 6 to 8 weeks and can be triggered by activities such as laughing or yawning. Adults with whooping cough usually have much milder symptoms than young children.

The disease can be diagnosed either from the symptoms, by taking samples from the sufferer's air tubes and growing the bacteria in culture, or by taking a blood sample to check for antibodies the body has produced against the disease.

Pathogenesis and treatments

Whooping cough bacteria attach to the cells lining the air tubes that lead to the lungs. The more severe symptoms of the disease are caused by toxins that the bacteria produce. Whooping cough also lays the body open to other infections, such as pneumonia. All these effects tend to be more severe in young children. About 1 in 500 young children with whooping cough dies, either from breathing difficulties or from other complications.

Young children with whooping cough need careful attention, especially to make sure they can breathe properly. Children may also be sick after a coughing fit and start to lose weight. Sometimes hospital admission is necessary. Treatment by antibiotics at an early stage, especially before the coughing fits begin, shortens the infection. Treating sufferers and those around them also makes them less infectious to other people.

Epidemiology and prevention

Whooping cough is spread by those infected coughing or sneezing water droplets into the air. Others then breathe in these droplets. The disease is far more common in unvaccinated communities. Because infants and young children are most at risk, vaccination starts at 2 months old, with further vaccinations later in infancy. Vaccination lasts only a few years, so adults can get whooping cough even if they were vaccinated as children. Vaccines are based on whole dead *Bordetella* cells or on the toxins. Cell-free vaccines produce fewer side effects and are the type used in the United States today.

Richard Beatty

KEY FACTS

Description
A bacterial disease of the upper air tubes.

Cause
Infection with the bacterium *Bordetella pertussis*.

Risk factors
Infants are more at risk of severe disease.

Symptoms
Violent coughing fits, usually with a characteristic "whooping" sound when breathing in.

Diagnosis
Usually by the symptoms; also by laboratory investigations.

Treatments
Antibiotics make the sufferers less infectious; symptoms and complications also need treatment.

Pathogenesis
Bacteria release toxins that irritate the respiratory system.

Prevention
Vaccination; avoiding contact with people who have the illness.

Epidemiology
Bacteria spread in air droplets produced by coughing and sneezing.

See also
• Childhood disorders • Croup • Infections, bacterial • Respiratory system disorders

Yeast infection

A yeast infection is a type of fungal infection that can cause a variety of skin infections, including dandruff. The fungus *Candida albicans* is one of the most common yeast infections. It causes vaginal infections in women, but it can also infect the mouth and cause diaper rash in babies.

Although many people think of yeast as just an ingredient for bakers and brewers, there are many yeasts that can cause infections in humans. Under normal, healthy conditions the growth of these microbes goes unnoticed. But when the body gets out of balance, the fungi can quickly grow out of control, causing infections, skin rashes, and even dandruff.

Types of yeast infections

Candida is a fungus that is found almost everywhere, including the digestive system and in the reproductive tract of women. Paronychia is an infection of the skin around the nails that can be caused by candida, bacteria, or other fungi. The infection can be acute or chronic, affecting the nail and cuticle as well as the surrounding skin.

Malassezia furfur (formerly called *Pityrosporum ovale*) is a common yeast that produces dandruff when it grows in abundance on the scalp. It is estimated that one in three people have experienced problems with dandruff. Seborrheic dermatitis is a more severe infection that can occur in infants or adults. In infants, the rash that often occurs on the scalp is commonly called "cradle cap." The rashes can spread to the eyebrows, eyelids, and folds in the skin. In infants, yeasts are one of the causes of diaper rashes.

Causes and risk factors

There are more than 150 species of candida, but only 10 of them can cause disease in humans. More than 90 percent of all infections are caused by a single species: *Candida albicans*. Women are at highest risk, and 75 percent of all women will have a vaginal yeast infection at some point in their life. These often occur when a woman takes antibiotics that destroy the normally beneficial bacteria growing in the vagina. Other risk factors include the use of birth control pills, corticosteroid medications, pregnancy, diabetes, and a depressed immune system. It is rarely transmitted by sexual activity.

Paronychia is common in people whose hands are often in water. Hairdressers and dishwashers are at higher risk. Other risk factors include nail-biting, improper nail care, and exposure to chemical irritants. Women are at higher risk, along with diabetics and patients with compromised immune systems.

The risk of seborrheic dermatitis varies greatly by age. Infants are at risk until about six months of age. After that, the risk is low until puberty. The incidence of dandruff and seborrheic dermatitis appears to peak

KEY FACTS

Description
A fungal infection of the genital tract, mouth, or the skin.

Causes
The fungus *Candida albicans*.

Risk factors
Pregnancy, diabetes, a suppressed immune system, and the use of antibiotics, birth control pills, or steroids. Women are at highest risk.

Symptoms
Vaginal itching, redness, pain while urinating, a thick white discharge from the vagina, or white patches in the mouth.

Diagnosis
Laboratory cultures from swabs of the infected area.

Treatments
Antifungal medicines can be taken orally or applied directly to the infected area.

Pathogenesis
Candida is normally present, but grows out of control during infections. In rare cases, an untreated infection can reach the bloodstream and spread throughout the body.

Prevention
Moist, warm conditions, and nylon underwear should be avoided; cotton is a better choice. Skin should be kept clean and dry.

Epidemiology
Roughly 75 percent of women will have a vaginal infection at least once in their lifetime. Genital infections in men are rare.

around age 40. Hormones appear to play a factor, because men are at greater risk than women. People with weakened immune systems are also at greater risk, as are patients with Parkinson's disease and epilepsy, although it is not clear why the disorders are linked. Dandruff is not caused by dry skin or frequent shampooing. In fact, oily skin is a known risk factor.

Symptoms, diagnosis, and pathogenesis

Vaginal yeast infections produce itching, redness, and a thick white discharge. Infections in the mouth and throat produce patchy white areas. This infection is commonly called "thrush." In babies, the moist damp skin inside a diaper is a prime breeding ground for the fungus. The rash causes weepy, red pustules. Candidemia is an invasive form of the disease. It is one of the most common bloodstream infections found in hospitalized patients and is potentially fatal.

Laboratory tests can identify the candida microbe, but the symptoms are often sufficient for a doctor to make a diagnosis.

Depending on the microbe responsible, paronychia can produce swollen, tender nails with pus-filled abscesses during an acute infection. Chronic infections can spread to include nail discoloration as well as redness and swelling of the nail folds. In rare cases, the infection can spread across the hand and throughout the body as a systemic infection.

Reddish patches with white crusts and oily skin are typical in patients with seborrheic dermatitis. In the milder case of dandruff, the major symptom is an itchy, flaky scalp. The infections can be persistent but are generally mild in nature.

Treatments and prevention

Keeping the skin clean and dry can prevent many yeast infections. Women should use cotton underwear and avoid nylon pantyhose and other tight-fitting clothes. Deodorants, bubble baths, and douches can irritate the vagina and should be avoided.

It is still not clear if eating yogurt can prevent vaginal yeast infections, but yogurt with active cultures does contain lactobacilli, which are beneficial bacteria that can normally be found in the vagina.

If an infection occurs, it can be treated with antifungal ointments or pills. Recurrent infections can be more troublesome if resistance occurs. In the case of candidemia, intravenous medication may be required.

Soaking the infected nails can help to relieve the pressure and infection in paronychia. However, in most cases, an antibacterial or antifungal agent will be

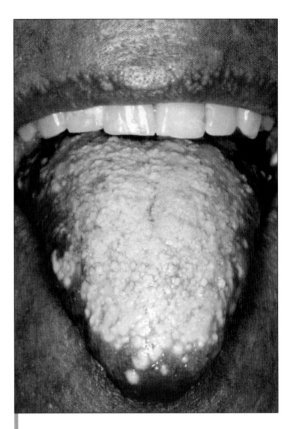

This thick, creamy coating on the tongue is a symptom of severe oral candidiasis (thrush). Candidiasis is an infection caused by a yeastlike fungus, usually Candida albicans.

required to clear up the infection. Chronic cases involving fungal infections can be very difficult to cure and require several weeks or even months of treatment. The best prevention is good nail care. This includes trimming nails regularly, avoiding the use of irritating cuticle removers, and not chewing or biting the nails. Rubber gloves with cotton liners should be used to protect the nails and hands from water and chemical irritants.

Dandruff is best controlled with a medicated shampoo that targets the yeast growing on the scalp. The shampoos need to be left on the scalp for several minutes and should be used regularly until the scalp recovers. Seborrheic dermatitis is usually treated with topical ointments ketoconazole, selenium sulfide, pyrithione zinc, and corticosteroids.

Chris Curran

See also

• Diabetes • Infections, fungal • Pregnancy and childbirth • Skin disorders

Yellow fever

Yellow fever is caused by the yellow fever virus (YFV). The virus is transmitted by mosquitoes. Infection can cause rapid liver failure, hemorrhage, and death within 10 days of onset. In the past, yellow fever occurred in coastal cities of the United States and in many European cities. However, as a result of mosquito eradication programs and the development of an effective live attenuated vaccine in the 1930s, it is now largely restricted to regions of tropical Africa and South America.

Yellow fever is a mosquito-transmitted viral disease occurring in tropical regions of Africa and South America. It may affect both genders equally at any age, although because of a forest cycle involving wild primates, in South America men are more at risk as a result of their occupation as forestry workers. Because of the occurrence of yellow fever in remote locations with poor communications, accurate information is difficult to obtain, and it is believed that official reports may greatly underestimate actual numbers. Between 2000 and 2005 there were 3,309 cases officially reported from Africa and 657 cases from South America. However, the World Health Organization estimates that there may be 200,000 human infections each year with 30,000 deaths, 90 percent occurring in Africa.

Causes and risk factors

The causative agent, yellow fever virus, is transmitted to people via the bite of infected mosquitoes. The most frequent mosquito vector in urban outbreaks is *Aedes aegypti*, a species that breeds in close proximity to humans, laying eggs in any small container that contains water. It feeds preferentially on people and has been responsible for large urban epidemics. Other species are involved in rural and jungle cycles. Not being vaccinated is a significant risk factor, especially for those entering endemic areas and likely to come in contact with infected mosquitoes. The recent development of the ecotourism industry is providing new opportunities for people to visit regions in which yellow fever may occur. Since 1996, at least six travelers (from Belgium, Germany, Switzerland, and the United States) have died of yellow fever virus infections acquired while visiting Africa or South America.

Symptoms, signs, and diagnosis

Symptoms of infection are variable, probably as a result of natural human resistance factors, and perhaps differences between virus strains. Less than 30 percent of people who are infected become sick. The incubation period is 3 to 6 days. Disease can be characterized into three phases. The "period of infection," which lasts 3 to 4 days, presents as mild nonspecific and flulike symptoms, with fever up to 105°F (40.6°C) lasting for three and half days with fatigue, headache, photophobia, back pain and general myalgia, nausea, vomiting, and disorientation and dizziness. In relation to the

KEY FACTS

Description

A viral disease that infects the liver.

Cause

Infection with yellow fever virus.

Risk factors

Mosquito bites, mainly in Africa but also in South America. Lack of vaccination.

Symptoms

Flulike symptoms progressing to fatal multi-organ failure. In severe cases, fatality rates range from 20 percent to over 50 percent, with death occurring 8 to 10 days after first symptoms.

Diagnosis

Examination by experienced medical personnel; tests of blood and tissue samples. Protocols for rapid diagnosis using polymerase chain reactions.

Treatments

No specific treatment is available. Where conditions permit, supportive care, including nutritional and fluid maintenance, dialysis, and transfusion, may be administered.

Pathogenesis

Liver damage. Eosinophilic degeneration also occurs in the tubular epithelium of the kidneys.

Prevention

Long-term protection is provided by vaccination with a live vaccine, recommended to travelers visiting areas where the disease is endemic.

Epidemiology

The virus is typically transmitted in a forest cycle between mosquitoes and primates. Although large-scale epidemics are infrequent due to vaccination and mosquito control, yellow fever is regarded as a reemerging disease because of an increasing number of cases over the last 25 years.

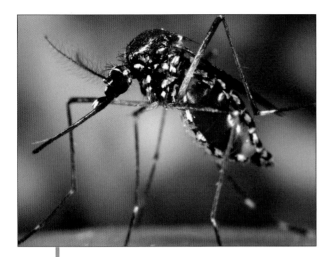

A female A. aegypti *mosquito is about to fly off a host's skin surface after obtaining a blood meal.*

fever, the pulse rate is slow. The tongue is characteristically bright red at the tip and sides, with a central white coating, and the liver may be tender and enlarged. The virus may be isolated from the blood at this stage, and serum transaminase levels are elevated. During the "period of remission" the fever and symptoms wane, and most patients continue to recover. However, after 48 hours, about 15 percent of patients progress to the "period of intoxication." Although anti-YFV antibodies can now be detected, and the virus disappears from the blood, fever and vomiting return, and the patient becomes jaundiced; hence the name *yellow fever*.

Specific diagnosis can now be made based on laboratory detection of viral antigen and specific antibodies using a variety of techniques including enzyme-linked immunosorbent assay (ELISA), hemagglutination inhibition, complement fixation, neutralization tests, immunofluorescence assays, and viral isolation in culture or mice. Polymerase chain reactions (PCR) assays to detect viral nucleic acids in blood and tissues have been developed and will accelerate detection in the future.

About 20 percent of patients with jaundice die as a result of multi-organ failure. Symptoms are complex, but patients can become delirious with convulsions, vomit blood that is blackened as a result of the action of gastric juices (so-called coffee-grounds vomit), and lapse into a coma prior to death. Postmortem diagnosis is based on unique liver pathology, including the detection of "councilman bodies," which are liver cells degenerated by white blood cells. In patients who survive, recovery may take several weeks.

Treatment and prevention

No specific treatment exists, although supportive measures, including nutritional maintenance, fluid replacement, aspiration to prevent gastric swelling, administration of oxygen and vasoactive drugs (affecting dilation or constriction of blood vessels), transfusion of plasma, and dialysis, may all be required to sustain life in severe cases. The live attenuated 17D vaccine, available from travel clinics and hospitals, is regarded as one of the safest and most effective vaccines available. Revaccination is advised at ten-year intervals, although a single dose may provide lifelong protection.

Epidemiology

Yellow fever probably arose in Africa and spread as a result of the slave trade. There is a jungle cycle in Africa that involves *A. africanus* and other mosquito species that feed upon wild primates, and there is a so-called intermediate cycle in moist savanna regions. In South America, a jungle cycle also exists, involving *Haemagogus* and *Sabethes* species of mosquito. The South American primates succumb to fatal infection.

For humans, the most important cycle is the urban cycle, involving transmission between *A. aegypti* and people. In the urban setting, transmission can be intense, and if not controlled can result in massive epidemics. Urban cycles have not been observed in tropical South America since 1942. A few cases have been reported from South American towns and cities, and urban transmission is still reported in Africa, especially in Nigeria. The continuing pattern of increasing numbers of yellow fever cases over recent years may be the result of several factors. In many countries, vaccination programs and mosquito control efforts have not been sustained because of economic reasons. More people are moving from rural areas to urban towns and cities, and most of these people are unvaccinated, so uncontrolled outbreaks occur before emergency vaccination campaigns can be organized. Because the principal mosquito vector, *A. aegypti*, is widely distributed and since the 1970s has become reestablished in many South American cities, the risk of urban transmission of yellow fever virus is also increasing in that continent.

Global warming may represent a new threat, since *A. aegypti* may expand its range into regions in which it has not previously occurred.

Stephen Higgs

See also
• Infections, viral

Resources for Further Study

General Reference Works

American College of Physicians. 2003. *Complete Home Medical Guide.* New York: DK Publishing, Inc.

American Medical Association. 2006. *Concise Medical Encyclopedia.* New York: Random House Information Group.

American Psychiatric Association (APA). 2000. *Diagnostic and Statistical Manual of Mental Disorders.* 4th ed. Washington, D.C.: APA.

Clayman, Charles, ed. 2005. *The Human Body.* New York: DK Publishing, Inc.

Gray, Henry, and H. V. Carter (illustrator). 2000. *Gray's Anatomy.* New York: Barnes and Noble.

Labrecque, Mary C., Robert Pantell, Harold C. Sox, Timothy B. Walsh, and John H. Wasson. 2002. *Common Symptom Guide.* Columbus, OH: McGraw-Hill.

Marks, Andrea, and Betty Rothbart. 2003. *Healthy Teens, Body and Soul: A Parent's Complete Guide to Adolescent Health.* New York: Simon and Schuster.

Sultz, Harry A., and Kristina M. Young. 2005. *Health Care USA: Understanding Its Organization and Delivery.* Sudbury, MA: Jones and Bartlett Publishers, Inc.

Infections

Bennett, John E., Raphael Dolin, and Gerald L. Mandell. 2004. *Mandell, Douglas, and Bennett's Principles and Practice of Infectious Diseases.* Philadelphia: Elsevier Churchill Livingstone.

Black, Samuel J., Peter J. Krause, Dennis J. Richardson, and Richard J. Seed, eds. 2002. *North American Parasitic Zoonoses.* Boston, MA: Kluwer Academic Publishers.

Bottone, Edward J. 2003. *An Atlas of Infectious Diseases.* Boca Raton, FL: CRC Press.

Callahan, Gerald N. 2006. *Infection: The Uninvited Universe.* New York: St. Martin's Press.

Chiodini, Jane. 2004. *Atlas of Travel Medicine and Health.* Ontario: B. C. Decker Inc.

Davidson, Robert, Michael Eddleston, Stephen Pierini, and Robert Wilkinson. 2004. *Oxford Handbook of Tropical Medicine.* Oxford, UK: Oxford University Press.

Fauci, Anthony S., John I. Gallin, and Richard Krause, eds. 2000. *Emerging Infections.* Burlington, MA: Elsevier Science.

Freeman-Cook, Kevin, Lisa Freeman-Cook, and Edward Alcamo, eds. 2005. *Staphylococcus Aureus Infections.* New York: Chelsea House Publishers.

Gittleman, Ann Louise, and Omar M. Amin. 2001. *Guess What Came to Dinner: Parasites and Your Health.* Wayne NJ: Avery.

Gualde, Norbert, and Steven Rendall (translator). 2006. *Resistance: The Human Struggle against Infection.* Washington, DC: Dana Press.

Hart, Tony. 2004. *Microterrors: The Complete Guide to Bacterial, Viral, and Fungal Infections That Threaten Our Health.* Toronto: Firefly Books, Ltd.

Heelan, Judith Stephenson. 2004. *Cases in Human Parasitology.* Herndon, VA: ASM Press.

Henderson, Gregory, Allan Warshowsky, and Batya S. Yasgur. 2002. *Women at Risk: The HPV Epidemic and Your Cervical Health.* Wayne, NJ: Avery.

Irving, William L., John W. McCauley, and Dave J. Rowlands, eds. 2001. *New Challenges to Health.* NY: Cambridge University Press.

Martin, Jeanne Marie. 2000. *Complete Candida Yeast Guidebook.* New York: Crown Publishing Group.

Mandell, Gerald L., John E. Bennett, and Raphael Dolin, eds. 2004. *Mandell, Douglas, and Bennett's Principles and Practice of Infectious Diseases,* 6th ed. Philadelphia: Elsevier Churchill Livingstone.

Molyneux, David H., ed. 2006. *Control of Human Parasitic Diseases.* Burlington, MA: Elsevier Science and Technology.

Regush, Nicholas. *The Virus Within.* 2000. New York: Penguin Group.

Richardson, Malcolm D., and David W. Warnock. 2003. *Fungal Infection, Diagnosis and Management.* Malden, MA: Blackwell Publishing.

Sfakianos, Jeffrey N. 2006. *Avian Flu,* edited by I. Edward Alcamo. New York: Chelsea House Publishers.

Sherman, Irwin W. 2006. *Power of Plagues.* Herndon, VA: ASM Press.

Shmaefsky, Brian Robert. 2004. *Meningitis,* edited by I. Edward Alcamo. New York: Chelsea House Publishers.

Superficial Fungal Infections. 2002. UK: Health Press.

Noninfectious disorders
Addiction

Bellenir, Karen, ed. 2002. *Drug Information for Teens: Health Tips about the Physical and Mental Effects of Substance Abuse,* Detroit, MI: Omnigraphics, Inc.

Brick, John, ed. 2004. *Handbook of the Medical Consequences of Alcohol and Drug Abuse.* New York: Haworth Press.

Carson-DeWitt, R., ed. 2001. *Encyclopedia of Drugs, Alcohol, and Addictive Behavior.* 2nd ed. Farmington Hills, MI: Macmillan Reference USA.

Conyers, Beverly. 2003. *Addict in the Family: Stories of Loss, Hope, and Recovery.* Center City, MN: Hazelden.

Ehrlich, Caryl. 2003. *Conquer Your Food Addiction.* New York: The Free Press.

Griffin, Kevin. 2004. *One Breath at a Time: Buddhism and the Twelve Steps.* Emmaus, PA: Rodale.

Nakken, Craig. 1996. *The Addictive Personality: Understanding the Addictive Process and Compulsive Behavior.* Center City, MN: Hazelden.

United Nations Office for Drug Control and Crime Prevention. 2003. *Alcohol and Drug Problems at Work: The Shift to Prevention.* Geneva: ILO.

Aging
Bullen, Timothy, and Anthony Campbell. 2004. *The Directory of Your Back, Your Bones, and Things That Ache.* Secaucus NJ: Chartwell Books, Inc.

Whitbourne, Susan Krauss. 2004. *Adult Development and Aging: Biopsychosocial Perspectives.* New York: John Wiley & Sons, Inc.

AIDS
Greene, Warner C., Merle A.Sande, and Paul Volberding, ed. 2007. *Global HIV/AIDS Medicine.* St. Louis, MO: Saunders Publishing.

Allergies
Mitchell, Dean. 2006. *The Allergy and Asthma Cure: A Revolutionary New Treatment Program for All Airborne Allergies and Asthma.* New York: Marlowe & Company.

Arterial disorders
Gersh, B. J. 2000. *Mayo Clinic Heart Book: The Ultimate Guide to Heart Health.* New York: W. Morrow.

Arthritis
Bruce, Debra Fulgham. 2003. *Pain-Free Arthritis.* New York: Henry Holt & Company, Inc.

O'Driscoll, Erin Rohan. 2004. *Exercises for Arthritis.* New York: Hatherleigh Press.

Vad, Vijay. 2006. *Arthritis Rx.* New York: Penguin Group.

Backache
Freedman, Janet, and Elaine Petrone. 2003. *The Miracle Ball Method.* New York: Workman Publishing Company, Inc.

Katz, Jeffrey N., and Gloria Parkinson. 2007. *Heal Your Aching Back.* Columbus, OH: McGraw-Hill.

Kubey, Craig, and Robin A. McKenzie. 2001. *Seven Steps to a Pain-Free Life.* New York: Penguin Group.

Blood disorders
Sutton, Amy L. 2005. *Blood and Circulatory Disorders Sourcebook.* Detroit, MI: Omnigraphics, Inc.

Cancer
Black, Peter, and Sharon Cloud Hogan. 2006. *Living with a Brain Tumor.* New York: Henry Holt & Company, Inc.

Mayer, Musa. 2003. *After Breast Cancer.* Sebastopol, CA: O'Reilly Media, Inc.

Tsupruk, Pavel. 2005. *Prevent Cancer Today.* Frederick, MD: PublishAmerica.

Weinberg, Robert A. 2006. *Biology of Cancer.* Oxford, UK: Taylor & Francis, Inc.

Chronic fatigue syndrome
Friedberg, Fred, and Jacob Teitelbaum. 2006. *Fibromyalgia and Chronic Fatigue Syndrome.* Oakland, CA: New Harbinger Publications.

Dental disorders
Sutton, Amy. 2003. *Dental Care and Oral Health Sourcebook: Basic Consumer Health Information about Dental Care, including Hygiene, Dental Visits, Pain Management, Cavities, Crowns, Bridges, Dental Implants, and Other Oral Health Concerns.* Detroit MI: Omnigraphics, Inc.

Diabetes
American Diabetes Association. 2000. *Diabetes and Pregnancy: What to Expect.* Alexandria, VA: American Diabetes Association.

Becker, Gretchen E. 2001. *The First Year —Type 2 Diabetes.* New York: Avalon Publishing Group, Inc.

Endocrinology
Gordon, John D., Dan I. Lebovic, and Robert N. Taylor. 2005. *Reproductive Endocrinology and Infertility.* Glen Cove, NY: Scrub Hill Press.

Kronenberg, Henry M., Reed P. Larsen, Shlomo Melmed, and Kenneth S. Polonsky. 2003. *Williams Textbook of Endocrinology.* Philadelphia, PA: Elsevier Health Sciences.

Environmental disorders
Brebbia, C. A., D. Fayzieva, and V. Popov. 2005. *Environmental Health Risk III*, Vol. 9. WIT Press.

Eye disorders
Billig, Michael D., Gary H. Cassel, and Harry G. Randall. 1998. *Eye Book: A Complete Guide to Eye Disorders and Health.* Baltimore, MD: Johns Hopkins University Press.

Mogk, Lylas G., and Daniel L. Roberts. 2006. *Age-Related Macular Degeneration: An Essential Guide to the Newly Diagnosed.* New York: Avalon Publishing Group, Inc.

Shaw, Kimberley Williams, and Amy Sutton. 2003. *Eye Care*

Sourcebook. Detroit, MI: Omnigraphics, Inc.

Genetic disorders and birth defects

Iannucci, Lisa. 2000. *Birth Defects.* Berkeley Heights, NJ: Enslow Publishers Inc.

Wynbrandt, James. 2007. *Encyclopedia of Genetic Disorders and Birth Defects.* New York: Facts on File.

Heart disease

Cohen, B. M., and B. Hasselbring. 2002. *Coronary Heart Disease: A Guide to Diagnosis and Treatment.* Omaha, NE: Addicus Books.

Esselstyn, Caldwell. 2007. *Prevent and Reverse Heart Disease.* New York: Penguin Group.

Gersh, B. J. 2000. *Mayo Clinic Heart Book: The Ultimate Guide to Heart Health.* New York: W. Morrow.

Katzenstein, Larry, and Ileana L. Pina. 2007. *Living with Heart Disease.* New York: Sterling Publishing.

Sheps, Sheldon G. 2003. *Mayo Clinic on High Blood Pressure.* New York: Mayo Foundation for Medical Education & Research.

Hepatitis

Wright, Lloyd. 2002. *Triumph over Hepatitis C.* Malibu, CA: Lloyd Wright Publishing.

Herpes

Connolly, Sean. 2002. *STDs.* Portsmouth, NH: Heinemann.

Stanberry, Lawrence. 2006. *Understanding Herpes.* Jackson, MS: University Press of Mississippi.

Hormonal disorders

Isaacs, Scott, Todd Leopold, and Neil Shulman. 2006. *Hormonal Balance: Understanding Hormones, Weight, and Your Metabolism.* Boulder, CO: Bull Publishing Company.

Immune system

Sompayrac, Lauren. 2003. *How the Immune System Works.* Malden, MA: Blackwell Publishing.

Kidney disorders

Cheung, Alfred K., and Arthur Greenberg, ed. 2005. *Primer of Kidney Diseases.* Philadelphia, PA: Elsevier Health Sciences.

Lupus

Wallace, Daniel J. 2005. *Lupus Book: A Guide for Patients and Their Families.* Oxford, UK: Oxford University Press.

Motor neuron disease

Eisen, Andrew, and Pamela Shaw, eds. 2007. *Motor Neuron Disorders and Related Diseases.* Philadelphia, PA: Elsevier Health Sciences.

Multiple sclerosis

Blackstone, Margaret. 2003. *The First Year—Multiple Sclerosis: An Essential Guide for the Newly Diagnosed.* New York: Avalon.

Hill, Beth, and Joanne Wojcieszek. 2003. *Multiple Sclerosis Q & A: Reassuring Answers to Frequently Asked Questions.* New York: Penguin Group.

Obesity

Brownell, Kelly, and Katherine Horgen. 2004. *Food Fight: The Inside Story of the Food Industry, America's Obesity Crisis, and What We Can Do about It.* Columbus, OH: McGraw-Hill.

Koplan, Jeffrey P., ed. 2005. *Preventing Childhood Obesity: Health in the Balance.* Washington, DC: National Academies Press.

Pain

Abelson, Brian, Kamali Abelson, and Michael P. Leahy. 2005. *Release Your Pain: Resolving Repetitive Strain Injuries with Active Release Techniques.* Berkeley, CA: North Atlantic Books.

Ballantyne, Jane C. 2005. *The Massachusetts General Hospital Handbook of Pain Management.* 2005. Baltimore, MD: Lippincott Williams & Wilkins Publishers.

Egoscue, Pete, and Roger Gittines. 2000. *Pain Free: A Revolutionary Method for Stopping Chronic Pain.* New York: Bantam Books.

Parkinson's disease

Schwarz, Shelley Peterman. 2006. *Parkinson's Disease: 300 Tips for Making Life Easier.* New York: Demos Medical Publishing, LLC.

Prostate disorders

Kelman, Judith, and Peter T. Scardino. 2005. *Dr. Peter Scardino's Prostate Book: The Complete Guide to Overcoming Prostate Cancer, Prostatitis, and BPH.* Wayne, NJ: Avery.

Psychotherapy and psychology

Leszcz, Molyn, and Irvin D. Yalom. 2005. *The Theory and Practice of Group Psychotherapy.* New York: Basic Books.

Reproductive system

DeZarn, Christine (foreword), Milton Hammerly, and Cheryl Kimball. 2003. *What to Do When the Doctor Says It's PCOS.* Gloucester, MA: Rockport Publishers.

Heffner, Linda, and Danny J. Schust. 2006. *Reproductive System at a Glance.* Malden, MA: Blackwell Publishing.

Manassiev, Nikolai, and Malcolm I. Whitehead. 2003. *Female Reproductive Health.* Boca Raton, FL: CRC Press.

Thatcher, Samuel S. 2000. *PCOS (Polycystic Ovarian Syndrome): The Hidden Epidemic.* Indianapolis, IN: Perspectives Press, Inc.

Respiratory disorders

Broaddus, Courtney V., Robert J. Mason, John F. Murray, and Jay A. Nadel. 2005. *Murray and Nadel's Textbook of Respiratory Medicine.* Philadelphia PA: Elsevier Health Sciences.

Sexual and gender identity disorders

Drescher, Jack, and Dan Karasic, eds. 2006. *Sexual and Gender*

Diagnoses of the Diagnostic and Statistical Manual (DSM). New York: Haworth Press, Inc.

Sexually transmitted diseases

Parker, James N., and Philip M. Parker, eds. 2002. *The Official Patient's Sourcebook on Bacterial STDs.* San Diego, CA: ICON Health Publications.

Skin disorders

Goroway, Patricia, and Richard H. Keller. 2006. *Facial Fitness: Daily Exercises and Massage Techniques for a Healthier, Younger Looking You.* New York: Barnes and Noble Books.

Mancini, Anthony J., and Amy S. Paller. 2005. *Hurwitz Clinical Pediatric Dermatology: A Textbook of Skin Disorders of Childhood and Adolescence.* 2005. Orlando, FL: W. B. Saunders Publisher.

SIDS

Byard, Roger W., and Henry F. Krous, eds. 2001. *Sudden Infant Death Syndrome: Problems, Progress, and Possibilities.* London, UK: Hodder Arnold.

Sleep disorders

Breus, Michael. 2006. *Good Night: The Sleep Doctor's 4-Week Program to Better Sleep and Better Health.* New York: Penguin Group USA.

Buysse, Daniel J., ed. 2005. *Sleep Disorders and Psychiatry*, Vol. 24. Arlington, VA: American Psychiatric Publishing, Incorporated.

Urinary system disorders

Datta, Shreelata. 2003. *Crash Course: Renal and Urinary Systems.* Philadelphia, PA: Elsevier Health Sciences.

Mental disorders

Abel, Kathryn M., David Castle, and Jayashri Kulkarni, eds. 2006. *Mood and Anxiety Disorders in Women.* NY: Cambridge University Press.

Andrews, Linda Wasmer, and Dwight L. Evans. 2005. *If Your Adolescent Has Depression or Bipolar Disorder: An Essential Resource for Parents.* 2005. Oxford, UK: Oxford University Press.

Attwood, Tony (foreword), and Isabelle Henault. 2005. *Asperger's Syndrome and Sexuality: From Adolescence through Adulthood.* London, UK: Jessica Kingsley Publishers.

Barkley, Russell A., and Eric J. Mash, eds. 2006. *The Treatment of Childhood Disorders.* New York: Guilford Publications, Inc.

Brown, Thomas. 2005. *Attention Deficit Disorders: The Unfocused Mind in Children and Adults.* New Haven, CT: Yale University Press.

Brownell, Kelly D., and Christopher G. Fairburn. 2005. *Eating Disorders and Obesity: A Comprehensive Handbook.* New York: Guilford Publications, Inc.

Buckman, Dana, and Charlotte Farber. 2006. *A Special Education: One Family's Journey Through the Maze of Learning Disabilities.* New York, NY: Da Capo Press.

Davidson, Larry D. 2003. *Living Outside Mental Illness: Qualitative Studies of Recovery in Schizophrenia.* New York: New York University Press.

Earley, Pete. 2007. *Crazy: A Father's Search through America's Mental Health Madness.* New York: Penguin.

Findling, Robert L., Elena Harlan, and Charles S. Schulz. 2000. *Psychotic Disorders in Children and Adolescents.* Thousand Oaks, CA: Sage Publications.

Guyol, Gracelyn, and Stephen T. Sinatra. 2006. *Healing Depression and Bipolar Disorder without Drugs.* New York: Walker & Company.

Handler, Lowell, and Elkhonon Goldberg (foreword) and Neal R. Swerdlow (afterword). 2004. *Twitch and Shout: A Touretter's Tale.* Minneapolis, MN: University of Minnesota Press.

Kingdon, David G., and Douglas Turkington. 2004. *Cognitive Therapy of Schizophrenia.* 2004. New York: Guilford Publications, Incorporated.

Kreisman, Jerold J., and Hal Straus. 2006. *Sometimes I Act Crazy: Living with Borderline Personality Disorder.* 2006. New York: John Wiley & Sons, Inc.

Le Grange, Daniel, and James Lock. 2004. *Help Your Teenager Beat an Eating Disorder.* New York: Guilford Publications, Inc.

Miklowitz, David J. 2002. *The Bipolar Disorder Survival Guide.* New York: Guilford Publications, Inc.

Nicholl, Malcolm J., and Jacqueline B. Stordy. 2000. *LCP Solution: The Remarkable Nutritional Treatment for ADHD, Dyslexia and Dyspraxia.* New York: Random House Publishing Group.

Notbohm, Ellen. 2005. *Ten Things Every Child with Autism Wishes You Knew.* Arlington, TX: Future Horizons, Inc.

Rosen, Gerald, ed. 2004. *Posttraumatic Stress Disorder.* New York: John Wiley & Sons, Inc.

Sarno, John E. 2006. *Divided Mind: The Epidemic of Mindbody Disorders.* New York: HarperCollins Publishers.

Tammet, Daniel. 2007. *Born on a Blue Day: Inside the Extraordinary Mind of an Autistic Savant.* New York: Simon and Schuster Adult Publishing Group.

Wagner, Aureen. 2004. *Up and Down the Worry Hill: A Children's Book about Obsessive-Compulsive Disorder.* Rochester: Lighthouse Press, Incorporated.

HEALTH HOTLINES

AIDS/HIV Treatment, Prevention, and Research   800-HIV-0440

Alcohol and Drug Abuse
800-729-6686

Alzheimer's Disease
800-438-4380

American Medical Association   312-645-5000

American Public Health Association
202-789-5600

Americans with Disabilities Act Information and Assistance Hotline   800-949-4232

Cancer   800-4-CANCER
800-422-6237

Centers for Disease Control and Prevention
404-639-3311

Child Health and Human Development
800-370-2493

Department of Transportation's Hotline for Air Travelers with Disabilities
1-800-778-4838 (voice)

Diabetes   800-860-8747

Digestive Diseases   800-891-5389

Drug Abuse   301-443-1124

Endocrine and Metabolic Disorders
888-828-0904

Eye Diseases   301-496-5248

Food and Drug Administration (FDA)
301-443-2410

Genetic and Rare Diseases   888-205-2311

Human Genome Research   301-402-0911

Mental Health and Mental Illness
301-443-4513

National Herpes Hotline   919-361-8488

National Mental Health Association
800-969-NHMA (6642)

National Pediatric and Family HIV Resource Center
973-972-0410
800-362-0071

National Suicide Prevention Lifeline
800-273-TALK (8255)

Neurological Disorders
800-352-9424

Ovulation Research   888-644-8891

Pharmaceutical Research and Manufacturer's Association (drug information)
202–835-3400

Schizophrenia Research
888-674-6464

SIDS (Sudden infant death syndrome)
800-505-CRIB

Smoking Cessation, NCI's Smoking Quitline
877-44U-QUIT

Stroke   800-352-9424

Teens AIDS Hotline   800-283-2473

WE CAN (Ways to Enhance Children's Activity and Nutrition)   866-35-WE-CAN

Weight Control   877-946-4627

Women's Health   301-496-8176

WEB RESOURCES

The following World Wide Web sources feature information useful for students, teachers, and health care professionals. By necessity, this list is only a representative sampling; many government bodies, charities, and professional organizations not listed have Web sites that are also worth investigating. Other Internet resources, such as newsgroups, also exist and can be explored for further research. Please note that all URLs have a tendency to change; addresses were functional and accurate as of April 2007.

American Academy of Family Physicians

www.familydoctor.org
The Web site supplies health information and an A–Z index of conditions that can be accessed with links for different groups of people.

American Academy of Orthopaedic Surgeons

www.orthoinfo.aaos.org
Information on growth plate fractures, knee ligament injuries, and impact of osteoarthritis of the knee.

American Cancer Society

www.cancer.org
A self-help Web site for patients, family, and friends to learn about cancer, treatment options, clinical trials, and coping with the disease. There are links to connect patients with cancer survivors and support programs.

American College Health Association

www.acha.org
ACHA aims to provide advocacy, education, communications, products, and services, as well as to promote research and culturally competent practices to enhance its members' ability to advance the health of all students and the campus community.

American Heart Association

www.americanheart.org
A comprehensive Web site including many suggestions for a better lifestyle to reduce the risk of a heart attack; warning signs; and explanations of diseases and conditions.

American Social Health Association

www.ashastd.org
ASHA aims to improve the health of individuals, families, and communities, with emphasis on the prevention of sexually transmitted diseases and infections (STDs/STIs). The site lists information about specific STDs/STIs, tips for reducing risk, and ways to talk with health care providers and partners.

Aurora Health Care

www.aurorahealthcare.org/aboutus/mission.asp
A not-for-profit organization with a mission to promote health, prevent illness, and provide state of the art diagnosis and treatment to meet individual and family needs.

Birth Defect Research for Children

www.birthdefects.org
This resource provides free information about birth defects and details about parent networking and birth defect research through the National Birth Defect Registry.

Centers for Disease Control and Prevention

www.cdc.gov
Government-compiled health information, including health statistics, links to other Web sites, and research and development.

Childhelp

www.childhelp.org
Childhelp is dedicated to meeting the physical, emotional, and spiritual needs of abused and neglected children by focusing on prevention, intervention, and treatment. The Childhelp National Child Abuse Hotline, 1-800-4-A-CHILD, operates 24 hours a day, 7 days a week.

Mayo Clinic

www.mayoclinic.com
A site produced by a collective of medical experts with the aim of helping people manage their health. Information is up to date and many health issues are discussed.

MedlinePlus

www.nlm.nih.gov/medlineplus
U.S. National Library of Medicine.

National Cancer Institute

www.cancer.gov

National Institutes of Health (U.S. Department of Health and Human Services)

www.nih.gov
Health information with an A–Z index of NIH resources, clinical trials, health hotlines, and drug information. Also includes MedlinePlus.

National Institute of Neurological Disorders and Stroke

www.ninds.nih.gov/disorders/stroke/stroke_needtoknow.htm#URGENT
Information about strokes.

National Mental Health Information Center

mentalhealth.samhsa.gov

All aspects of mental health are covered on this site, which provides links to a large spectrum of topics. A drop-down menu allows users to look for mental health and substance abuse services by state.

Nutrition Source

www.hsph.harvard.edu/ nutritionsource

The site supplies clear tips for healthy eating and dispels nutrition myths. Gives advice on what foods to eat and why.

TeenGrowth

www.teengrowth.com

Health information specifically for teens; debates on relevant topics.

U.S. National AIDS Hotlines and Resources

www.thebody.com/hotlines/ national.html

This site supplies hotline numbers for every group of people who are affected by AIDS or HIV.

U. S. National Library of Medicine (National Institutes of Health)

www.nlm.nih.gov

This Web site provides links to authoritative health information resources on hundreds of diseases, conditions, and health topics.

World Health Organization (WHO)

www.who.int/about/en

WHO is the United Nations' specialized agency for health. WHO's mission is the attainment by all peoples of the highest possible level of health. Health is defined as not just the absence of disease but a positive state of physical, mental, and social well-being.

Specific disorders

Alcohol and Bone Health

www.niams.nih.gov/bone/h/ fitness_bonehealth.htm

Arthritis/Scleroderma Fact Sheet

www.mayoclinic.com/health/ scleroderma/DS00362

Carpal Tunnel Syndrome Fact Sheet

www.ninds.nih.gov/disorders/carpal _tunnel/detail_carpal_tunnel.htm

CDC Travelers' Health: Yellow Book

www2.ncid.cdc.gov/travel/yb/utils/ ybGet.asp?section=dis&obj= aftrypano.htm

Center for the Evaluation of Risks to Human Reproduction, National Toxicology Program, Department of Health and Human Services

cerhr.niehs.nih.gov

Emergency Preparedness and Response: Fact Sheet

www.bt.cdc.gov/radiation/ars.asp

Kids and Their Bones

www.niams.nih.gov/hi/topics/ osteoporosis/kidbones.htm

Maintain a Healthy Back

www.nih.gov/od/ors/ds/ ergonomics/wellbackhealth.html

National Institute of Diabetes, Digestive, and Kidney Diseases

www.niddk.nih.gov/index.htm

North American Spine Society

www.spin.ors/fsp/anatomy-functions
Details the anatomy of the spine.

Oral and Throat Cancer

www.mayoclinic.com/health/ oral-and-throat-cancer/DS00349

Peptic Ulcer

www.mayoclinic.com/health/ peptic-ulcer/DS00242

Polio Eradication

www.who.int/mediacentre/ factsheets/fs114/en
www.polioeradication.org/history.asp

Public Health Emergencies: Radiological Hazards

www.in.gov/isdh/bioterrorism/ manual/section_11.htm

Questions and Answers about Scoliosis in Children and Adolescents

www.niams.nih.gov/hi/topics/ scoliosis/scochild.htm

Questions and Answers about Knee Problems

www.nimas.nih.gov/hi/topics/ kneeprobs/kneeqa.htm

Radiation Sickness

www.britannica.com

Radiation Sickness

www.mayoclinic.com/health/ radiation sickness/DS00432/ DSECTION=2

Scleroderma Fact Sheet

www.medicinenet.com/ scleroderma/article.htm

Scleroderma Research Foundation

www.srfcure.org/srf/patients/ whatis.htm

Sleeping Sickness

www.who.int/mediacentre/ factsheets/fs259/en/

Toxoplasmosis Fact Sheet

www.cdc.gov/ncidod/dpd/ parasites/toxoplasmosis/ factsht_toxoplasmosis.htm

Glossary

achondroplasia
Genetic disorder causing severe limitation of skeletal growth.

acromegaly
Abnormal enlargement of face, hands, and feet as a result of a tumor of the pituitary gland.

acute
A term that describes an illness of sudden onset, which may or may not be severe but is usually of short duration.

affective flattening
A lack of emotional response.

AIDS
Acquired immunodeficiency syndrome. Caused by HIV (human immunodeficiency virus), AIDS leads to potentially fatal depression of the immune system.

albinism
A condition characterized by a lack of pigment in the hair, eyes, and skin.

alcoholism
Addiction to alcohol, which can lead to deterioration in physical and psychological health, family life, and social position.

allergen
A substance that causes an allergy.

allergy
Hypersensitive reaction, such as wheezing or a rash, to a foreign substance that stimulates the immune system.

alogia
A lack of appropriate speech. Unless prompted by the questioner, someone with alogia will give minimal responses.

alopecia
A lack or loss of bodily hair that is most obvious on the scalp, which tends to develop patchy hair loss.

alternative medicine
Medical systems, therapies, or techniques that are used in place of conventional medicine.

amebic dysentery
Inflammation of the intestines caused by infestation with the amoeba *Entamoeba histolytica*, characterized by blood-flecked diarrhea.

amenorrhea
Lack of menses (the flow of blood that occurs during menstruation) by age 16 is called primary amenorrhea; the absence of menses for more than three cycles is called secondary amenorrhea.

amniocentesis
A procedure in which a sample of the amniotic fluid around the fetus is removed from the mother's uterus for testing.

amyotrophic lateral sclerosis (ALS)
A form of motor neuron disease, characterized by weakness in the muscles, caused by degeneration of cells in the spinal cord.

analgesic
A drug that relieves pain.

anaphylactic shock
Severe allergic reaction; often includes respiratory symptoms.

anemia
A disorder of the blood in which there is a deficiency or disorder of hemoglobin, the oxygen-carrying pigment in red blood cells.

aneurysm
A dilatation (stretching) of a blood vessel, often filled with clotting blood, as a result of its wall becoming weakened.

angina
A cramplike pain, often felt in the chest, arms, and legs, resulting from narrowing of the arteries. This narrowing starves the heart muscle of oxygen.

anorexia nervosa
Anorexia nervosa is an eating disorder in which people perceive that they are too heavy, even though they are underweight. This perception results in a refusal or inability to maintain normal body weight.

antibiotic
A drug that selectively attacks microorganisms by breaking down bacteria and prevents

the growth of bacteria. Specific antibiotic drugs will work only against certain bacteria, leaving other bacteria unharmed.

antibody
A protein produced in the blood that inactivates invading organisms (or other foreign substances) and makes them susceptible to destruction by immune system cells such as phagocytes.

anticoagulant
Any drug that delays or prevents coagulation (clotting) of the blood.

antigen
A substance that can trigger the immune system into producing antibodies as a defense against infection and invading organisms.

antipruritic
A drug that relieves persistent itching, or pruritis, by reducing inflammation or numbing nerve impulses.

appendicolith
A calcified deposit within the appendix.

arrhythmia
Any variation in the normal rhythm or rate of the heartbeat.

arteriole
The smallest vessel of the arterial system.

artery
Blood vessels carrying oxygen-rich blood from the heart to the tissues.

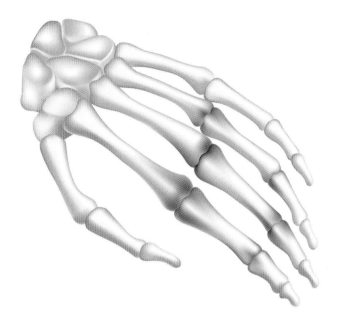

Arthritis has affected the joints of the bones in this hand. The red areas denote swelling and inflammation of the joints.

arthritis
Inflammation leading to pain and swelling of joints.

artificial insemination
The insertion of sperm into the vagina or uterus by mechanical means rather than by sexual intercourse.

astigmatism
A condition that occurs because the cornea (outer lens of the eye) is not the correct spherical shape. As a result, light rays from an object do not focus on the retina but focus either in front of or behind the retina, so that the object appears blurred.

atheroma
Fatty deposit, also called arterial plaque, which is laid down in the inner lining of the artery walls. Atheroma causes narrowing of the lining of the arteries and reduced blood flow, leading to heart attacks or strokes.

atherosclerosis
Formation of deposits of plaques consisting of cholesterol and lipids in the arteries, causing narrowing of the arteries.

atrophy
Wasting away of tissue or an organ.

autoimmune
The term refers to any disorder caused by the body's immune system reacting against its own tissues and cells.

autonomic nervous system
The part of the nervous system that controls automatic functions, such as heartbeat and sweating.

autosome
Any chromosome that is not a sex chromosome; in each cell, 22 pairs of chromosomes are autosomes.

avolition
Avolition is a condition in which a person lacks energy, spontaneity, and initiative. It is one of the symptoms noted in people who are suffering from schizophrenia.

bacteria
Small unicellular microorganisms. Bacteria exist in many areas in the body, but they are usually restrained by the immune system. Many bacteria cause life-threatening diseases.

benzodiazepine drugs
A class of drugs used as sedatives and mild tranquilizers and for the short-term treatment of insomnia. They have largely replaced barbiturates for these purposes. The advantage of using benzodiazepines is that, at smaller doses, they have a calming effect and allay anxiety, without the sleep-inducing effects of barbiturates.

beta-blockers
A family of drugs that block the effects of epinephrine, beta-blockers are principally used to treat heart disorders and high blood pressure.

bile
Greenish-brown fluid produced by the liver that carries away the liver's waste products and helps to break down fats in the small intestine. Bile enters the duodenum, the first part of the small intestine, through the bile duct.

bipolar disorder
Also called manic depression and manic depressive disorder. Someone with this disorder fluctuates between feeling deep depression and excessive euphoria.

bladder
The hollow, muscular organ situated in the lower abdomen. The bladder is protected by the pelvis and holds urine until it is excreted.

botulism
A dangerous form of food poisoning that is caused by a toxin produced by the bacterium *Clostridium botulinum*. Botulism can occur in preserved food that has been contaminated by the toxin, and can cause paralysis of the muscles.

bradycardia
An abnormally slow heartbeat, below 60 beats per minute.

bronchoscope
Instrument used via the trachea to examine the main airways of the lungs.

calorie
A unit used by dieticians to express the amount of energy taken into the body from digested food. A calorie is defined as the amount of heat that will raise 1 gram of water by 1 degree Celsius.

cancer
A group of diseases in which there is unrestrained growth of abnormal cells in tissues and organs of the body.

carcinoma
A tumor that occurs in the lining membrane of organs, such as the lungs, breasts, and stomach.

cataract
An area of opaque tissue that develops in the internal lens of the eye. If a cataract is not treated, it leads to impaired sight.

celiac disease
A condition caused by sensitivity of the intestinal lining to gluten, that leads to malabsorption of food from the intestines.

central nervous system
The brain and the spinal cord comprise the central nervous system (CNS), which receives sensory information from organs and sensory receptors in the body, analyzes the information, and produces an appropriate response.

cervical smear
A test in which a small sample of cells is removed from the surface of the cervix to detect abnormal changes in the cervix.

cervix
The lower part and neck of the uterus. The cervix separates the uterus from the vagina. The cervix is composed of smooth muscle tissue to form a sphincter or circular muscle that expands during childbirth.

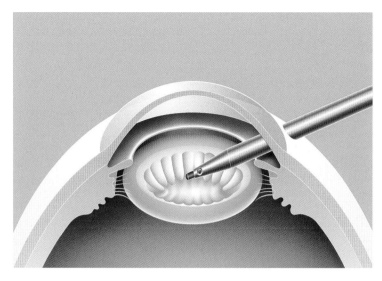

Cataracts can be treated using a simple procedure. A new lens is inserted into a tiny incision, which does not require stitching.

cesarean section
Surgery to remove a baby from the uterus through an incision in the abdominal wall.

chemotherapy
Treatment using anticancer drugs to destroy cancer cells or stop them from multiplying. Normal tissues are also affected; side effects can be severe.

chicken pox
A common infectious disease usually contracted during childhood. The symptoms are mild fever and a rash of fluid-filled spots.

cholesterol
A fatty substance that is essential to the structure of cell walls. However, when cholesterol is present in the blood in excessive quantities (usually owing to a diet too rich in animal fats), there is the risk of atherosclerosis. Cholesterol can also crystallize as gallstones in the bladder.

chromosomes
Structures in the cell nucleus that carry genetic information. Each human cell has 23 pairs of chromosomes; 22 pairs are autosomal, that is, they are the same in both sexes. The other pair are sex chromosomes, which are either XX (female) or XY (male).

chronic
Term used to describe an illness that persists over a long period of time.

cirrhosis
Long-term damage to the liver that causes scarring and impairment of liver function.

color blindness
Inability to distinguish between colors such as red and green.

coma
A state of profound unconsciousness, as a result of brain damage from head injuries, blood clots, poisoning, or strokes.

complementary medicine
Therapies or treatments used in conjunction with conventional medicine.

compound fracture
A fracture in which a broken bone breaks through the skin.

concussion
A brief loss of consciousness owing to a head injury; often followed by temporarily disturbed vision and loss of memory.

congenital
Term used to describe a disease or abnormality that is present from birth but is not necessarily hereditary.

conjunctiva
The transparent mucous membrane lining the inner surface of the eyelids and the white part of the eyeball.

conjunctivitis
Inflammation of the conjunctiva due to infection or allergy, causing red eyes and a thick discharge.

contrast medium
A radiopaque substance injected into the body in order to enhance detail on X-rays.

cornea
The transparent outer covering of the eye, which is composed of five layers. The

cornea has a dual role in the eye; it protects the eye from damage and foreign bodies, and it also helps focus light rays onto the retina.

coronary thrombosis
A condition in which a clot, or thrombus, blocks one of the coronary arteries, thus preventing oxygen from reaching the heart muscle. When a coronary artery is blocked in this way, the result can be a heart attack.

CT (computed tomography) scan
An X-ray technique that creates detailed pictures of the body's internal structures by producing detailed cross-sectional images of tissue composition.

cystic fibrosis
A genetic disorder that affects the lungs and digestive system. Cystic fibrosis appears in infancy and is characterized by excessive mucus, breathing difficulties, and abnormal secretion and function of many of the other secretory glands of the body. Treatments are available, but so far there is no cure.

cystoscopy
A procedure to examine the urethra and bladder by inserting an instrument called a cystoscope into the urethra. Sometimes the end of the cystocope carries a camera and a small cutting instrument.

cytotoxic drugs
A number of anticancer drugs that are used to kill cancer cells.

dementia
A set of symptoms that result in impaired intellectual functioning, with loss of memory, confusion, and disorientation.

depression
This state of mind, characterized by a loss of interest in life and feelings of sadness, may be caused by a life event, such as a bereavement, or may be a symptom of a depressive disorder.

diabetes
A disease in which the cells of the body do not get enough insulin, usually because the pancreas is producing too little or no insulin. In other cases, the pancreas produces sufficient insulin, but the cells in the body become resistant to its effects. There are two types of diabetes: type 1, which is insulin dependent, and type 2, which is non-insulin dependent.

Diagnostic and Statistical Manual of Mental Disorders
Also known as the DSM-IV, this reference work is published by the American Psychiatric Association and gives information on mental health disorders affecting children and adults. It also supplies lists of causes of disorders, useful statistics, and

prognoses. The manual is used by professionals to make diagnoses in the United States and other countries.

dilatation (dilation)
A condition in which a body opening is stretched, such as during childbirth, during a medical procedure, or as a result of disease.

DNA (deoxyribonucleic acid)
The genetic material from which chromosomes are formed. DNA is involved in protein synthesis and in inheritance. Because of DNA's structure (a double helix),

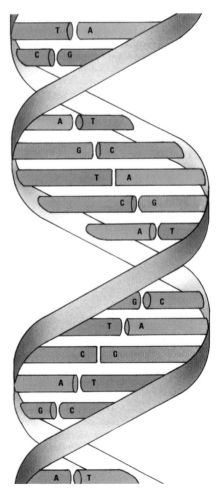

The DNA double helix has a ladder shape; the sides are sugars and phosphates, the rungs are paired complementary bases.

exact replication occurs during cell division.

dysfunction
Any impairment of social, psychological, or physiological function.

ECG (electrocardiogram)
A graph showing the sequence of electrical changes occurring in the heart during a succession of heartbeats. Characteristic changes in the graph can help diagnose heart disorders.

echocardiogram
An ultrasound technique used to build a moving picture of the heart.

eclampsia
An uncommon complication of pregnancy characterized by high blood pressure and seizures.

ECT (electroconvulsive therapy)
An electric shock to the brain given under anesthesia in order to produce a convulsion. Used to relieve symptoms of clinical depression.

ectopic pregnancy
A pregnancy developing outside the uterus, usually in one of the fallopian tubes.

eczema
Superficial dermatitis, characterized by a red, scaly, itchy, and often weeping skin rash.

edema
Any swelling of tissues due to an increase in fluid content.

EEG (electroencephalogram)
A multi-channel recording of electrical activity of the brain.

electrolytes
Soluble mineral compounds that conduct electrical currents; these include sodium, potassium, calcium, magnesium, and chloride, which must be kept within narrow limits for the normal function of cells, especially nerve cells.

elephantiasis
Massive swelling of the legs or areas of the trunk or head due to blockage of the lymph vessels by a tiny worm called *Wuchereria bancrofti.*

embolism
The result of a blood vessel becoming blocked by an embolus.

embolus
A foreign object, usually part of a thrombus, a tumor, or other tissue, or a mass of air, that drifts in the bloodstream until it becomes lodged in a blood vessel. *See also* embolism.

embryo
The early stages of a baby's development in the uterus, from the second week or so after conception until the seventh or eighth week of pregnancy. *Compare with* fetus.

emphysema
A chronic lung disease, resulting from overenlargement of the lung's air spaces, resulting in the destruction of the lung tissue.

encephalitis
Inflammation of the brain.

endemic
Term used to describe a disease that is native to a particular area or population. *Compare with* epidemic, epizootic, *and* pandemic.

endocarditis
Infection on the inner surface of the heart, usually occurring only when there is already some minor abnormality of structure.

endocrine system
The system of endocrine glands (pituitary, thyroid, parathyroid, and adrenal) that produces the body's hormones.

endoscopy
Examination of any part of the interior of the body by a narrow, rigid, or flexible optical viewing device, which is introduced via a natural anatomical opening or through a short incision.

enteritis
Infection of the intestines, leading to diarrhea and abdominal colic.

enzyme
A protein molecule that acts as a catalyst in chemical reactions in the cells of the body, without being altered itself.

epidemic
Term used to describe a widespread outbreak of an infectious disease. *Compare with* endemic, epizootic, *and* pandemic.

epidemiology
The study of the incidence and prevalence of disease among a population. Statistical markers such as the variables of gender, age, race, and occupation are counted. Over a period of time, changes are calculated and information is gathered about the distribution of diseases.

epilepsy
A disease of the nervous system that causes recurrent convulsions due to an overwhelming electrical discharge in the brain.

epinephrine
A hormone produced by the adrenal glands that has many effects. The hormone produces a bodily state appropriate for coping with sudden physical emergency. The hormone is produced synthetically as a treatment for cardiac arrest, anaphylactic shock, and acute asthma. Epinephrine is also known as adrenaline.

epizootic
An outbreak of infectious

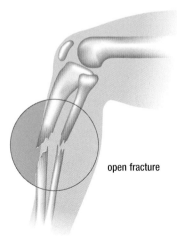

open fracture

disease that spreads through an entire species of animal in the same geographic area.

esophagus
The muscular canal that leads from the back of the throat down to the stomach.

estrogen
One of the two important female hormones. Variations in estrogen levels occur during the menstrual cycle and are responsible for many of the changes that occur in the uterus.

fallopian tubes
The two tubes arising out of the uterus and ending near the ovaries, through which eggs produced in the ovaries normally pass on their way to the womb. Also called oviducts.

fertilization
The process whereby a sperm enters an egg and fuses with it to start the process of cell division that may end in the production of an embryo.

fetal alcohol syndrome
Physical and mental abnormalities in a baby as a result of excessive alcohol intake by the mother during pregnancy.

fetus
Human conceptus growing in the uterus—usually called a fetus from the seventh or

The type of fracture depends on the force applied and the injury incurred; stress fractures (right) are caused by unusual stress on a bone. Open fractures (left) are those in which an exterior wound leads to a broken bone.

eighth week of pregnancy. *Compare with* embryo.

fever
A high body temperature, above the normal 98.6°F (37°C). Most infectious illnesses cause fever, which is a sign that the body's temperature-regulating mechanism has been affected by the infection.

fibroids
Benign fibromuscular tumors that grow in the uterus and that may cause heavy menstruation and problems in urination.

fissure
A split in the skin or other surface.

fistula
An abnormal channel leading from one body cavity to another, or from an internal organ to the skin.

fomites
Objects that harbor infectious organisms and are able to transmit an infection from one person to another. Examples

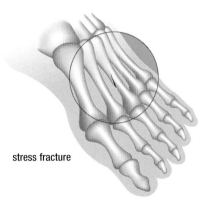

stress fracture

of fomites are books, clothes, handles, telephone receivers, and towels.

forensic medicine
The branch of pathology that investigates unnatural deaths and deaths by criminal injury.

fracture
Term used to describe an injury to a bone in which the continuity of the tissue is broken.

frostbite
Traumatic tissue injury due to cold.

frozen section
Tissue taken during surgery on which a very rapid microscopic examination is carried out in order to determine the course of the operation.

gallbladder
A saclike organ, attached to the liver, that collects bile and then discharges it into the intestine in response to a fatty meal.

gangrene
Death of tissue following a breakdown in the blood supply.

gastrectomy
The surgical removal of the stomach.

gastric ulcer
A break in the inner lining of the stomach, usually resulting from the effects of stomach acid.

gastritis
Inflammation of the mucosa of the stomach, causing pain and vomiting.

gastroenterology
The branch of medicine concerning the stomach, intestines, liver, and pancreas.

gastroscopy
Inspection of the stomach and duodenum using a flexible endoscope that is swallowed through the mouth. On its tip, the endoscope has a camera and a small cutting implement that is used to take a biopsy of tissue.

genes
Biological units that contain hereditary information. A gene is a tiny segment of DNA. The chainlike structure of DNA is composed of intertwined strands; each strand has thousands of pairs of genes, arranged on 23 pairs of chromosomes.

genetics
Genetics is the science of genes, heredity, and the variation of organisms. Modern genetics is based on the understanding of genes at the molecular, or DNA, level.

German measles
A viral infection. Also called rubella.

gerontology
The study of aging from a medical, psychological, and biological perspective.

gingivitis
Painful ulceration of the gums that causes inflammation.

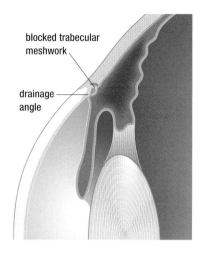

blocked trabecular meshwork

drainage angle

The diagram shows chronic glaucoma, in which the meshwork through which fluid flows out of the eye is blocked.

gland
A group of cells that produce secretions, which may be enzymes or hormones. The adrenal glands, the pituitary, and the thyroid are examples of endocrine glands, which release secretions into the bloodstream. Exocrine glands include salivary and sebaceous glands, which release secretions into the mouth and skin.

glandular fever
See infectious mononucleosis.

glaucoma
An eye disease caused by excessive pressure of fluid in the eye, which may lead to gradual loss of vision.

glucose
A simple sugar produced by the digestion of starch and sucrose. Glucose is the main source of energy for the body's cells.

gluten
A protein constituent of wheat and wheat products. Celiac disease results from sensitivity to gluten.

glycogen
A form of glucose stored in the liver and muscles. Glycogen is released when it is needed for energy.

goiter
A visible swelling of the thyroid gland.

gonorrhea
A sexually transmitted disease that produces a greenish yellow urethral or vaginal discharge.

gout
Swollen painful joints. Gout especially affects the joint at the base of the big toe; it is caused by excessive accumulation of uric acid.

greenstick fracture
A partial fracture of a child's bone, which, because the bone is so pliable, splits rather than breaks.

group therapy
Treatment of psychological problems by discussion within a group of people and under the direction of a trained therapist.

growths
Popularly used to refer to tumors both benign and malignant.

gynecologist
A specialist in the diseases of the female reproductive system.

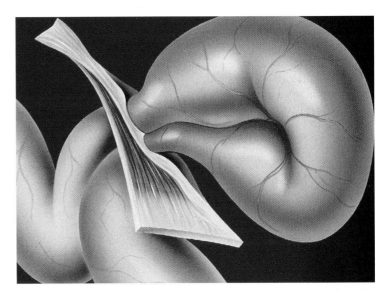

In this strangulated hernia, part of the intestine (orange) has breached the abdominal wall. Swelling may cut off the blood supply, leading to a danger of gangrene.

hallucination
An imaginary sensation perceived through any of the five senses; the result of drug use, alcohol withdrawal, severe illness, or schizophrenia.

hallucinogenic
Term describing a drug that produces hallucinations.

hay fever
Runny nose and coldlike symptoms caused by pollen allergy.

heart attack
A sudden, acutely painful, distressing, and often fatal event in which part of the heart muscle is deprived of its blood supply and dies because of the blockage of a branch of one of the coronary arteries. In those who survive, the dead tissue is replaced by scar tissue, but the pumping power of the heart is usually weakened.

heartburn
A burning sensation behind the sternum, caused by stomach acid in the esophagus.

heart failure
A condition in which the heart can no longer pump enough blood to meet the metabolic requirements of the body.

heart murmur
Any of several sounds heard in addition to the regular heartbeat.

heat exhaustion
Condition caused by loss of body fluids due to prolonged exposure to high temperature, causing cramps, nausea, and finally loss of consciousness. *Compare with* heatstroke.

heatstroke
The medical term for sunstroke. A severe and sometimes fatal condition resulting from the collapse of the body's ability to regulate its temperature, due to prolonged exposure to hot sunshine or high temperatures. Also called heat hyperpyrexia.

hematoma
A trapped mass of blood in the tissues of an organ or in the skin.

hematuria
Blood in the urine.

hemiplegia
Paralysis of one side of the body caused by damage to nerves in the opposite side of the brain.

hemodialysis
The use of a kidney machine to remove waste products from the blood after a patient's kidneys have ceased functioning.

hemoglobin
The oxygen-carrying substance in red blood cells.

hemophilia
An inherited disorder of blood clotting due to absence of one of the factors needed for clotting (factor VIII). Generally only males are affected, but females may be carriers.

hemorrhage
Medical term for bleeding.

hemorrhoids
Varicosity in the blood vessels of the anus that can give rise to bleeding and discomfort. Also called piles.

hemostasis
Arrest of bleeding or hemorrhage.

hepatitis
Inflammation of the liver, usually caused by one of the hepatitis viruses.

hernia
A weakness in the muscular wall of the abdomen that allows tissue (often the small intestine) to push through.

herpes
A group of viruses responsible for cold sores, chicken pox, shingles, and genital sores.

hiatus hernia
Condition in which the stomach pushes up through the diaphragm via the orifice normally occupied by the gullet (esophagus). There may be no symptoms, or the person suffers pain and heartburn.

HIV
The human immunodeficiency virus (a retrovirus), which can lead to AIDS. The immune system makes antibodies in an attempt to combat the virus; the presence of these antibodies in the blood confirms the presence of HIV.

Hodgkin's disease
Cancerlike disease of the lymph nodes.

holistic
An approach that attempts to treat the whole body and mind.

homeopathy
Treatment of disease using tiny doses of a substance that produces symptoms similar to those of the disease itself.

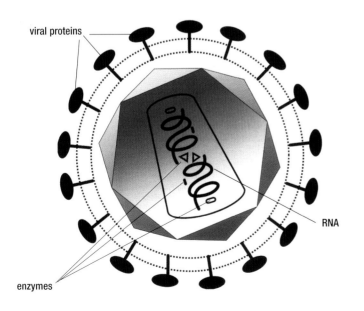

viral proteins

RNA

enzymes

When HIV invades a cell, enzymic action alters the RNA of the virus to DNA. The viral DNA can then invade and infect the chromosomes of the host cell.

homologue
Any organ that is similar to another organ, for example the hands and feet.

hormone
A chemical messenger released from tissue or a gland to alter the activity of tissues elsewhere in the body. Hormones control processes of metabolism, sexual development, and growth.

hormone replacement therapy (HRT)
Synthetic or natural hormones that are used to counteract hormonal deficiency during menopause. HRT carries a slightly higher risk of heart disease, strokes, breast cancer, and ovarian cancer.

hydatid disease
A disease caused by larval forms of tapeworms, characterized by cysts in the liver and other organs, and sometimes in muscle.

hydrocephalus
Increase in volume of the cerebrospinal fluid within the brain's ventricles. In children hydrocephalus can lead to enlargement of the head, and the condition is often associated with spina bifida.

hyperactivity
A term used to describe excessive activity in children. Associated with brain damage, epilepsy, and psychiatric problems, but only very rarely with food allergy. Also known as attention deficit hyperactivity disorder.

hyperparathyroidism
An excessive production of parathyroid hormone that is often caused by a noncancerous tumor called an adenoma.

hypertension
Raised blood pressure, which puts extra strain on the heart and arteries, thereby increasing the risk of heart attacks, strokes, and kidney damage.

hyperthyroidism
Overactivity of the thyroid gland that can lead to weight loss, tremor, protrusion of the eyes, hyperactivity, moist skin, and jumpiness.

hypertrophy
Abnormal enlargement of an organ or tissue in order to meet extra demands made on it by the body.

hyperventilation
Abnormally rapid breathing, leading to dizziness, tingling in the hands, or even sometimes loss of consciousness. Hyperventilation can be caused by anxiety.

hypochondria
Neurotic preoccupation with one's own health and with disease.

hypoglycemia
An abnormally low level of sugar in the blood, which can cause such symptoms as confusion, coma, trembling, sweating, and even death.

hypotension
Low blood pressure.

hypothalamus
The area at the base of the brain that coordinates part of the nervous and endocrine (hormonal) systems.

hypothermia
Abnormally low body temperature—below 95°F (35°C)—usually caused by prolonged exposure to cold, leading to a faint heart rate, pallor, and eventual collapse.

hypothyroidism
Underactivity of the thyroid gland, leading to fatigue, weight gain, and thick, dry skin.

hypoxia
A low level of oxygen in the tissues as a result of lung or heart disease.

hysterectomy
Removal of the uterus.

iatrogenic
A disorder caused by medical treatment.

ichthyosis
A skin condition in which the skin is abnormally thick and scaly.

idiopathic
Denoting a disease or symptom for which the cause is unknown.

immune system
The complex system by which the body defends itself against infection.

immunization
Preparing the body to fight

and prevent an infection through the injection of material from the infecting organism, or by using an attenuated (non–disease-causing) strain of the organism itself.

immunoglobulin
See antibody.

immunomodulatory
An agent that can stimulate or reduce immune responses.

immunosuppressive drugs
Drugs that suppress the immune system. They are used to treat autoimmune disorders such as rheumatoid arthritis, and after transplant surgery.

impetigo
An acute staphylococcal skin infection characterized by pustules with yellowish crusts.

impotence
Failure to achieve or sustain an erection of the penis.

incontinence
Failure to control the bladder or bowel movements, or both.

incubation period
The period between exposure to a contagious or similar infection and the first appearance of any symptoms of the disease.

infectious mononucleosis
Viral infection that causes swollen lymph nodes and a sore throat. Also called glandular fever.

infertility
Inability of a couple to conceive and reproduce after a reasonable period of time (about 1 year to 18 months).

inflammation
A reaction of the body's tissues to injury or illness, characterized by redness, heat, swelling, and pain. A mechanism of defense and repair.

inoculation
Administration of a vaccine in order to stimulate the immune system to produce antibodies and, hence, immunity to disease.

insulin
A hormone, secreted in the pancreas, that regulates blood sugar levels.

interferon
A protein produced by the body cells when triggered by a virus infection. The activity of killer cells is increased by interferon. It is also produced artificially as a drug to treat certain diseases.

intrauterine device (IUD)
A small device inserted into the uterus in order to prevent pregnancy.

intravenous (IV)
Within or into a vein. The term describes a procedure by which drugs, or fluids such as blood, can be introduced into the body either by injection or by infusion.

in vitro fertilization (IVF)
A method of enabling women who are unable to conceive to bear children; egg cells are fertilized with sperm outside the body ("in vitro" literally means "in glass," that is, in an artificial environment), and then some of the fertilized eggs are inserted in the uterus.

irradiation
Exposure to any form of radiant energy, such as light, heat, and X rays, for therapeutic or diagnostic purposes.

irritable bowel syndrome
A common condition that is characterized by episodes of abdominal pain and disturbance of the intestines (constipation or diarrhea). Also called irritable or spastic colon.

ischemia
Condition in which tissues receive an inadequate blood supply.

isotope scanning
A diagnostic technique based on the detection of radiation emitted by radioactive isotopes introduced into the body. Also called radionuclide scanning.

keyhole surgery
Surgery performed via an endoscope through small incisions rather than one large incision. Also known as minimally invasive surgery.

kwashiorkor
A disease in children, caused by a protein-deficient diet, resulting in retarded growth, edema, lassitude, and diarrhea. It is common in many parts of Africa.

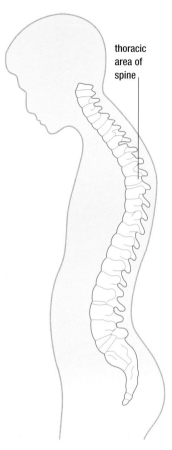

thoracic area of spine

The thoracic area of the spine has an exaggerated curve, giving a stooped appearance. The condition, called kyphosis, has a number of causes, including tuberculosis of the spine, poor posture, and rickets.

kyphosis
Outward curvature of the thoracic part of the spine, which can be caused by a congenital abnormality.

laparoscopy
The use of a special endoscope that is passed through the abdominal wall in order to view the abdominal organs.

laparotomy
Surgical incision to open the abdominal cavity for diagnostic purposes or surgical treatment.

laryngitis
Inflammation of the mucous membrane lining the larynx, caused by an infection or irritation, and accompanied by hoarseness or loss of voice.

lassa fever
A frequently fatal viral disease occurring in sub-Saharan Africa.

leptospirosis
Acute infectious disease caused by the organism *Leptospira interrogans*, which is transmitted to humans via the urine of rats and dogs. Symptoms include jaundice and fever. The most serious form is Weil's disease.

lesion
An area of tissue in which the structure and function are altered or impaired owing to injury or disease.

leukemia
A blood disease in which cancerous changes in the bone marrow produce abnormal numbers and forms of immature white blood cells.

leukocytosis
An excess of white cells in the blood, often due to infection.

leukopenia
Lack of white blood cells, often the result of blood disease or a side effect of anticancer drugs, causing a reduced resistance to infection.

leukoplakia
A condition featuring white patches of thickened mucous membrane, especially in the mouth. Leukoplakia can proceed to cancer.

lupus erythematosus
A chronic inflammatory autoimmune disease of the connective tissue, affecting the skin and internal organs.

lymphatic system
A network of vessels that transfer lymph from the tissue fluids to the bloodstream. Lymph nodes occur along the lymphatic vessels.

lymph node
A small structure that filters infection; part of the lymphatic system.

lymphocyte
A type of white blood cell that is produced in bone marrow and is present mainly in lymph and blood. Lymphocytes are part of the immune system and fight infection and cancer.

malabsorption
Failure of the small intestine to absorb nutrients properly.

malaria
Serious infectious illness that is common in the tropics. It is caused by four species of the organism *Plasmodium*, which is passed to humans via an infected anopheles mosquito. Typical symptoms are fever and an enlarged spleen.

malignant
Term used to describe tumors that spread into surrounding

tissues and elsewhere in the body. The term is also used to describe other dangerous diseases or states.

malnutrition
A nutritional deficiency, usually brought on by a severe food shortage, but which can also be caused by inadequate absorption of food or an intake of inappropriate food. The term *malnutrition* increasingly refers to the type of excessive eating that causes obesity.

malocclusion
Improper alignment of the upper and lower teeth, which affects the bite and the appearance of the teeth.

mammography
X-ray of the breast, used to help detect tumors.

mania
A state of excessive excitement, in which patients lack insight into their behavior.

manic depression
See bipolar disorder.

Mantoux test
A skin test used to determine exposure to infection with tuberculosis.

Marfan's syndrome
A genetic disorder of the connective tissue that causes elongation of the bones. It is often accompanied by heart, eye, and spinal abnormalities.

mastoiditis
Inflammation of the air cells in the bone behind the ear.

measles
An acute, highly contagious viral disease that occurs principally in childhood, characterized by red eyes, fever, and a rash. Also called morbilli and rubeola.

melanin
The black or dark brown pigment that is present in the skin, hair, and eyes.

membrane
Any thin layer of tissue.

Ménière's disease
A chronic disease of the inner ear, found in older people who have recurrent deafness, buzzing in the ears, and vertigo.

meninges
This is composed of three membranes that surround the brain and spinal cord.

meningitis
Any infection of the meninges.

meningocele
A hernial protrusion of the meninges or covering of the spinal cord.

menopause
The cessation of ovulation and menses, which in the majority of women occurs between the ages of 45 and 55.

menorrhagia
Excessive bleeding during menstrual periods.

menses
The flow of blood that occurs during menstruation.

menstruation
Periodic bleeding as the uterus sheds its lining each month during a woman's reproductive years. Menstruation begins at puberty and ends at menopause.

mental retardation
A low level of mental ability, which is usually congenital.

metabolism
The various vital processes that are necessary for bodily functions. These processes include the breakdown of complex molecules to produce energy (catabolism) and building up complex molecules, such as proteins, from simpler components (anabolism).

metastasis
The process by which cancerous cells spread from a tumor to remote sites in the body. *Metastasis* also refers to a secondary tumor.

microsurgery
Surgery on tiny structures, such as blood vessels or eyes, using a microscope and miniature instruments.

migraine
Recurrent severe headaches that are associated with nausea and visual disturbance.

minerals
Metallic elements, such as sodium, that are vital to many bodily functions.

miscarriage
Loss of an embryo or fetus from the uterus before 28

weeks of pregnancy, but usually occurring during the first 16 weeks. The medical term is *spontaneous abortion*.

mitogen
A chemical that triggers a cell to commence mitosis (cell division).

mitral stenosis
An obstructive lesion in the valve between the left atrium and ventricle, usually as a result of rheumatic fever.

MMR vaccine
A combined vaccine that protects children against measles, mumps, and rubella. The MMR vaccine is first given to a child between 12 and 15 months. Follow-up booster doses occur when the child is between 3 and 5 years old. Large-scale administration of the vaccine in the developed world has greatly reduced the occurrence of mumps.

mole
A pigmented spot on the skin.

MRSA (methicillin-resistant *Staphylococcus aureus*)
A bacterium that is difficult to treat, particularly in hospitals, where it may be fatal for already ill patients.

mumps
An acute viral disease that primarily affects the parotid glands in the cheeks.

narcotic
A drug that dulls the senses. Used to induce sleep or as a painkiller.

naturopathy
A system of health care or therapies that relies on natural substances, exercise in water, and a natural environment to maintain health and attempt to effect cures.

nausea
The sensation of wanting to vomit.

necrosis
Death of tissue.

neurology
Branch of medicine concerned with the treatment of diseases of the nervous system.

neuron
A nerve cell. The nervous system is made up of billions of neurons, each comprising a cell body, a long fiber called an axon, and shorter projections, or dendrites. There are three main types of neurons: sensory neurons that transmit information from sense receptors toward the brain; motor neurons that transmit signals toward the muscles and glands; and interneurons that transmit signals within the central nervous system.

neurosis
An emotional disorder such as mild depression, anxiety, or any of the phobias.

over-the-counter (OTC) drug
A drug sold lawfully without a prescription in a pharmacy or drugstore. Painkillers, such as acetaminophen and aspirin, are available in this way.

pandemic
Any disease that spreads over a very wide area, sometimes worldwide. *Compare with* epidemic.

pap smear
A simple method of detecting cervical cancer. The test involves the staining of a sample of exfoliated cells taken from the cervix. Also called Papanicolaou smear.

pediatrics
The branch of medicine concerned with the treatment of children and childhood diseases.

phocomelia
A defect in which the legs or hands are joined to the body by short stumps. Phocomelia occurred in many children as a result of their mothers taking the drug thalidomide during pregnancy.

prophylaxis
Any procedure to prevent a disease from developing or from becoming worse.

psychosis
Any psychiatric disorder, such as schizophrenia or bipolar disorder, in which the person has distorted beliefs that are inappropriate and disconnected from reality. Delusions or hallucinations can occur.

retrovirus
A type of virus that has RNA (ribonucleic acid) as its genetic material and that uses an enzyme (reverse transcriptase) to produce DNA from the RNA.

The viral DNA thus produced is then incorporated into the DNA of the host cell. HIV is an example of a retrovirus.

RNA (ribonucleic acid)
Genetic material in animal and plant cells that transmits the coded instructions held in DNA to the protein-synthesizing system of the cell. In some viruses, RNA is the genetic material, not DNA.

sarcoma
A malignant tumor arising in muscle, bone, or other connective tissue.

scabies
Skin infection caused by mites that burrow into the skin.

schistosomiasis
A tropical parasitic infestation, afflicting over 200 million people worldwide. The disease can damage the bladder and liver. Also called bilharzia.

schizophrenia
A group of psychiatric disorders in which thinking, emotions, and behavior are disrupted and the person is often delusional. Symptoms are hallucinations, which are often auditory (a person "hears voices") rather than visual.

septicemia
A condition in which bacteria multiply in the bloodstream. Also called blood poisoning.

side effect
An unwanted result that occurs as a consequence of a medication or therapy.

syncope
The medical term for fainting.

syndrome
A collection of symptoms or signs that occur together to indicate a specific disorder.

synthesize
To produce a substance by building it from smaller components. Proteins are synthesized in the body from smaller units called amino acids.

tachycardia
An abnormally fast heartbeat of more than 100 beats per minute, which can be experienced by a healthy person during exercise. If someone is resting and experiences tachycardia, it can indicate hyperthyroidism, fever, anxiety, or coronary artery disease.

tachypnea
An abnormally fast rate of breathing, induced by exertion, anxiety, or heart or lung problems.

tamponade
Breathlessness and sometimes collapse as a result of fluid buildup and pressure in the double membrane surrounding the heart (pericardium). It can occur after heart surgery, from inflammation of the pericardium, or after a chest injury.

teratogen
Any agent that causes abnormalities in a fetus. The agent may be a virus, a drug (for example, thalidomide), or an environmental factor such as radiation.

trisomy
The condition of having three of a certain chromosome instead of just two.

The diagram below shows the life cycle of schistosomiasis.

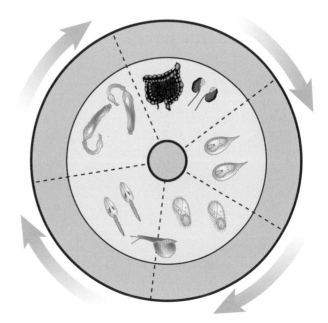

Subject Indexes

Mental disorders

Health care

Comprehensive Index